Psychosocial Care of the Adult Cancer Patient

Psychosocial Care of the Adult Cancer Patient

Evidence-Based Practice in Psycho-Oncology

DONALD R. NICHOLAS

OXFORD
UNIVERSITY PRESS

OXFORD
UNIVERSITY PRESS

Oxford University Press is a department of the University of Oxford. It furthers the University's objective of excellence in research, scholarship, and education by publishing worldwide.

Oxford New York
Auckland Cape Town Dar es Salaam Hong Kong Karachi
Kuala Lumpur Madrid Melbourne Mexico City Nairobi
New Delhi Shanghai Taipei Toronto

With offices in
Argentina Austria Brazil Chile Czech Republic France Greece
Guatemala Hungary Italy Japan Poland Portugal Singapore
South Korea Switzerland Thailand Turkey Ukraine Vietnam

Published in the United States of America by
Oxford University Press
198 Madison Avenue, New York, NY 10016

Library of Congress Cataloging-in-Publication Data
Nicholas, Donald R.
Psychosocial care of the adult cancer patient : evidence-based practice in psycho-oncology / Donald R. Nicholas.
pages cm
Includes bibliographical references and index.
ISBN 978-0-19-974444-2 (hb : alk. paper)
1. Cancer—Social aspects. 2. Cancer—Psychological aspects. 3. Cancer—Patients—Family relationships. 4. Physician and patient I. Title.
RC262.N54 2016
616.99'40651—dc23
2015014035

This book is dedicated to the many cancer patients and families who have allowed me to participate in their illness—their personal and unique human experience of cancer. It has been a privilege to be a part of what is both one of life's greatest challenges, while also one of life's greatest learning experiences. I have learned much from you and hope that this book passes on some of those lessons to other cancer care professionals.

CONTENTS

FOREWORD

Don Nicholas and I have spent the last 30 years working in our young and evolving field of psycho-oncology, he plowing the field in the Midwest, and I turning the furrows in the Northeast. We have never met, though I have heard colleagues sing his praises as a gifted teacher and clinician. From his base of operation as professor of psychology at Ball State University and through his clinical work at the Indiana University (I.U.) Health Ball Memorial Cancer Center, over many years Don has developed, synthesized, and published the key facts that a beginning psycho-oncologist must know to adequately care for patients with cancer. The organizing principle of the book is evidence-based medicine, which he has applied to the critical components of psycho-oncology. I particularly like that he points out that one cannot take care of cancer patients psychologically if one does not have some basic knowledge of the disease. He gives background that is important to know. He treats psychotherapy in the same way, examining the evidence base for our therapies in research and real-world settings, with excellent background information about individual, group, couples, and family interventions. But we also learn that research findings are not always readily accepted into clinical practices, which are manned by professionals who have their own long-held beliefs and attitudes. Psycho-oncology is in the process of learning this lesson as we attempt to implement evidence-based psychosocial and psychopharmacologic interventions in routine cancer practice. We are fortunate that implementation science has arrived to guide this complex step of research geared toward change in clinical practice. Bench to bedside can be a long and tortuous route.

This is a "must-have" book for the budding psycho-oncologist, assuring knowledge of the basics while also providing an overview of the history, present state, and future challenges we face. I look forward to meeting Don and telling him in person how important a contribution his book will be. I suspect I will just be one of many attempting to tell him this.

Jimmie Holland, MD
New York, NY
February 2015

PREFACE

The evidence-based practice (EBP) of adult psycho-oncology is the application of a series of key competencies that formulate clinically relevant questions; access and critically evaluate relevant scientific literature; translate and integrate the identified literature to the needs of a particular cancer patient, couple, family, or group of patients; and evaluate the overall process. Once a psychosocial health service intervention and any needed adaptations are determined, collaboration with a patient to consider patient preferences occurs before the intervention is skillfully provided, with attention to both fidelity—providing the service in a manner consistent with prior research—and flexibility—attending closely to the needs of the particular patient. This highly complex, recursive process is not easy to do! It requires a broad range of scientific and clinical skills, resources for quick and accurate electronic literature searching, as well as an attitude that appreciates and values the combined importance of both science and practice. At present, "there is little evidence that EBPs are yet effectively disseminated or implemented in the vast majority of real-word practice settings, or that EBPs are implemented in ways that are likely to support wider dissemination efforts" (Frueh, Ford, Elhal, & Grubaugh, 2012, p. 8). Recognizing these problems, this book has been written to provide a resource that explains the application of EBP to psychosocial health service interventions in oncology and demonstrates how an experienced clinician uses the core competencies.

As I write this preface, nearly 4 years from when I started this project, I realize that this is not the book I set out to write. Much has changed during its writing. My understanding of the constructs of EBP and translational research has evolved. A sense of urgency to more quickly bring what is discovered by science to practice has only grown stronger, both personally and professionally, as evidenced by new developments such as the growth of the field of implementation science. And most recently, the United States is entering a time of change and uncertainty as health care enters the era of the Affordable Care Act with many unknowns regarding its impact on all components of health care.

When I first considered writing such a book, I thought I could offer something new to the psycho-oncology literature from my nearly 30 years of clinical experience, editorial work, and training of PhD students in counseling psychology. I knew I had enjoyed the work and had learned a lot that I thought would be valuable to pass on to others. I figured I would mostly write about my clinical experience, highlighting key concepts, ideas, and successful outcomes that would add some structure to the still relatively young discipline of psycho-oncology (Holland & Weiss, 2010). I knew the literature well from serving on the National Cancer Institute's (NCI) Palliative and Supportive Care PDQ Editorial Board for a number of years and prided myself on staying current with relevant literature. But then I was introduced to the concept of EBP (Norcross, Hogan, & Koocher, 2008), and the direction of this book changed. I saw EBP as the structure around which this book could not only be written but also add more to the existing literature. I wasn't aware of any other attempts to write such a book, and I felt like I could do that—explain to others in the field of psycho-oncology first what EBP is and then how an experienced clinician might implement the core EBP competencies via four (individual, group, couples, and family) different treatment modalities. Thus, structuring it around EBP significantly altered the book.

As I wrote, I also came to realize that this book can be a part of a growing set of solutions to the problem of how to narrow the gap between science and practice. It has been noted (McHugh & Barlow, 2012a) that there are primarily two strategies for narrowing this gap—both ultimately assist clinicians in their decision making about what treatments to provide. Developing and promoting clinical practice guidelines that synthesize and summarize the literature for clinicians is one method, while teaching clinicians the skills for accessing, appraising, evaluating, and ultimately integrating best available evidence to the needs of individual patients is the second method. This book is an example of this second method.

Part I includes Chapters 1 through 4 and provides background knowledge for the psycho-oncologist. Chapter 1 introduces the need for quality psychosocial services for cancer patients by noting the many calls for action and available practice guidelines. Chapters 2 and 3 provide essential background knowledge needed for the EBP of psycho-oncology—Chapter 2 on the basics of cancer and Chapter 3 on psychotherapy. Chapter 4 concludes Part I with a detailed explanation of EBP in psycho-oncology. For the more experienced clinician not familiar with EBP, Chapter 4 may be a good place to begin, and it may also serve as a detailed stand-alone chapter on how to do EBP.

Part II describes the EBP of psycho-oncology in the delivery of psychosocial *health services*. The health services of screening, assessment, individual, group, couples, and family interventions are described. Screening for psychosocial distress, with its goal of identifying those in need of further services—and assessment, with its goal of evaluating patients' and/or families' overall psychosocial adaptation—are described and explained in Chapter 5. Chapters 6 through 9 describe psychosocial health services focused on the needs of individual patients, couples, and families/caregivers, as offered via four different treatment modalities. These chapters are organized around the four most common modalities of face-to-face, in-person (1) individual, (2) group, (3) couples, and (4) family.

Each of these chapters has three sections: background knowledge, best available research evidence, and a case example(s). Consistent with the competencies of EBP, the psycho-oncologist's first encounter with a new patient often results in a number of general-knowledge background questions. Thus, the first section of Chapters 6 through 9 summarizes background knowledge regarding each treatment modality and its use with cancer patients. The second section provides an overview of some best available evidence organized around tables of exemplar studies, chosen for their research design and generally positive outcomes, as examples of well-done individual, group, couple-focused, and family-focused research. Each table includes study characteristics (type cancer, stage, sample size, and results) and information about dissemination and implementation (intervention description, theory, accessibility of treatment manual, therapist characteristics, patient acceptability, and trainability). The use of exemplar studies as examples of best available evidence is consistent with the focus of this book on EBP, as it is beyond the scope of this book to do a comprehensive, detailed review of the literature.

The third and most detailed section of each of these four chapters is a case example(s) that shows how to do EBP by use of the six competencies of Asking, Accessing, Appraising, Translating, Integrating, and Evaluating—AAA TIE (Norcross, Hogan, & Koocher, 2008) for each of the four treatment modalities. Thus, by the end of each chapter the reader will

- have been introduced to general background knowledge about the use of each treatment modality with adult cancer patients,
- be provided a table that describes study characteristics and their ease of dissemination of a number of high-quality intervention exemplars, and
- see how to do evidence-based practice by following the six, sequential EBP competencies.

Throughout all four chapters, the case examples are written to show different procedures for adopting, adapting, or abandoning best available evidence. They describe a personal, internal, and recursive process. The goal is to communicate the thought processes, clinical decision making, and internal self-reflection of the psycho-oncologist as you work your way through the steps of EBP. Communicating this personal process, from the speaker (author) to the listener (reader)—both of whom are clinicians involved in an ongoing clinical decision-making process—is done more effectively by using second-person, as has been done in other EBP training efforts (Council for Training in Evidence-Based Behavioral Practice [EBBP], 2009). Thus, each case example is written in second-person, with use of second-person pronouns—*you* and *your*—to highlight this internal, working, clinical perspective and thereby acknowledging that the reader is also the clinician. As a result, these case examples are presented in a more personal and individualized manner that also recognizes that individual practitioners may make different decisions as they strive to provide evidence-based care; care that is always faced with multiple limitations in (a) the quality of the evidence, (b) the clinical expertise, and (c) the needs, preferences, and idiosyncrasies of each patient.

Please also note as you work your way through the book, that EBP is a fluid and recursive process. It changes as new research is published. Online databases and their search engines evolve. New resources for background knowledge and filtered and unfiltered information emerge and become more efficient and user-friendly than earlier ones. The availability of resources also changes as organizations purchase, renew, and choose not to renew subscriptions to databases and other clinical decision support tools. Given these changes, it is clear that no single book could include all potentially relevant resources for searching the extant literature. Plus, searches done at one time will necessarily change when done at a later date or time. This is the nature of online searching and should be anticipated. Thus, what is most important is that the competent psycho-oncologist learn and use the EBP core competencies with the goal of bringing effective, evidence-based interventions to front-line, day-to-day care in the comprehensive cancer care setting.

Don Nicholas
May, 2015

ACKNOWLEDGMENTS

Although at times the writing of this book felt like a solitary, sometimes lonely endeavor, as I look back I have many people to thank and to acknowledge. First and foremost is my family, to whom I want to express my appreciation for their understanding and support for time away. Since this was not written during some time period free from other professional responsibilities, it was written on weekends, evenings, and during those days when I could carve out time from an otherwise busy professional life. Thanks Pam, Leah, AJ, Jacob, Jon, and Calvin for your love, support, and understanding. I hope to return to a more normal daily routine now!

Next, I would like to thank those cancer care professionals from whom I have learned the most about the field of psycho-oncology. My friend and colleague Steve Passik, with whom I served on the NCI's PDQ Editorial Board for many years, offered me the opportunity to be involved in one of the most rewarding experiences of my professional life by serving on the board. Thanks Steve, as well as Jean Kristeller, Robin Baldwin, Danny Montgomery, Myra Glajchen, Deb Barton, Larry Cripe, Jay Kamath, Lillian Nail, Barry Eagel, and the many other palliative and supportive care board members who collectively taught me much of what I have included in this book.

My local cancer care professionals with whom I work on a routine basis have also been instrumental in supporting my work as a counseling psychologist and professor. They have allowed me the opportunity to do the work of a psycho-oncologist in an excellent local cancer care setting—I.U. Health Ball Memorial Cancer Center in Muncie, Indiana. Thanks to Melody Stanley, Anurita Sarin, Steve Tilmans, Trish Avila, Terry Pence, Amy Upchurch, Ruth Ann Tolle, Rod Stephens, Bill Fisher, Yunjie Xie Lin, Michael Williamson, Sulfi Ibrahim, Joe Spahr, Dejuania Brown, Abby Koons, and all of the exceptional cancer center staff.

I have also called upon many of our doctoral students in counseling psychology at Ball State University for their help. Many have been instrumental in assisting me with various tasks of this book. Erin Sadler has created nearly all of the figures throughout the book, completing one that was first drawn by my nephew Nicholas Shank. Thanks Erin and Nick. James Van Hoven and Meredith

Berry worked hard on seeing that some complicated tables were readable and understandable; and Courtney Ryan, Jill Sullivan, Summer Ibarra, Aikaterina Psarropoulou, Kodee Walls, and Sean Jones all helped with organizing references, reviewing articles, and reading chapters of the book. My friend and local colleague Bill Frederick did an excellent and detailed review of the entire book. Thanks everyone.

Finally, none of this would have ever been completed if not for the exceptional work of the editors at Oxford University Press, Sarah Harrington, Andrea Zekus, Kate Scheinman, and the helpful comments of blind reviewers. Thank you all for your time, expertise, and professionalism.

PART I

Psycho-Oncology Background

1

Case Examples and Calls for Action

> *Cancer care today often provides state-of-the-science biomedical treatment, but fails to address the psychological and social (psychosocial) problems associated with the illness.*
>
> —Institute of Medicine (2008)

Psychosocial Care of the Adult Cancer Patient: Evidence-Based Practice in Psycho-Oncology focuses on the evidence-based practice of adult clinical psycho-oncology in the local cancer care setting. The human experience of cancer is often emotionally, socially, and spiritually distressing. Patients, along with their families and loved ones, encounter situations that, for the most part, they have never before encountered. They face pain, nausea, fatigue, and difficulties in sleeping, along with multiple and varied losses—from the loss of hair, to loss of appetite, to even the loss of their assumptions about how life was to unfold. Changes to daily routines, financial concerns, and practical concerns, such as transportation to treatments or how to get household chores done, are often problematic. The frequency with which cancer patients encounter these and other distressing experiences makes it essential that cancer care professionals be knowledgeable about the psychological, social, and spiritual aspects of the human experience of cancer, and understand that psychosocial care can be provided as evidence-based practice. The three cases that follow illustrate typical scenarios that health care professionals working with cancer patients may encounter.

CASE EXAMPLE 1

Penny is a 50-year-old mother of three children, ages 9–16 years. In the past she has struggled with anxiety related to parenting and caring for her elderly parents. Two years ago, you were her psychotherapist. The last you saw her, after a successful course of cognitive-behavioral treatment, Penny reported that she was doing much better with controlling her worry, and she had developed the skill of "calming herself" when needed. Together you mutually decided to end treatment, with the provision that she could always call and reschedule if needed.

Penny called last week to schedule an appointment. She comes today with news that she was recently diagnosed with Stage I colon cancer following a recent colonoscopy—her first ever—done when she turned 50. You recognize how stressful this period is and will continue to be, particularly given her past history of anxiety. Even before her diagnosis of cancer, Penny was prone to lots of "catastrophizing" about events that, although possible, were highly improbable. You wonder how she will ever be able to control the very realistic worries and concerns about cancer-related issues. At times in the past, her worries were so strong that she was nearly paralyzed into a state of inaction and would fear even the most common everyday stressors. As you begin thinking about ways you can help, you recognize that although you have had a few clients with family members diagnosed with cancer, this will be your first client that you will be seeing throughout her time while receiving cancer treatments. You wonder if there is specific, cancer-related knowledge that you should have. You already can identify a number of relevant questions:

- *How serious is colon cancer?*
- *How does it compare to breast cancer in women? Is it more or less serious?*
- *Is this a very common cancer in women?*
- *What is its typical prognosis?*
- *What does Stage I mean? Is it better than Stage II or higher?*
- *Will Penny require surgery?*
- *What other treatments will she be going through?*
- *If she receives chemotherapy, what will the side effects be?*
- *Will Penny's history of anxiety influence any of her treatments?*
- *Will she be more prone to any side effects because of her anxiety?*
- *How much do her children already know about her disease?*
- *How will she deal with talking to her children about her disease?*
- *How much anxiety is considered "normal" or typical in these circumstances, given that there are realistic and understandable things about which to be worried?*
- *What are the differences between normal or typical amounts of anxiety and a level of anxiety that would be considered abnormal?*
- *Will Penny automatically become depressed as well? Do most cancer patients experience depression?*

CASE EXAMPLE 2

As part of the primary oncology team, you have provided oncology-nursing care to William, a 62-year-old married truck driver who was originally diagnosed with

Stage IIA non-small cell lung cancer 12 months ago. After surgery, he completed a course of chemotherapy and recently began to experience bone pain. After a series of scans, it has been determined that William has metastatic disease to his clavicle, as well as a few other "spots" on his sternum and humerus (upper arm). He comes today, accompanied by his wife of almost 40 years and two adult children, to get the results of these scans. You realize the results will be devastatingly bad news for this likeable family, and you try to anticipate how William will feel and react, as well as what his experience of receiving this news will be like for him and his family. A number of questions come to mind about what you might be able to do to help him and his family:

- *What are the most common emotional reactions when receiving such bad news?*
- *Will William react with "denial" of the reality of his situation?*
- *How can you tell the difference between a "normal" reaction in these circumstances and denial?*
- *What is the best thing for you to say to him, and to his wife and adult children?*
- *Should you consider referring William to a mental health professional? If so, what is the best way to explain why you think such a referral would be helpful?*
- *You worry that he may not completely understand the implications of this new information and you want to be sure he and his family understand what this means for his future. What is the best way for you to try to see that this happens?*

CASE EXAMPLE 3

In your role as the hospital chaplain you have a regular routine of visiting patients in the chemotherapy suites and waiting area. As you "round," you have come to know most of the patients in general ways, while others you have come to know more closely. They trust you and seem to find it very easy to talk to you about many aspects of their lives—medical, social, family, spiritual, and religious practices and beliefs. Recently, you were visiting with Jane, a very intelligent, religious woman with whom you have developed a close relationship of trust and respect. Two years ago, at age 42, she was diagnosed with Stage II breast cancer. She completed a lumpectomy and combination chemotherapy/radiation therapy and is back today for a follow-up appointment with her medical oncologist. Most of the times when you visit Jane, she is optimistic and in a positive mood. Oftentimes she is even inspirational to others with how well she has coped with her illness and its treatments. You have often thought that she represents the "ideal patient" and would be a good role model for other breast cancer patients.

Today you are visiting with Jane as she waits to see her oncologist. You notice she is not nearly as cheerful as usual and, in fact, looks and acts down and discouraged.

As you talk, she shares with you her doubts about her faith, her anger toward God, and, for the first time since you met her, some thoughts that maybe she "won't make it" in her "battle with cancer" and even that she is not sure she wants to "continue the fight." You are quite surprised, and a number of questions come to mind.

- *Is this depression? How do you differentiate between normal frustration and discouragement from more serious clinical depression?*
- *Are these feelings really that different to the "usual Jane," or is it that she is just now feeling trustful enough to share these thoughts with you and, thus, maybe this is a good sign that your relationship with her is improving?*
- *Are any of these thoughts suicidal ideation? If so, what is your responsibility in terms of asking Jane more about them and/or to referring her to a mental health professional?*
- *What is her past history of mental health? Has she ever felt this way before?*
- *Are you competent to deal with her situation, or are you "in over your head"?*
- *If you were to refer Jane to a mental health professional, how would you do that?*

The purpose of this book is to educate mental health and cancer care professionals about the evidence-based practice of adult psycho-oncology. As will be elaborated in upcoming chapters, despite significant advances in biomedical treatments for cancer, much progress remains in providing high-quality psychological and psychosocial evidence-based care. These ideas are not new; in recent years there have been multiple calls for action and ongoing development of clinical practice guidelines.

CALLS FOR ACTION AND PRACTICE GUIDELINES

A number of recent reports (Institute of Medicine & National Research Council, 2004, 2006) note the lack of high-quality psychological and social care for the cancer patient. As one key example, the 2008 Institute of Medicine (2008) report, *Cancer Care for the Whole Patient: Meeting Psychosocial Health Needs* highlights the following:

The extensive reach of cancer

- Fully 41% of all Americans can expect to be diagnosed with cancer at some point in their life. (p. 23)
- More than 10.5 million people in the United States live with a past or current diagnosis of some type of cancer. (p. 24)

The increase in length of life for many cancer patients and the reconceptualization of cancer as a chronic illness

- . . . substantial progress in the early detection and treatment of multiple types of cancer has significantly extended the life expectancy of patients to the point that many people diagnosed with cancer can be cured, and the illness of many others can be managed as a chronic disease. (p. 23)

and the lack of high-quality psychosocial care

- . . . the remarkable advances in biomedical care . . . have not been matched by achievements in providing high-quality care for the psychological and social effects of cancer. (p. 23)

This and other reports (Institute of Medicine & National Research Council, 2004, 2006) have emphasized the need for a discipline to focus on the psychological and social aspects of cancer. With the publication of the first handbook of psycho-oncology in 1989 (Holland & Rowland, 1989) followed by a much expanded version in 1998 (Holland, 1998), and its second edition in 2010 (Holland, Breitbart, et al., 2010), the field of psycho-oncology has advanced with the hope of addressing these needs. In recent years, researchers, clinicians, and policy makers have focused efforts on identifying, understanding, and addressing the psychological, social, emotional, spiritual, existential, and practical components of life, as affected by the human experience of the cancer illness by patients, families, caregivers, friends, and even professional health care providers.

Paralleling the growth and development of the field of psycho-oncology, there have been multiple "calls for action," both within the United States and internationally, to provide high-quality psychosocial services to all affected by cancer. Within the United States, most of these reports have been under the auspices of the National Academy of Science's Institute of Medicine. One of these reports, *Cancer Care for the Whole Patient: Meeting Psychosocial Health Needs* (Institute of Medicine, 2008) lists 15 related reports relevant to the provision of psychosocial services to cancer patients. Table 1.1 contains highlights of these reports and the clear need for the provision of high-quality psychosocial services.

Clinical practice guidelines, as defined by the Institute of Medicine as "systematically developed statements to assist practitioner and patient decisions about appropriate health care for specific clinical circumstances" (Field & Lohr, 1992, p. 2), have also been developed. Table 1.2 contains lists and explanations of clinical practice guidelines in psycho-oncology developed in the United States, Australia, and Canada.

PURPOSE, FOCUS, AND ORGANIZATION OF THIS BOOK

This book has a number of purposes:

- To introduce psychologists, psychiatrists, social workers, mental health counselors, marriage and family counselors, oncology nurses, chaplains, and other cancer care professionals to the importance of evidence-based practice of psycho-oncology

Table 1.1. MAJOR CALLS FOR HIGH-QUALITY PSYCHOSOCIAL SERVICES IN PSYCHO-ONCOLOGY

Reference	**Summary**
Crossing the Quality Chasm: A New Health System for the 21st Century (Institute of Medicine, 2001)	This was a broad-based report investigating health care in the United States. This report proposed a five-part agenda for "crossing the chasm" between (a) the dramatic growth in medical science and technology and (b) the provision of quality health care. Ten rules for redesigning health include these three: "continuous healing relationships," "evidence-based decision making," and "customization based upon patient needs and value." Within one specific recommendation the need for better infrastructure to support evidence-based practice and an emphasis on use of information technology are highlighted. Thirteen recommendations were offered; among them one specifically focuses on applying evidence to health care delivery.
Improving the Quality of Health Care for Mental and Substance-Use Conditions (Institute of Medicine, 2006)	This report notes a successful application of the earlier *Crossing the Quality Chasm* format to the unique aspects of mental and substance-use treatments. Among the nine recommendations offered, five are directly relevant to psychosocial care: reduction of stigma, improved strategies for suicide prevention, improved access and accountability, culturally competent care, and equity in addressing mental health problems (equal to physical health). In addition, specific mention of advancing evidence-based practice by demonstration projects and efforts to enhance dissemination of available evidence are also recommended.
Ensuring Quality Cancer Care (Institute of Medicine, 1999)	This was an early report that focused on the state of the entire cancer care system (all cancer types, all forms of treatment and delivery models), defining quality cancer care and problems evident through the mid-1990s. The report concluded that some individuals with cancer do not receive care that is known to be effective for their disease. Ten recommendations were offered, one of which focused on "elements of quality care" that included "psychosocial support services and compassionate care."

Meeting Psychosocial Needs of Women With Breast Cancer (Institute of Medicine & National Research Council, 2004)	This report focused specifically on psychosocial needs of women with breast cancer. Five questions regarding psychosocial distress in women with breast cancer were addressed: frequency, effectiveness of interventions, delivery of interventions, barriers to receiving services, and what steps can be taken to improve psychosocial care? Relevant conclusions: About 30% of women show significant distress, particularly at transition points in their care (e.g., time of diagnosis, recurrence, etc.). There is strong evidence of effectiveness of interventions, from randomized trials and meta-analyses sufficient to support the inclusion of psychosocial services in routine care. However, the availability of services is quite variable and largely unknown since there is no systematic monitoring. A number of barriers impede availability of care (e.g., outpatient care, often in private practice facilities without psychosocial staff; fragmented, uncoordinated care across multiple specialists). Three categories of recommendations were offered that focused on improving clinical practice, professional education/training, and research.
From Cancer Patient to Cancer Survivor: Lost in Transition (Institute of Medicine & National Research Council, 2006)	This report estimates that in 2002 there were "10 million Americans alive with a personal diagnosis of cancer" (p. 1). It focused on the transition from the active phase of treatment to posttreatment care, highlighting the need for improved survivorship care. Four components make up survivorship care: *prevention* of recurrent and new cancers, *surveillance* for cancer spread, *intervention* for consequences of cancer and its treatment, and *coordination* between specialist and primary care providers. This report had three goals: (a) raise awareness of the medical, functional, and psychosocial consequences of cancer treatment; (b) define quality health care for cancer survivors; and (c) improve quality of life by focusing on access to care, fair employment practices, and health insurance. In addressing these goals, ten recommendations were made, two of which are directly relevant to evidence-based, psychosocial care: provide a written survivorship care plan and develop evidence-based clinical practice guidelines.

(*Continued*)

Table 1.1. Continued

Reference	Summary
Improving Supportive and Palliative Care for Adults With Cancer (National Institute for Clinical Excellence, 2004)	The National Institute for Clinical Excellence (NICE) is an independent organization charged with providing guidance on health issues in the United Kingdom. These guidelines define supportive care as that which "helps the patient and their family to cope with cancer and treatment of it—from pre-diagnosis, through the process of diagnosis and treatment, to cure, continuing illness or death and into bereavement" (p. 18). The guidelines are similar to the NCCN, encompassing psychological, social, and spiritual support, as well as the importance of coordinated care, provision of information to patients and families, and open face-to-face communication, while also distinguishing general palliative care by the primary care team from more specialized palliative care.
Standards of Psychosocial Health Services for Persons With Cancer and Their Families (CAPO, 2010)	These Canadian standards are updated from an early statement in 1999. They are organized into four sections. Section I introduces key definitions of terms, including *psychosocial health services*, *psychosocial oncology*, and *supportive*. Section II explains the scope of the standards as they apply to all cancer patients and their families/caregivers, across various health care settings (i.e., tertiary care, community oncology program, primary care providers, community-based cancer agencies) and the requirement for routine, regular screening and assessment of health care needs. Section III explains key principles guiding the development of the standards, and Section IV presents the actual standards of care organized into four sections specifying standards for organizational structure, professional education, and patient care. Key principle 6 is on evidence-based care and Standards of Care II–VI specify that patients are entitled to psychosocial screening, treatment, palliation, survivorship, and grief/bereavement services across the continuum of cancer care.

Table 1.2. Clinical Practice Guidelines in Psycho-Oncology

Reference	Summary
National Comprehensive Cancer Network (NCCN) Distress Management Guidelines (National Comprehensive Cancer Network, 2014)	The NCCN is a nonprofit alliance of 21 of the leading, comprehensive cancer centers in the United States. They offer clinical practice guidelines for many components of cancer care, one of which is focused on the management of distress. These guidelines are based on categorized levels of evidence that are a combination of consensus and strength of scientific evidence. For distress management, all recommendations are listed as Category 2A—lower level of scientific evidence, but full NCCN consensus. The guideline proposes standards of care in which distress should be screened for regularly (at initial visit, any change in status such as recurrence/progression, and at other times as clinically indicated), and appropriate referral made to qualified professionals. This guideline also calls for availability of licensed and appropriately trained mental health professionals and chaplains; reimbursement for such services; inclusion of psychosocial assessment in any health outcomes measurement; and education of patients, families, and treatment providers that the management of distress is a part of total medical care. Algorithms outlining the evaluation and treatment process of a number of problems involving mental health, social work, and chaplaincy services are provided. Guidelines are updated annually.
Clinical Practice Guidelines for the Psychosocial Care of Adults With Cancer (National Breast Cancer Centre and National Cancer Control Initiative, 2003)	These Australian-developed guidelines, applicable to all adult cancers, are an extension of earlier guidelines developed for breast cancer. They specify levels of evidence, where Level I evidence is from systematic literature reviews (e.g., meta-analyses) and Level II are from randomized controlled trials. These guidelines acknowledge the stress experienced by health care professionals providing services to cancer patients. They then summarize the 41 specific statements with the appropriate corresponding level of evidence rating. Guidelines are presented in three sections focused on (a) care provided to all patients by the primary oncology team, (b) referral for specialized psychosocial care, and (c) consideration of special issues. In part one, the importance of good communication between patient and clinician (e.g., empathy, active listening, open questions); the provision of accurate information (e.g., telling of the diagnosis, discussing prognosis, treatment options, preparation for stressful medical procedures); awareness of and attention to emotional, social, practical, and financial support; and continuity of care and support at end of life are emphasized. In part two, specialty referrals to psychology, psychiatry, social work, and other services are explained and encouraged by providing summaries of the evidence of the efficacy of such services. Part three attends to special issues of diversity (cultural, linguistic, age, gender, geography, and sexual orientation). These guidelines are unique in their recognition of the stress experienced by health care professionals.

(*Continued*)

Table 1.2. Continued

Reference	Summary
A Pan-Canadian Clinical Practice Guideline: Assessment of Psychosocial Health Care Needs of the Adult Cancer Patient (Howell et al., 2009)	"This guideline provides professional health care providers with recommendations regarding routine, systematic and standardized assessment of psychosocial health care needs for adult populations affected by cancer. Recommendations are informed by empirical evidence embedded in international guidelines, systematic reviews, and consensus of interdisciplinary psychosocial experts" (p. 6). They offer 12 recommendations based upon expert consensus, regarding adult psychosocial health care needs.
A Pan-Canadian Practice Guideline: Screening, Assessment, and Care of Psychosocial Distress (Depression, Anxiety) in Adults With Cancer (Howell et al., 2010)	Closely related to the guideline above, this guideline focuses on screening for depression and anxiety in adult cancer patients. It provides detailed information about the optimum screening, assessment, and psychosocial-supportive care of patients identified as experiencing depression and/or anxiety. It follows recommended procedures for guideline development and provides detailed information about the development methodology. Detailed information is provided distinguishing between screening (a "snapshot" to flag a problem), comprehensive assessment (a combination of procedures to identify specific problems and contributing factors), and focused assessment (a targeted appraisal, typically by practitioners with specialized training) of both anxiety and depression. Detailed flow diagrams illustrating the screening and assessment processes and subsequent care pathways are provided.
Cancer Care Ontario (CCO) Psychosocial Health Care for Cancer Patients and Their Families (Turnbull et al., October 2012)	These guidelines were developed by determining the applicability of the Institute of Medicine's (2008) *Cancer Care for the Whole Patient* recommendations, for the cancer care context of Ontario. Eight of the Institute of Medicine recommendations were adapted, from which 31 recommendations for high-quality psychosocial care were made.

Oncology Nursing Society (ONS, 2008b). *Putting Evidence Into Practice (PEP): Depression*	These guidelines are focused on oncology nurses and what types of interventions they could use, in daily clinical practice, to assist patients with depression.
Oncology Nursing Society (ONS, 2008a). *Putting Evidence Into Practice (PEP): Anxiety*	These guidelines are focused on oncology nurses and what types of interventions they could use, in daily clinical practice, to assist patients with anxiety.
An American Society of Clinical Oncology Guideline Adaptation: Screening, Assessment and Care of Anxiety and Depressive Symptoms in Adults with Cancer (Andersen et al., 2014)	These ASCO Guidelines were adapted from the Pan-Canadian Guidelines on Screening, Assessment, and Care of Psychosocial Distress in Adults (Howell et al, 2010) to fit the health care context of the United States. Detailed algorithms for screening and assessment of depression and anxiety are provided, along with care maps that detail pathways for varying levels of symptoms. A list of selected measures for screening is also provided.

- To educate readers about the necessary steps and competencies for doing evidence-based practice
- To demonstrate how to do evidence-based practice in psycho-oncology by providing detailed case examples, organized around four treatment modalities: individual, group, couples, and family
- To contribute to the growing field of resources about dissemination and implementation of evidence-based psychological treatments in health care
- To provide a resource that will increase the capacity of clinicians to deliver evidence-based psychosocial interventions—an important component of the proposed *push-pull infrastructure* for translating research to practice (Jacobsen, 2010)

To achieve these purposes, this book is to be:

- Both *introductory*—Part I introduces relevant literature in oncology, evidence-based practice, and psychotherapy—and *advance*d. Part II demonstrates how to use the evidence-based competencies for individual, group, couples, and family-focused interventions.
- *Clinically useful* with detailed case examples of evidence-based practice
- *Accessible* in format by providing tables and figures throughout
- *Current* with recommended exemplars of best available evidence and a discussion of issues in translational research, and processes of diffusion→ dissemination→implementation

Cancer has an extensive impact on the lives of millions of people. Improved biomedical treatments have extended lives, increasing the number of cancer survivors, and yet most cancer patients do not receive adequate psychological and psychosocial care. As cancer care settings increase efforts to identify psychosocial distress, knowledgeable and well-trained professionals, prepared to provide evidence-based psycho-oncology, are needed. A comprehensive resource with background knowledge and detailed case examples, illustrating how to do evidence-based care, will contribute to the development of well-qualified providers of psychosocial health services in oncology.

2

Background Knowledge of Oncology

This chapter focuses on the general background knowledge that health care professionals working with cancer patients will need to understand regarding the evidence-based practice (EBP) of adult psycho-oncology. EBP begins by asking general-knowledge questions to first acquire an understanding of relevant background literature. *General* background knowledge ultimately guides the formation of a clinically relevant question about a *particular* individual patient. To proceed with EBP, an understanding of both the general and the particular is needed. Chapters 3 and 4 provide general background knowledge.

This chapter contains three sections:

- The basics of cancer
- Terms and definitions most relevant to the EBP of adult clinical psycho-oncology
- A review and critique of the psycho-oncology evidence base

THE BASICS OF CANCER

To function in the multidisciplinary oncology setting, the psycho-oncologist needs to have a basic understanding of oncology. Communication with other cancer care professionals assumes a level of basic shared knowledge. This section provides that basic information by providing answers to specific, relevant questions.[1]

1. The information for this Basics of Cancer section was taken from three primary sources: The APOS "Cancer 101 for Mental Health Professionals" online educational modules (http://www.apos-society.org/professionals/meetings-ed/webcasts/webcasts-ican3.aspx); the National Cancer Institute Web site for basics of cancer (http://www.cancer.gov/cancertopics/cancerlibrary/what-is-cancer); and the NCI's general information about cancer treatments (http://www.cancer.gov/cancertopics/treatment/types-of-treatment).

What Is Cancer?

The human body is made up of millions of cells, each containing 23 pairs of chromosomes that carry genetic information within the DNA that directs the growth and functioning of each cell. Cells divide and grow through a multiphase process known as the *cell cycle*, in which specific activities occur at each phase of the cycle. In normal cell development, cells reproduce through a process of *mitosis*. Likewise, over time, cells die via a normal process of programmed cell death known as *apoptosis*. This process of cell growth and death allows new cells to replace old cells, with a turnover rate of more than a billion cells per day. Cancer is a disease that originates from normal, healthy cells losing their ability to control growth. As mitosis and apoptosis malfunction, cells divide and grow without control or order. Such abnormal cell growth can result in a malignant tumor (growth, lesion, mass, or lump) known as cancer. Cancer is not a single disease, but rather a group of more than 200 different diseases.

Etiology: What Causes a Normal Cell to Be Transformed Into a Cancer Cell?

Various genetic and environmental processes are thought to cause gene mutations that transform a gene into an oncogene. An *oncogene* is a mutated form of a gene involved in the process of cell growth. Oncogenes may cause cancer cells to grow. *Carcinogenesis* is the process by which normal cells are transformed into cancer cells. It begins with an initiation phase in which damage to the DNA occurs such that a gene is altered or mutated and becomes an oncogene. After this initial process of carcinogenesis, further cell growth is promoted and encouraged, which may result in the process of *progression* in which abnormal cellular growth continues. In the earliest stages of growth, cancer cells are confined to the particular layer of cells in which they first develop. This is known as *carcinoma* in situ, or noninvasive cancer. As cancer cells continue to grow, however, they can invade other layers of cells and destroy surrounding healthy tissues. Uncontrolled growth can proceed to compress, invade, and damage normal tissues, producing debilitating local and distant effects.

Cancer Types: How Are the Many Types of Cancer Organized?

One system for organizing the variety of types of cancer is based on the types of cells that make up the cancer. Two categories of cell types result in two groups of cancers: solid tumors and hematologic tumors. *Solid tumors* are abnormal masses of tissue that *do not* contain liquids or cysts. Solid tumors consist of cell types further subdivided into two categories: sarcomas and carcinomas. *Sarcomas* are tumors that develop in bone, cartilage, fat, muscle, blood vessels, or other connective or supportive tissues. *Carcinomas* are tumors that form in the skin or in epithelial tissue that lines or covers internal organs and account for the majority (80%–90%) of all cancers. The second broad category is *hematologic* tumors or cancers of the blood, plasma cells, bone marrow, or lymphatic system, such as the leukemias or lymphomas.

Beyond organization by cell type, cancers are also categorized by the site, location, or organ system where they are located, such as breast, colorectal, lung, and prostate. A particular organ system can have a solid tumor that is either a sarcoma or a carcinoma, as many sites have both connective or supportive tissue as well as tissue that lines or covers organs.

Mortality: How Many People Die From Cancer?

Cancer is the second leading cause of death in the United States, after heart disease. In 2014, it is estimated that more than 310,000 men and 275,000 women will die from cancer—with lung cancers accounting for about 28% of those deaths in men and 26% in women. In men, prostate and colorectal cancers account for an additional 10% and 8% each, while in women breast cancer is the second most common, accounting for an additional 15% (American Cancer Society, 2014). The good news is that the overall death rates from cancer have been declining since the early 1990s for both men and women, with rates reported in 2005 being 19.2% lower in men and 11.4% in women and in 2010 as a 20% decline in all cancer deaths (Siegel, Ma, Zou, & Jemal, 2014). There are important differences in death rates between Whites and African Americans in the United States. Death rates from cancer in African Americans continue to be higher than in Whites, although rates have dropped in both populations, with declines in death rates dropping faster in African Americans.

Incidence: How Many New Cases of Cancer Are Being Diagnosed?

It is estimated that approximately 1.6 million new cases of cancer will be diagnosed in 2014. Of these, about 855,000 will be in men and 810,000 in women. In men, prostate (27%), lung (14%), and colorectal (8%) are expected to be the three most common types of new cancers, while in women it will be breast (29%), lung (13%), and colorectal (8%). Men have a lifetime probability of being diagnosed with cancer of 1 in 2 and women have a 1 in 3 lifetime prevalence. Risk of developing cancer increases with age. More optimistically, it is important to note that the overall incidence of cancers is declining for both men and women: declining 1.5% per year from 2001 to 2005 and 0.6% per year from 2006 to 2010 for men and dropping 0.6% per year from 1998 to 2005 and remaining steady during 2006–2010 for women (Siegel et al., 2014).

Severity: Once Diagnosed, How Are Cancers Determined To Be More or Less Severe?

A system of both staging and grading of tumors determines the relative severity of a newly diagnosed cancer. *Staging* is a system designed to organize the size, location, and extent of the cancer into a stage ranging from 0 to IV, with increasing stage indicative of a more severe cancer. The stage of a cancer is also critical in determining the appropriate treatment options. There are various staging systems that depend upon the type of cancer, but one common system is organized around three components: primary tumor (T), regional lymph nodes (N), and metastasis (M). In the TNM system, the T (primary tumor) indicates the tumor location (e.g., breast, prostate, lung), size, extent, and depth of invasion. The N (lymph nodes) indicates the regional lymph nodes and the presence or absence of cancer cells in the lymph nodes or lymphatic system, and M (metastasis) indicates whether there is or is not any evidence of cancer cells anywhere throughout the body other than at the primary tumor or regional lymph nodes. A number is added after each of these three components indicating increases in size, depth, involvement, or extent of disease. The TNM information is then converted to a specific stage ranging from 0 to IV. For example, a breast cancer where the primary tumor was between 2 and 5 centimeters, there were no cancer cells in any lymph nodes, and no evidence of any metastases would be staged as T2N0M0, which is Stage IIA. Treatments are determined by stage.

Grading is a system for classifying cells in which it is determined how much a cell looks like or does not look like a normal, healthy cell when examined under a microscope. A "well-differentiated" cancer cell is a cell that looks a lot like a healthy cell (although it is still a cancer cell), and this appearance is helpful in knowing from what part of the body this cell originated (e.g., breast, lung, prostate). A grade can provide information about how likely a cell is to grow and spread, and this information has implications for decisions about treatment. Different grading systems are used for different types of cancers, and thus the meaning of a particular grade depends on the type of cancer. However, in general, the more a cancer cell is like known healthy cells (i.e., well-differentiated), the better the overall scenario.

Prognosis: Which Types of Cancer Have Better or Worse Prognoses Than Other Types?

In addition to stage or grade, the site, or type of cancer is predictive of prognosis. Cancer types differ in long-term prognoses, and their overall severity can be estimated by considering 5-year relative survival rates (American Cancer Society, 2014). Cancer types, organized by 5-year survival rates from highest to lowest likelihood of survival, provide a *continuum of severity* from least severe at the top of the list to most severe at the bottom. This severity continuum is shown in Table 2.1.

Table 2.1. Cancer Severity Continuum as Based on 5-Year Relative Survival Rates

Very high likelihood (>90%) of 5-year survival

- prostate (99%), thyroid (98%), testis (97%), melanoma (93%)

High likelihood (80%–90%) of 5-year survival

- female breast (90%), Hodgkin's lymphoma (88%), uterine corpus (84%), bladder (80%)

Moderate likelihood (60%–80%) of 5-year survival

- kidney (73%), non-Hodgkin's lymphoma (71%), rectal (68%), colon (65%), oral cavity/pharynx (65%), larynx (63%)

Low likelihood (20%–50%) of 5-year survival

- leukemia (59%), myeloma (45%), ovarian (44%), brain (35%), stomach (29%)

Very low likelihood (<20%) of 5-year survival

- esophageal (19%), lung/bronchus (18%), liver (18%), pancreas (6%)

NOTES: This continuum ranges from *least severe* disease at the top of the table to *most severe* at the bottom of the table, based upon 5-year relative survival rates. Five-year survival rates provide only a general introductory information about severity and prognosis. Many other variables influence prognoses and, thus, this information should be used cautiously when considering their relevance to an individual cancer patient's prognosis.

Note that 5-year survival rates can vary considerably based on other variables such as stage, grade, presence of metastases, and other individual patient differences. This continuum provides general introductory information about severity and should thus be used cautiously when considering an individual cancer patient's prognosis.

Survival: How Many and Who Are the People Surviving After a Diagnosis of Cancer?

Survival rates for all cancers have improved over the past 30 years. The 5-year relative survival rate for all cancers diagnosed between 2002 and 2009 is 68%, which is up from 49% in 1975–1977. This increase is thought to be due mostly to improvements in early detection and treatment. In 2014 it is estimated that there are nearly 14 million Americans currently living with a prior diagnosis of cancer. The following types of cancers and their estimated percentage of all survivors, as reported in 2009 (American Cancer Society, 2009) provide a better idea of who current survivors are.

- In men, 42% are prostate cancer survivors, 11% colorectal, 8% bladder, 7% melanoma, 4% non-Hodgkin lymphoma, 4% lung/bronchus, 3% oral cavity and pharynx, 3% kidney and renal pelvis, 3% leukemia, 2%

Hodgkin lymphoma, and all other cancers account for the remaining 13% of male survivors.

- In women, 41% are breast cancer survivors, 9% uterine corpus, 9% colorectal, 6% melanoma, 4% uterine cervix, 3% non-Hodgkin lymphoma, 3% lung/bronchus, 3% ovarian, 2% bladder, 2% kidney and renal pelvis, and all other cancers account for the remaining 18% of female survivors.

As survival rates have increased, the associated medical and psychosocial issues have become increasingly important and attention to the needs of survivors of cancer has increased (Feuerstein, 2007; Institute of Medicine & National Research Council, 2006).

Treatment: What Are the Major Methods of Treating Cancers?

Surgery

Surgery is both the oldest and most common form of cancer treatment for solid or nonhematologic tumors. The goals of surgical procedures for cancers are varied, with the obvious goal being to remove the tumor. Other surgeries are for diagnostic purposes, such as obtaining a portion of the tumor cells for an accurate histologic diagnosis, which entails examining tissues under a microscope. Surgical procedures are also used for reconstruction (e.g., in breast cancer) and for prevention of future cancers (e.g., in the decision of a woman with a genetically high risk of breast cancer who chooses a prophylactic, bilateral mastectomy—surgery to remove both breasts). As a local procedure, side effects from surgery are generally contained to the area of the body where the surgery occurred. Patients' overall health status prior to the surgery will influence the severity of side effects and recovery time. In the past, surgery was usually the first line of treatment, with chemotherapy and/or radiation administered after. However, in recent years, chemotherapy and/or radiation treatments have often been done prior to surgery, with the goal of shrinking the tumor to make surgery less invasive and, hopefully, more successful. Treatments given prior to the main treatment, like surgery, are known as *neoadjuvant* therapies.

Chemotherapy

Chemotherapy is the treatment of malignant tumors with medications. It works by killing or slowing the growth of cancer cells as they grow and develop through the stages of the cell cycle. Chemotherapy is a systemic form of treatment administered (e.g., intravenously) so that its effects can be felt throughout multiple physical systems of the body (e.g., throughout the gastrointestinal, dermatologic, cardiovascular, and immune systems). It is used in the treatment of both solid and hematologic cancers. The goals of chemotherapy treatments for cancer are to stop or slow the growth of cancer cells. Chemotherapy is used to cure cancers, to control the spread of cancer cells, and to ease symptoms. As a systemic treatment, chemotherapy has multiple side effects. One of the more common effects is *bone marrow suppression*, which is the decreased production of white cells, red cells, and platelets by the marrow (the sponge-like tissue in the center of most bones) responsible for production of these cells. Bone marrow suppression can result in anemia caused by a decreased number of red cells; an increased risk of infection due to a decrease in white cells to fight off infections; and an increased risk of excessive bleeding or poor wound healing due to the decrease in platelets. The most common side effect of chemotherapy is fatigue. Alopecia (hair loss) is another common side effect, as are nausea and vomiting. These side effects are common because chemotherapy drugs have their strongest effect on those cells with the shortest half-lives—those that reproduce the most quickly—such as cells of the inner lining of the gastrointestinal system and hair cells. Recent years have seen improvement in methods for controlling these side effects, and it is important to note that chemotherapy drugs differ in terms of how minimal or strong their side effects can be. A specified period or number of chemotherapy treatments, followed by a specified period of rest, is considered a cycle of treatment. Chemotherapy protocols vary by the number and pattern of a cycle and are determined by the type of cancer, its stage, and other patient and disease characteristics. The medical oncologist's overarching goal is to administer the full recommended dose of chemotherapy and closely attend to and manage treatment-related side effects.

Radiation Therapy

Radiation therapy is the use of high-energy radiation to kill cancer cells and shrink tumors by damaging the cells' genetic material. Radiation can be administered in the form of an external beam coming from a machine outside the body or as an implant in the form of radioactive materials placed inside the body (brachytherapy) near the tumor site. Radiation therapy differs by how deeply it can penetrate and how accurately it can be targeted to a small area in the body. The overall goal is to kill cancer cells while keeping healthy cells unaffected. Radiation is administered to about 60% of all cancer patients and is used for both local and hematologic cancers. Fatigue and skin changes are the most common side effects. The cause of fatigue is often unknown but when identified (e.g., anemia) can be treated. As a symptom, fatigue is often thought to be part of other problems such as depression, anxiety, overall distress, or lack of activity. Energy conservation measures are recommended to help manage the fatigue. As a local treatment, most side effects of radiation therapy are contained to the area of the body receiving the radiation. Thus, a common side effect is skin changes, such as redness, sunburn, itchiness, dryness, and peeling. In areas of the body where there are skin folds, it may become moist, wet, sore, and infected. Other local side effects vary by the location of the treatment, such as diarrhea for treatments to the abdomen, or dry mouth, mouth sores, and loss of taste sensations with radiation to the head and neck.

Biological Therapies

Biological therapies (also called biologic response modifiers, biotherapy, and immunotherapy) are cancer treatments that use substances made from a living organism or its products (i.e., biologic agent) in the prevention, diagnosis, or treatment of cancers. These naturally occurring biologic agents are reproduced in the laboratory. Examples include monoclonal antibodies, interleukins, growth factors, and vaccines. These treatments work by boosting or restoring the immune system's ability to fight cancer and infections. Side effects include fatigue, depression, and flu-like symptoms. Depression is associated primarily with the use of the interleukins and interferons and can be quite severe. Many biological therapies are being researched for use in new ways. The use of biological therapies for cancer treatments include interleukin-2 for the treatment of metastatic kidney cancer and interferon alpha for treatment of hairy cell leukemia, chronic myeloid leukemia, melanoma, and AIDS-related Kaposi's sarcoma. In efforts to control some side effects from bone marrow suppression, colony-stimulating factors (CSFs, also called hematopoietic growth factors) encourage growth of new bone marrow stem cells that, in turn, will produce more white blood cells, red blood cells, and platelets. One example is the use of erythropoietin to increase the number of red blood cells to treat anemia and decrease the need for red blood cell transfusions.

Antibodies are proteins created as part of an immune response to substances within the body known as antigens. Another form of biological therapy involves monoclonal antibodies (MOABs)—antibodies created in a laboratory that are specific to a single antigen. If MOABs can be created to "find" specific antigens that are involved in tumor growth, then malignant cells can be "targeted." The MOAB can then deliver an anticancer drug directly to a tumor. MOABs can also be built to react against certain growth factors that are involved in the regulation of cell division and survival.

Vaccines are another form of biological therapy that work by enhancing the immune response following injection of a small and weaker form of an antigen. Efforts are underway to identify effective vaccines for both prevention and treatment of cancers.

A term closely related to biological therapies is *targeted cancer therapies*. These are drugs or other substances that block the growth and/or spread of cancer by interfering with specific molecules and molecular processes known to be involved in the growth and progression of cancer cells. These various forms of therapies are labeled "targeted" because they are focused on identified molecular and cellular processes specific to cancer cells and target these processes only, rather than systemic treatments that affect normal cells. Thus, they are often less harmful to normal, noncancerous cells, resulting in fewer side effects than traditional chemotherapy and radiation therapy. Three types of drugs (and other substances that interfere with specific molecules involved in cancer cell growth) have been developed for use as targeted therapies: small molecules, antibodies, and vaccines. They work in a variety of ways to affect cancer cells:

- They interfere with the signaling mechanisms involved in cellular growth.
- They interrupt and prevent the development of blood vessels to cancer cells (i.e., angiogenesis).
- They promote known mechanisms that enhance cell death (apoptosis).

- They stimulate the immune system to destroy cancer cells.
- They are a part of the transport system that delivers specific toxic drugs to kill cancer cells.

A number of targeted therapies have FDA approval for treatment of specific types of cancers such as breast cancer, lymphomas/leukemia, multiple myeloma, and prostate cancer, with more in development and in ongoing clinical trials. One well-known example in breast cancer involves various drugs (e.g., tamoxifen, toremifine, fulvestrant) that interfere with the hormone estrogen from binding to estrogen receptors within the cell—a process that normally triggers molecular processes that result in increased cell/tumor growth. As the drugs interfere with estrogen from binding with estrogen receptors, these processes of cancer cell growth are interrupted. Thus, for those breast cancers that are determined to be responsive to the hormone estrogen (i.e., ER positive), this type of targeted treatment is used.

Transplantation: Bone Marrow and Peripheral Blood Stem Cells
Bone marrow, the soft, sponge-like material inside bones, contains immature cells known as hematopoietic (blood-forming) stem cells. Stem cells divide and grow to produce more stem cells, which mature into red cells, white cells, and platelets, all of which are essential for energy, fighting infections, and healing. Most stem cells are found in bone marrow, but some are also found in the bloodstream and are thus known as peripheral blood stem cells. High doses of chemotherapy and other treatments can be given to severely damage and even destroy the bone marrow such that it stops or fails to produce these stem cells. Patients then undergo a bone marrow transplant. The actual transplant is done as an intravenous procedure in which previously "harvested" healthy stem cells are transplanted via a regular intravenous injection, following very heavy doses of chemotherapy. The intent is (1) to "kill off" cancer cells with a heavy dose of chemotherapy, and then (2) to transplant healthy stem cells with the intent that these new stem cells will produce healthy red cells, white cells, and platelets. There are two main types of transplant procedures, one in which the patient receives his or her own stem cells (autologous) and the other in which the patient receives stem cells from another person (allogeneic). Cells are harvested from a donor, who is typically a close family member. Transplantation is most commonly used in the treatment of leukemias and lymphomas. The major risk of both of these treatments is increased susceptibility to infection and bleeding as a result of the very-high-dose chemotherapy given prior to the transplant. Short-term side effects include nausea, vomiting, fatigue, loss of appetite, mouth sores, hair loss, and skin reactions, while long-term risks are mostly the result of the pretransplant chemotherapy and radiation and include infertility, cataracts, damage to major organ systems (kidney, liver, heart, lungs), and an increased risk, over the life span, of new cancers. Graft versus host disease (GVHD) is a potential complication of allogeneic transplants where the patient receives stem cells from another person.

Hormonal Therapy

A *hormone* is a chemical made by the endocrine glands of the body that circulates throughout the bloodstream, to control the actions of certain cells and organs. *Hormonal therapy* is treatment that adds, blocks, or removes certain hormones. It is a systemic treatment and is used for solid tumors. Side effects are related to the particular type of hormone used and whether it is adding, removing, or blocking the production of natural hormones. The most common side effects include hot flashes, breast enlargement in men, and the induction of early menopause in younger women. Breast and prostate cancers are two types in which hormonal therapy is common. In prostate cancer, male sex hormones such as testosterone can cause cancer cells to grow. Thus, hormonal therapy is used to stop or block the effect of male sex hormones on the growth of cancer cells. In breast cancer, the drug tamoxifen inhibits the binding of estradiol (a natural estrogen) to estrogen receptor cells, causing the reduction of the actions of estrogen. This hormonal therapy has been used both to prevent the initial occurrence of breast cancer as well as to prevent its recurrence in already diagnosed women.

Treatment Goals: Are There Goals for Treatment Other Than Cure?

Whether administered individually, or in a wide variety of combinations, the treatments mentioned earlier can be provided for varying goals:

- Cure is the goal of all patients and health care providers.
- Cure is not always possible, however, and thus a secondary goal of treatment is to control the disease. This goal is increasingly achievable and results in more types of cancers being considered chronic conditions/diseases. A *chronic disease* is usually defined by its permanence, nonreversible pathology, and need for ongoing, long-term care.
- Palliation, another goal of treatment, focuses on relief of symptoms and suffering and enhanced quality of life. The goal of palliative care is not cure, but symptom relief, avoidance of suffering, and improved quality of life.
- One final goal is prevention. Here treatments are provided prior to a diagnosis of cancer in an effort to prevent its occurrence. One example is the use of bilateral mastectomy or tamoxifen as chemotherapy prevention in women with the *BRCA1* and *BRCA2* genetic mutations.

Cancer Care Trajectories

The IOM report *Cancer Care for the Whole Patient* (Institute of Medicine, 2008) organizes the varieties of the clinical course into four trajectories. All trajectories begin with *diagnosis and staging* and, given availability of a curative primary treatment, proceed to *treatment with intent to cure*. Figure 2.1 provides an illustration of four cancer care trajectories.

These four trajectories include the following:

- *Curative treatment*—treatment with intent to cure and long-term survivorship
- *No curative treatment available*—palliative treatment and death
- *Cancer as a chronic illness*—managed chronic, intermittent disease/treatments
- *Treatment with intent to cure, cancer-free survival followed by recurrence/metastasis, secondary treatment, and palliative care*

There is, of course, the potential for any individual patient to have some variation, or mixed combination, of these trajectories, but these descriptive labels are designed to provide a schema to help organize information about where a particular patient might be along the particular disease continuum.

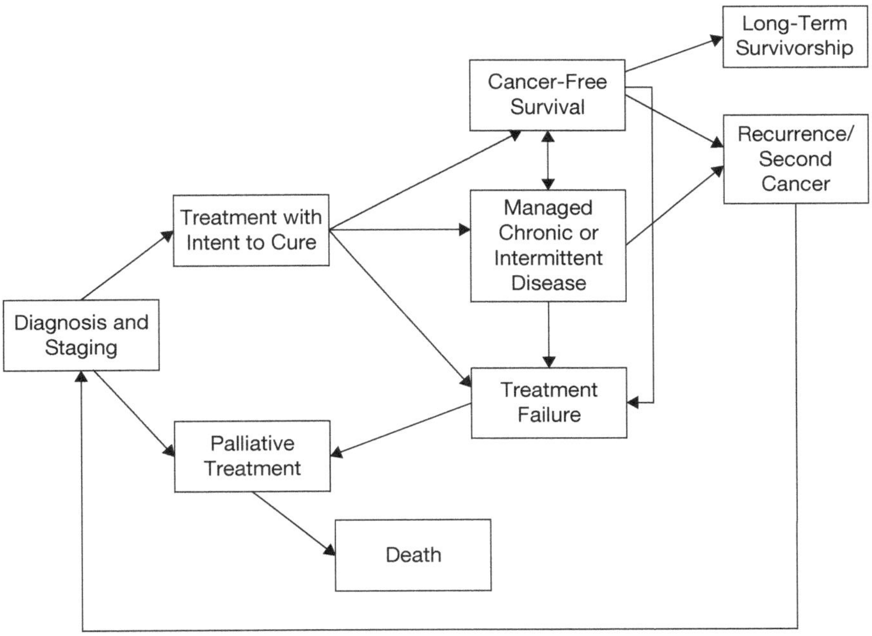

Figure 2.1 Cancer care trajectories.
SOURCE: Institute of Medicine (IOM). (2008). *Cancer care for the whole patient: Meeting psychosocial health needs*. Washington, DC: The National Academies Press. Adapted from Institute of Medicine (IOM) and National Research Council (NRC). Reprinted with permission from the National Academies Press, Copyright 2006 National Academy of Sciences.

TERMS AND DEFINITIONS FOR THE EVIDENCE-BASED PRACTICE OF ADULT, CLINICAL PSYCHO-ONCOLOGY

What follows are explanations and definitions of key terms and concepts relevant to the primary focus of this book: the evidence-based practice of adult, clinical psycho-oncology in the local cancer care setting.

Evidence-Based Practice

EBP has been defined as "the integration of best research evidence with clinical expertise and patient values" (Institute of Medicine, 2001, p. 147). EBP in psycho-oncology, as a multidisciplinary subspecialty, has been influenced by its parent disciplines of oncology, psychology, psychiatry, social work, and oncology nursing. In each of these parent disciplines, EBP has been variously defined, but all have maintained the three components of best available research with clinical expertise in the context of patient preferences. Chapter 4 provides a much more detailed explanation and discussion of EBP.

Adult Clinical Psycho-Oncology

In the context of cancer care, an *adult* is one whose physiology and anatomy are fully developed and matured; its relevance is to the selection and method of administration of appropriate cancer treatments. Most cancer care professionals receive specialized training in either adult or child oncology, but rarely for both populations. *Clinical* refers to the observation and treatment of actual patients, rather than theoretical or basic research. Clinical questions are those faced by an active clinician, who needs practical answers for real-world problems. In EBP, clinical questions are mostly focused on screening, assessment, diagnosis, treatment planning, interventions, and successful outcome (Straus, Richardson, Glasziou, & Haynes, 2005).

Psycho-oncology is a subspecialty of oncology concerned with the psychological and social issues related to cancer (Holland, 1992). This subspecialty has attracted interest from multiple disciplines and has thus become a multidisciplinary field consisting of two components: (a) the psychobiological or behavioral and (b) the psychosocial. These two components differ by their primary location along a typical health continuum, ranging from premature death to optimal health. The *psychobiological and behavioral* component focuses mostly on prevention of cancer. These factors influence the onset and severity of cancers, including risk factors to a diagnosis, treatment, and progression of cancer—typically those variables located along the health continuum *prior to* an actual cancer diagnosis. This first component focuses on behaviors such as smoking, diet, sun exposure, adherence to screening recommendations, and compliance to treatment regimens as related to issues of morbidity and mortality (Holland & Weiss, 2010).

The second component of psycho-oncology—the *psychosocial*—focuses on the psychological and social responses of patients, families, and caregivers, to the variety of factors that influence coping and adjustment at all phases of the illness experience—typically those variables located along the health continuum *after* a cancer diagnosis (Holland & Weiss, 2010). Adaptation or adjustment to cancer, prevalence of mental disorders, symptom management, psychosocial health services, and interventions for persons affected by cancer (Holland & Weiss, 2010) are all examples of the primary focus of the psychosocial component. This book's primary focus is on the psychosocial in psycho-oncology.

Psychosocial

No consensus exists on a definition of the term *psychosocial* as related to cancer care (Institute of Medicine, 2008). The psychological, social, behavioral, emotional, spiritual, existential, and practical components of life that are related to the experience of cancer have all been included, as have specific descriptions of types of psychosocial services. Noting this lack of consensus, the Institute of Medicine (2008) offered the following definition of "psychosocial" in the context of the provision of health services for cancer care[2]:

> Psychosocial health services are psychological and social services and interventions that enable patients, their families, and health care providers to optimize biomedical health care and to manage the psychological/behavioral and social aspects of illness and its consequences so as to promote better health. (pp. 359–360)

Some important components of this definition need further explanation. First, note the emphasis on *health*. Psychosocial *health* services are services aimed at health-related outcomes that optimize and promote health—not other worthy psychosocial outcomes (e.g., decreased child abuse, violence, or poverty). Next, note the distinction between health *services* and health *interventions*. Psychosocial health *services* involve the direct provision of formal activities such as psychotherapy and psychoeducational programs designed to meet specified psychosocial needs, such as help in coping with emotions or managing role changes; the emphasis is on direct (often face-to-face) provision of help to patients. In contrast, psychosocial health *interventions* are defined as specific health care delivery models (e.g., collaborative or integrative care, chronic care model) that when effectively utilized result in the provision of quality psychosocial health services. Thus, in the Institute of Medicine (2008) definition, *psychosocial health services* are the direct provision of *activities* designed to meet psychosocial needs, while

2. A more recent modification, by the Canadian Association of Psychosocial Oncology (http://www.capo.org) of this definition added "spiritual care" along with psychological and social services.

psychosocial health interventions are broader *models* for delivering such activities. This distinction becomes important when evaluating the current ability to provide evidence-based psycho-oncology in the local setting. There is no single agreed-upon psychosocial health intervention model in psycho-oncology. Some (Jacobsen & Jim, 2008) have suggested the NCCN guidelines for screening for distress or integrated care, as developed in many primary care settings, could serve as models. Others (Fann, Ell, & Sharpe, 2012) have suggested adaptation of a chronic care model as a psychosocial health intervention model. Only a few trials of specific models have been tested (Meijer et al., 2011). Most local oncology practices are just beginning to consider how to effectively provide interprofessional collaborative care in which psycho-oncologists are routinely integrated.

THE EVIDENCE BASE IN PSYCHO-ONCOLOGY: A REVIEW AND CRITIQUE

Knowledge of the evidence base in psycho-oncology is essential to the process of appraising *the best available research*. Psychosocial health services in psycho-oncology include the following:

- Psychotherapy
- Psychoeducational interventions
- Peer support programs
- Self-management/self-care programs
- Patient education
- Family/caregiver education
- Others (Institute of Medicine, 2008)

As the evidence base has matured, more literature reviews have been published, clinical practice guidelines are being developed, and the importance of translating the research to use in the local cancer care setting has become paramount.

Translational research is concerned with moving knowledge from basic research ("the bench") to applied research ("the bedside") to routine clinical use ("the trench"). As translational research becomes more important, models have been developed that provide a perspective from which to see the progression of an area of study (Thornicroft, Lempp, & Tansella, 2011). Research progresses from *basic research* during which opportunities to impact problems in health care are identified, through the discovery and development of *effective interventions* that address identified clinical problems, to their designation as *evidence-based interventions* and their inclusion in *clinical practice guidelines*, to efforts to *disseminate and implement* them in local settings, with the ultimate goal of having an impact on health outcomes of a specific population of study. A five-phase model (Institute of Translational Health Sciences, 2013) as described in Table 2.2, will be used to guide the following overview of the status of the evidence base in psycho-oncology.

Table 2.2. Five-Phase Model of Translational Research: Definitions, Types of Research, and Examples

Phase	Definition	Type of Research	Psycho-Oncology Examples
T0	Identification of opportunities to impact health care problems	Basic research questions (not yet translational research at this phase)	Is there a unique subjective experience in cancer (e.g., "existential plight")? Is there a greater prevalence of anxiety/depression in cancer patients than in the general population? Can we validly and reliably measure quality of life in cancer patients?
T1	Discovery of potential health service interventions (candidate interventions)	Phase I and II clinical trials; observational studies; randomized trials of absolute efficacy; quasi-experimental; replications	Does progressive muscle relaxation + imagery reduce anticipatory nausea/vomiting? Does a MCGP intervention improve quality of life? Does CBSM reduce symptoms of anxiety/depression, fatigue/distress? Does SEGT extend life? Can prior results be replicated?
T2	Assess value of interventions to development of evidence-based recommendations/guidelines	Phase III clinical trials; evidence syntheses/filtered literature such as systematic reviews/meta-analyses; guideline development; cost-benefit analyses	How many patients might benefit from the intervention? How much does it cost to provide the intervention? How many patients report a problem for which the intervention is designed? Is the intervention without any harm?
T3	Move evidence-based guidelines into local community practice settings	Diffusion, dissemination, and implementation research	Can local psycho-oncologists be trained to competently provide the intervention? Can the intervention be successfully provided at the local cancer setting? Are patients willing to participate in the intervention?

(*Continued*)

Table 2.2. Continued

Phase	Definition	Type of Research	Psycho-Oncology Examples
T4	Practice to population health impact in the "real world"	Outcomes research at population level; monitoring of prevalence, morbidity, benefits	Are fewer now reporting the problem? Are more patients now able to successfully complete their cancer treatments? Are all patients reporting distress screened, identified, and referred for care when willing?

CBSM, cognitive-behavioral stress management; MCGP, meaning-centered group psychotherapy; SEGT, supportive-expressive group therapy.
SOURCE: Adapted by permission from Macmillan Publishers Ltd: *Genetics in Medicine.* Khoury, M. J., Gwinn, M., Yoon, P. W., Dowling, N., Moore, C. A., & Bradley, L. (2007). The continuum of translation research in genomic medicine: How can we accelerate the appropriate integration of human genome discoveries into health care and disease prevention? *Genetics in Medicine: Official Journal of The American College of Medical Genetics, 9*(10), 665–674. Copyright, 2007.

The history of research on anticipatory nausea and vomiting (ANV) in cancer chemotherapy serves as a good example to explain the model. In Phase T0, the earliest discoveries of classical conditioning by Pavlov from the 1940s became relevant to an important health care problem when researchers conceptualized ANV as a classically conditioned response interfering with compliance to chemotherapy (Redd & Andrykowski, 1982). As described in Phase T0, basic research on classical conditioning was found to have an impact on an important health care problem. In Phase T1, initial studies investigated its prevalence (Nicholas, 1982) and potential interventions were developed (Lyles, Burish, Krozely, & Oldham, 1982; Morrow & Morrell, 1982; Redd, Andresen, & Minagawa, 1982). Various "candidate" interventions were tested first in efficacy trials, often with quasi-experimental or uncontrolled, single-group designs (Redd et al., 1982). Later, promising interventions were compared against a "usual care" or no-treatment control group (Lyles et al., 1982) in randomized trials (Morrow & Morrell, 1982). Potential health service interventions were being discovered.

In Phase T2, as multiple interventions were being tested and found to have adequate efficacy, their value as possible evidence-based recommendations were investigated. Next, relevant literature became synthesized and filtered reviews began to be published (Carey & Burish, 1988; Roscoe, Morrow, Hickok, Mustian, & Shelke, 2004), as questions were asked if they should be included in evidence-based guidelines. At present, the current status of the evidence base for ANV involves Phase T3 questions about transportability to the local community cancer setting (Morrow & Rosenthal, 1996).

As with all areas of the evidence base in psycho-oncology, Phase T3 involves the transfer of science to practice via processes of diffusion → dissemination → implementation (Schoenwald, McHugh, & Barlow, 2012). *Diffusion* is the provision of relevant information to the practitioner, typically via primary, unfiltered sources such as journal articles. It is a passive process in which the practitioner is mostly responsible for consuming relevant literature. No specific active mechanisms are in place to facilitate the process, and thus it is most likely only effective for the highly motivated practitioner (i.e., early adopters) who seeks out the information and uses it when it has direct clinical implications.

Dissemination is defined as a more active and targeted process in which filtered, secondary literature such as systematic reviews, meta-analyses, or practice guidelines are made available to the practitioner. More targeted and tailored information, often endorsed by reputable professional organization, is then influential in the development of clinical practice guidelines that then may become the standard of care.

Finally, *implementation* is defined as the most active of the three processes in which barriers to accessing the knowledge are identified, and broader organizational issues are addressed to identify incentives to the busy practitioner "in the trenches" to maximize the chance that clinical practice will be evidence based. Note that the recursive or iterative use of new knowledge in a phase model is another important characteristic, where newer findings and more recent research alters prior standards of care. In the example of ANV, more recent literature has reinvestigated the prevalence and continued need for psychological treatments in light of a new generation of antiemetic drugs (5-HT3), concluding that it continues to remain a prevalent side effect to highly emetic chemotherapies and that psychosocial interventions are still warranted (Morrow, Roscoe, Kirshner, Hynes, & Rosenbluth, 1998). This five-phase model as explained in Table 2.2 is used to structure an historical review of the status of the evidence base in psycho-oncology.

Basic Research and Opportunities to Impact Problems (Phase T0) (1970s)

Research in the relatively young discipline of psycho-oncology—formally established in the mid-1970s when basic research questions of Phase T0 dominated—might best be characterized as having passed through infancy and early childhood (Phase T1) and is now in its adolescence (Phases T1, T2, and T3). In its infancy, questions were being asked regarding how to develop valid and reliable ways to measure subjective, phenomenological experiences of cancer patients, often symptoms such as pain and quality of life. Basic research on the psychometric properties of self-report questionnaires—taken from prior knowledge about test construction and instrument development—was used to design studies to develop reliable and valid self-report questionnaires (Holland & Weiss, 2010). As cancer chemotherapy trials began to investigate quality of life, many of the same psycho-oncology researchers (Aaronson, 1991; Cella et al., 1993) developed valid, reliable, and brief measures of health-related quality of life and its components. The field used basic research strategies to investigate the prevalence and incidence of mental disorders (depression, anxiety, posttraumatic stress disorder) in cancer patients (Derogatis et al., 1983), comparing them to the general population to establish baseline knowledge of the impact of cancer on mental/emotional status. One other early area of study used qualitative research methods designed to identify the subjective experiences of cancer patients such as "the existential plight" (Weisman & Worden, 1976). These early Phase T0 studies focused on basic questions and relied on research strategies previously developed in the behavioral sciences and public health.

Discovery of Potential Health Service Interventions (Phase T1): Initial Development and Methodological Problems (1980–1995)

As the field developed into early childhood, a variety of nonpharmacologic interventions were developed. Over time, methodologies improved and research questions broadened to include the relative efficacy of psychosocial interventions, typically compared to "usual care." By the mid-1990s, a number of reviews of the efficacy of these interventions were published (Devine & Westlake, 1995; Fawzy, Fawzy, Arndt, & Pasnau, 1995; Meyer & Mark, 1995). This synthesized or filtered literature was representative of Phase T2 and concluded that a variety of interventions appear to help cancer patients. Not all reviews agreed on the meaningfulness or the strength of the evidence (Andrykowski & Manne, 2006; Coyne, Lepore, & Palmer, 2006; Lepore & Coyne, 2006; Manne & Andrykowski, 2006), with opinions differing on how to interpret their overall efficacy. There were concerns about inconsistent findings, and a number of methodological weaknesses were noted (Newell, Sanson-Fisher, & Savolainen, 2002). However, most reviews concluded that many psychosocial interventions resulted in positive outcomes such as decreases in anxiety and depression, improved quality of life, improved coping skills, and improved immune system indicators.

Prior to the 1980s, most psychosocial health services (about 70%) were case studies with only a few cohort studies or nonrandomized trials (i.e., quasi-experimental designs). From the 1980s to the 1990s, the number of randomized trials increased from 45% in the 1980s to 55% in the 1990s (Newell et al., 2002). Despite these improvements, in one of the most comprehensive systematic reviews of studies published prior to 1998 (Newell et al., 2002), it was concluded that a number of methodological problems remained. This systematic review evaluated 155 identified studies on 10 indicators of internal validity (Mulcrow & Oxman, 1997). Each trial was evaluated on how well it fulfilled recommendations for each of these 10 indicators and was given a score ranging from 0 to 30. Only one trial was classified as a "good" trial, achieving a score greater than 20, while the overall median score for the 155 trials was 9, classified as "poor." The overall conclusion was that the vast majority of randomized controlled trials (RCTs) prior to 1998 had significant methodological problems.

Problems With Randomization, Specifically the Process of Recruiting, Accruing, and Allocating Patients to Groups

Most studies (96%) failed to conceal the method for randomly assigning participants to groups, and secondly, only a small percentage (27%) randomly selected from a clearly specified population (clearly stated inclusions/exclusion criteria) or from all consecutive, eligible patients.

Problems With Describing the Interventions

More than half of the studies (52%) failed to provide an adequate description of the intervention used and/or failed to monitor adherence to the integrity of how the intervention was provided. Similarly, reviews have noted tremendous variability and the lack of any agreed-upon operational definitions for many psycho-oncology interventions (Jacobsen & Jim, 2008).

Problems With Patients Lost to Follow-Up and Data Analyses

Many studies (16%) either failed to provide the actual numbers of patients lost or failed to provide both the number lost and the reasons for the loss (23%). As a result, in 43% of studies from the 1990s, it was not possible to calculate the percent of patients lost to follow-up. More than half of all studies failed to do intent-to-treat analyses. This is problematic because it becomes impossible to distinguish how those who did complete the study might be different from those who did not complete.

Problems With the Outcome Measures

Potential bias is inherent in the use of outcome measures that call for a subjective judgment. Thus, it is best to have some mix of objective and subjective outcome measures. If raters are used to measure outcome, they should be unaware (i.e., blind) to which group (experimental or control) a particular patient was assigned. In 12% of these trials all outcome was measured by unblinded, subjective measures, while in another 59% only subjective measures were used and if raters were used, it was unclear if they were blinded to group assignment or not. Other reviews (Andersen, 2002; Jacobsen & Jim, 2008) noted additional methodological problems.

The Failure to Prescreen Participants, Prior to Selection and Randomization, for the Presence of Elevated Scores on Measured Outcome Variable(s)

Interventions that fail to screen and assess for heightened levels of the dependent variable (e.g., anxiety, depression) simply took all cancer patients regardless of their preintervention status. In such studies, the research question becomes, Is this intervention effective *for any* cancer patient, rather than for those reporting elevated or even clinical levels of distress? One review found that only 5% of studies selected participants on the basis of clinical levels of anxiety, depression, or distress (Jacobsen, Donovan, Swaine, & Watson, 2006). The result is that the overall power of the statistical analyses to find significant group differences is weakened.

A Lack of Consideration of Demographic and Disease Status Variables

The vast majority of intervention studies in psycho-oncology are focused on women with breast cancer, men diagnosed with prostate cancer, or participants diagnosed with mixed cancer types. Such studies fail to adequately investigate the role of many important demographic (e.g., age, ethnicity) and disease-related variables (e.g., prognosis, time since diagnosis). As a result, there are significant gaps in the evidence base about the efficacy of a wide variety of potential interventions designed to address specific demographic or disease-related variables.

The Failure to Specify Theoretical or Empirical Support for Theoretically Derived Hypotheses

Too many intervention studies are not based upon theory or prior empirical evidence to support specific hypotheses (Andersen, 2002). Theories are needed to specify mechanisms of change. Theories provide guidance on proposed mediators and moderators. When studies are developed without adequate theoretical support, it becomes more difficult to identify mediators or moderators. Despite this general failure, there are notable exceptions. Many cognitive-behavioral, supportive-expressive, and problem-solving interventions specify hypothesized mechanisms of change, as do thorough models of change such as Andersen's biobehavioral model (Andersen, Kiecolt-Glaser, & Glaser, 1994).

Continued Development, Evidence-Based Recommendations, and Clinical Practice Guidelines (Phases T1 → T2) (1990 to Present)

As psycho-oncology matured from childhood to early adolescence, Phase T2 studies have predominated (Jacobsen, 2013). Reviews have noted improvements over past methodological problems and improved outcomes. Multiple meta-analyses have been published and reviewed in recent summaries (Faller et al., 2013; Jacobsen & Jim, 2008). One of the first meta-analyses in psycho-oncology (Meyer & Mark, 1995) reported significant, yet small effect sizes for improved emotional adjustment ($d = .24$), functional adjustment ($d = .19$), treatment and disease-related symptoms ($d = .26$), and global outcomes ($d = .28$) in RCTs of a variety of psychosocial interventions for adults.

A recent meta-analysis of 198 RCTs covering more than 22,000 adult cancer patients investigated outcomes by six types of intervention: individual psychotherapies, group psychotherapies, couples therapies, psychoeducation, relaxation training/imagery, and information only. Psychoeducational interventions included comprehensive components such as health education, coping skills, stress management, and social support. The psychotherapies included coping skills training, cognitive-behavioral therapies, and supportive-expressive psychotherapy. Results found significant medium effect sizes (see Appendix A) for emotional distress (d = .48), anxiety (d = .49), depression (d = .35), and quality of life (d = .47) for a variety of *individual psychotherapies*; small to medium effect sizes for distress (d = .23), anxiety (d = .44), depression (d = .48), and quality of life (d = .14) for *group psychotherapies*; and a small but significant effect for emotional distress (d = .16) in *couples therapy*. For *relaxation training and imagery*, significant small to medium effects were reported for emotional distress (d = .29), anxiety (d = .53), depression (d = .37), and quality of life (d = .35); and for *psychoeducational interventions* significant small effects were noted for emotional distress (d = .18), anxiety (d = .22), depression (d = .14), and quality of life (d = .20). No effects on any outcome measures were noted for *information only*.

In an important finding that confirmed earlier concerns about not prescreening patients, large positive effects were reported in those studies where patients were chosen based on increased distress at pretest. In the 11 individual and 4 group psychotherapy studies that prescreened, large effect sizes for emotional distress (d = 1.01) and quality of life (d = .89) were reported, and medium effect sizes for anxiety (d = .56) and depression (d = .53). As anticipated, the effects of the interventions were greater in these prescreened patients, with larger effect sizes at posttreatment. Thus, as interventions have improved and participants have been those in more distress, and probably more in need of the interventions, effect sizes have grown from small/medium to medium/large.

Evidence-Based Recommendations and Clinical Practice Guidelines

The development of evidence-based recommendations and clinical practice guidelines (Phase T2) has also been an important development of the 1990s through 2010. As reviewed in Chapter 1 (see Table 1.2), clinical practice guidelines have been defined as "systematically developed statements to assist practitioner and patient decisions about appropriate health care for specific clinical circumstances" (Field & Lohr, 1992, p. 2). A number of guidelines have been developed to guide practice in the United States, Canada, and Australia. The National Comprehensive Cancer Network (NCCN), an alliance of 23 of the world's leading cancer centers, has, over the past 15 years, developed a comprehensive set of evidence-based, consensus-driven clinical practice guidelines designed to promote the provision of effective preventive, diagnostic, treatment, and supportive services for all cancer patients. The NCCN guidelines for supportive care serve as standards of care in psycho-oncology (Holland et al., 2010).

The NCCN distress management guidelines are most relevant to the function of the psycho-oncologist, and the implementation of routine distress screening procedures is now being required for accreditation by the Commission on Cancer (CoC) of the American College of Surgeons (ACOS), the accreditation body for nearly 70% of all cancer care in the United States (American College of Surgeons, Commission on Cancer, 2012). These NCCN guidelines could represent how to best organize and provide psychosocial health services and could serve as a model of health service interventions. However, although these guidelines are widely disseminated and recognized as important to the provision of psychosocial care, they have not been promoted as a model of health service delivery. No studies have directly tested the NCCN Guidelines as a mode for effective delivery of health services (Fann et al., 2012; Jacobsen, 2009). This is one of many gaps in the current evidence base. Much remains to be done before distress screening, identification, and referral will be routine in most local community cancer settings (see Chapter 5 for more details).

Many barriers remain, but the new CoC Standards have initiated more efforts at the local level. How to translate this evidence to local cancer care settings, with a well-planned, successful implementation strategy, remains unknown. From 2012 to 2015 most community cancer programs are trying to develop and implement "a process to integrate and monitor on-site psychosocial distress screening and referral for the provision of psychosocial care" (American College of Surgeons, Commission on Cancer, 2012, p. 76) despite the lack of consensus on how to best organize such screening (Bidstrup, Johansen, & Mitchell, 2011).

As mentioned earlier, although the NCCN Guidelines have had a significant influence on efforts to implement psychosocial services, they have been relatively neglected by researchers and much of the evidence base has neglected the NCCN guidelines as a model of health service delivery (Jacobsen, 2009). Thus, the impact of the NCCN guidelines on the efficacy of the provision of psychosocial services remains unknown. Efforts to address this gap in the evidence base have recommended the need for more studies in psycho-oncology modeled after the literature on another, more widely researched model of health service delivery: collaborative or integrated care (Jacobsen & Jim, 2008).

Collaborative or Integrated Care

Collaborative or *integrative care* in oncology is care in which multiple medical and nursing specialists routinely collaborate with psycho-oncologists. All providers understand their respective roles, the roles of others, and how to collaborate within a single health care system. All providers share responsibility for patient care that demonstrates enhanced patient outcomes. The need for collaborative care has been widely recognized (Institute of Medicine, 2001, 2008, 2011; Institute of Medicine & National Research Council, 2006) and yet rarely happens. This form of well-coordinated, multidisciplinary care is far from routine and in most settings remains an aspirational goal. The development of such systems is just beginning—most notably in the specification of core competencies for interprofessional collaboration (Interprofessional Education Collaborative Expert Panel, 2011).

Reviews have found a lack of clarity in definitions of basic terms and role awareness among practitioners, as well as a lack of structure and other support tools (e.g., user-friendly electronic health records) (Gagliardi, Dobrow, & Wright, 2011). The adaptation of a *chronic care* model as a *collaborative care* model in oncology has been recommended (Fann et al., 2012; Institute of Medicine, 2011), and a few randomized trials have tested variations of this model (Fann et al., 2012). Much remains to be known about how best to implement collaborative care in the specialty care setting of community oncology, particularly in local cancer care settings where resources are limited.

Oncology care can learn about effective collaborative/integrative care from examples in primary care, where the integration of mental and behavioral health has a longer history (Gilbody, Bower, Fletcher, Richards, & Sutton, 2006; Heath, Wise, Romero, & Reynolds, 2013; Miller, Kessler, & Peek, 2011). The research on screening for depression in primary care, where collaborative/integrative models have been implemented, provides a model for testing the efficacy of screening guidelines in psycho-oncology (Jacobsen, 2009). One randomized trial of an integrated care approach to the management of depression in an oncology setting provides an example of positive outcomes that can come from high-level collaboration (Strong et al., 2008). In this study of 200 patients with mixed types and stages of cancer, a systematic management of depression intervention was provided by nurses to those identified as meeting criteria for major depressive disorder, following routine screening for depression. The manualized intervention—supervised by psychiatrists—included up to 10 (mean of 7) individual sessions of education about depression, problem-solving therapy, antidepressant medications, and communication with the patient's primary care physician. Results indicated a reduction in symptoms of depression at 3, 6, and 12 months. Undoubtedly, more such trials testing this and other related models of integrated care in oncology are needed. In Chapter 5 of this book more detailed explanations of the process of screening and assessment in psycho-oncology will be offered.

Throughout the first two decades of the 21st century, translational research has become an increasing priority in psycho-oncology (Jacobsen, 2010). Focus has been on Phases T1 and T2, as researchers have developed, among other outcomes, evidence-based interventions to relieve emotional distress and to improve quality of life (Jacobsen, 2013). Primary literature investigating a range of questions related to distress screening, prevalence of mental disorders, efficacy and effectiveness of interventions, symptom management, palliative and end-of-life care, survivorship, caregiver stress, and many others are being diffused through peer-reviewed journal outlets and some online review summaries (e.g., NCI PDQ statements). Literature reviews synthesize and summarize the evidence in an effort to quickly disseminate knowledge to practitioners. An increasing number of systematic reviews, meta-analyses, and clinical practice guidelines are appearing as dissemination efforts increase. Consistent with Phase T3 of the model, efforts to move evidence-based guidelines into the local community cancer settings are increasing.

The Future of the Psycho-Oncology Evidence Base

Future studies should be based upon *stronger theoretical and conceptual models* in order to improve the ability to investigate possible mediators or moderators of positive outcomes. One exemplar is Andersen's biobehavioral model (Andersen et al., 1994), which has guided over 20 years of research on a psychological treatment for women with early-stage breast cancer. The model proposes that psychological variables, such as stress and quality of life, affect disease course via their direct effect on immune system functioning and their indirect effects on treatment compliance and relevant health behaviors. Such a model provides a strong theoretical and conceptual foundation on which to build both effective interventions and knowledge about possible mediators and/or moderators of change.

Future research should *continue to prescreen for the presence of distress.* Future studies should indicate if their goals are *prevention* of the development of negative emotions such as distress or *treatment* of already existing distress. When presecreened, patients can then be appropriately referred to the needed intervention: either one to prevent the development of distress or one to treat already existing distress.

Future research needs *greater attention to relevant demographic and disease status variables.* A large percentage of the existing evidence base has been focused on women with breast cancer and men with prostate cancer. However, more attention is being given to the impact of cancer type, stage, and prognosis (McLean & Jones, 2007) on the unique needs of specific populations. Couples (Baik & Adams, 2011), families (Zaider & Kissane, 2010), caregivers (Candy, Jones, Drake, Leurent, & King, 2011), and partners (Lewis et al., 2008) have all been targeted as relevant populations for whom to develop specific interventions. As greater attention is given to demographic and disease characteristics and the evidence base grows in understanding of relevant differences, it will also be important to consider interventions and their ability to generalize across populations, cancer types, and stages. It is not feasible to develop, test, disseminate, and implement unique interventions for every cancer type, stage, prognosis, or location along the clinical course. There will be a limit to how many interventions can be developed for the many demographic and disease-related characteristics. New, unique, or modified interventions should be designed when uniquely defined cancer-related experiences are identified and described.

Future research needs to *continue improvements made in the quality of reporting of studies.* Close attention to appropriate journal reporting standards such as the CONSORT statement for nonpharmacologic interventions or Journal Article Reporting Standards (JARS) for research in psychology needs to continue. As more and more journals adopt these standards, consistency and transparency in reporting of results should continue to improve, and concerns about the quality of the methodology should decrease.

Future research also needs to *include more replications* of highly effective interventions. Although a number of interventions have been identified as showing overall efficacy, replications by other research groups are needed to confirm initial findings as well as to demonstrate their ability to be implemented in more than one setting or by more than one research group.

As an important component in dissemination and implementation, future intervention research needs to *pay close attention to issues related to ease of translation to the local cancer care setting* (Jacobsen & Jim, 2008). The availability of local staff and resources, the acceptability and likelihood of patient participation, and the availability of intervention materials needs to be considered. For example, the total number of sessions in a particular intervention will affect how many patients will be willing to devote time to participate. Similarly, the availability of local professional staff competent to provide the intervention and the accessibility of treatment manuals will influence dissemination and implementation. Recommended parameters used to select interventions for implementation (Jacobsen & Jim, 2008) in clinical settings are those with fewer than 12 sessions, those able to be implemented by one qualified staff person, and those most acceptable to patients. Use of translational models such as Reach, Effectiveness, Adoption, Implementation, Maintenance (RE-AIM), designed to facilitate the translation of research to practice (Glasgow, Davidson, Dobkin, Ockene, & Spring, 2006; Glasgow, Klesges, Dzewaltowski, Bull, & Estabrooks, 2004) will continue to be needed in the future. Without attention to these important components of translational research, a highly effective intervention may never be provided to local cancer patients.

It has also been suggested that for effective dissemination and implementation of health service interventions attention be given to the *need for increased demand by both providers and patient groups* (Jacobsen, 2010). To date, most of the attention in translational research has been on efforts to diffuse, disseminate, and implement the evidence base to competent providers, with no particular focus on efforts to educate and advocate for access among patient and provider groups. Greater emphasis has been placed on efforts to "push" knowledge to providers, with little effort to develop a greater demand by consumers and providers that could result in a "pull" for greater availability of services.

Finally, future research should be guided by *more clearly articulated theoretical models and constructs*. Theory is critical to all science as it provides a conceptual structure from which to develop potential, testable hypotheses. It is also a very common component in the training of many psycho-oncologists.

CHAPTER SUMMARY

This chapter provided important information about (a) the basics of cancer for the nonmedical, mental health professional; (b) an introduction to key terms and concepts in EBP of adult clinical psycho-oncology; and (c) a review and critique of the evidence base in psycho-oncology organized by a model of translational research. This information is essential background knowledge for the EBP of psycho-oncology. The evidence-based practitioner of psycho-oncology also needs knowledge of the psychotherapy research literature, theories of psychotherapy as adapted to cancer care, and the important role of supportive psychotherapy in psycho-oncology. This is the focus of Chapter 3.

3

Background Knowledge of Psychotherapy

The evidence-based practitioner in psycho-oncology encounters a frequent dilemma when there are gaps in the evidence base. The busy psycho-oncologist has to make decisions about how to intervene in clinical situations where no evidence exists. In such situations, there *is* no best available research—the research base does not exist, or the clinical decision called for falls within one of the many gaps in the evidence base. Practitioners cannot wait; they must act based upon the *best available* evidence.

PSYCHOTHERAPY OUTCOME RESEARCH: AN OVERVIEW

The ability to evaluate the evidence base in psycho-oncology will be strengthened by a general understanding of findings from the psychotherapy outcome research and its application to cancer care. The history of psychotherapy research (Lambert, 2011b) has highlighted a number of important achievements.

The General Efficacy of Psychotherapy for Adults

One of the first and most important accomplishments of psychotherapy outcome research is the demonstration that psychotherapy does have a positive general effect—it does work and thousands of studies, with continuously improving research methods over the past 50–60 years (Lambert & Ogles, 2004), have demonstrated this general effect. In general, those people who receive psychotherapy are better off than those not receiving it. Effect sizes mostly range between .4 and .8 (Lipsey & Wilson, 1993; Shadish et al., 1997; Smith & Glass, 1977), indicating that by the end of treatment, the *average patient* who received treatment is better off than 64% to 80% of those who did not receive treatment (see Appendix A for further explanations). The change that happens is both statistically significant and, most important, clinically meaningful. Evidence of change that is considered meaningful or clinically significant—typically defined as change in outcome that is both larger than the standard error of the instrument and empirically indistinguishable from scores of "normal" populations (Jacobson, Roberts, Berns, & McGlinchey, 1999)—has accumulated (Lambert & Ogles, 2004). Long-term maintenance of treatment gains is less clear, although research indicates that treatment gains are maintained for many specific disorders such as some of the anxiety disorders, while less so for disorders that tend to recur such as depression and substance use.

In the mid-1990s, the accumulated findings of positive research on psychotherapy efficacy culminated in an important endeavor to highlight and emphasize those specific approaches with sufficient research support to be labeled as *empirically supported therapies (ESTs)*. This effort of a task force of the American Psychological Association (APA)—the Empirically Supported Therapies movement—took on the task of identifying all of the approaches for specific presenting problems, usually taken from the diagnostic criteria for mental disorders, that had accumulated sufficient research to be labeled "probably efficacious," "efficacious," or "efficacious and specific" (Chambless & Hollon, 1998; Compas, Haaga, Keefe, Leitenberg, & Williams, 1998). The results of these ongoing efforts include three editions of *Treatments That Work* (Nathan & Gorman, 1998, 2002, 2007) and a Web site that maintains updated lists of ESTs (currently referred to as "psychological treatments") (http://www.div12.org/PsychologicalTreatments/index.html).

The Effectiveness of Psychotherapy for Adults

Another important achievement in psychotherapy outcome research is the ability to translate positive outcomes in highly controlled research settings to everyday real-world clinical settings—Phase T3 translational research. In psychotherapy research, this process has been formulated as a distinction between *efficacy and effectiveness*, where *efficacy* refers to those studies in highly controlled, research settings where a very high degree of internal validity is paramount, while *effectiveness*—concerned with external validity—is all about generalization of findings to the local setting. Many positive outcomes in psychotherapy have been shown to generalize to the real-world everyday context (Howard, Moras, Brill, Martinovich, & Lutz, 1996; Minami et al., 2008; Shadish, Navarro, Matt, & Phillips, 2000), and most interventions with strong efficacy have also shown good effectiveness.

Patient-Focused Research

Despite positive outcomes in questions of overall efficacy and effectiveness, such results come from comparisons of mean differences between groups on measured outcome variables—evidence of improvements in *the average* patient.

Consequently, such results can guide therapists to select treatments with empirical support for patients with specified diagnoses or presenting problems. However, results from group studies fail to address many of the routine daily questions of most practitioners—questions that look for application of the general laws to the individual client, for example:

- Is my approach working with this particular patient?
- Is it time to consider termination?
- Is my patient improving as should be expected, or is she getting worse?

These questions have been the focus of patient-focused research (Howard et al., 1996; Lambert, 2001; Lambert, Duncan, Miller, Wampold, & Hubble, 2010). Patient-focused research provides for routine client feedback as a method of tracking patient change and a mechanism for prevention of treatment failures (Lambert, 2010). Routine collection of client feedback has been identified as a *demonstrably effective* general element of effective psychotherapy relationships (Lambert, 2011a). In psycho-oncology, the direct application of patient-focused research has not yet begun but is needed. The routine clinical application of frequent assessment of outcomes is needed to answer the many questions of practitioners "in the trenches."

Lack of Differential Treatment Efficacy

The question of whether some psychotherapy approaches are better than others has been another important research question that has generated both decades of research findings and considerable controversy (Duncan, Miller, Wampold, & Hubble, 2010; Wampold, 2008). Interestingly, of the many psychotherapy approaches that have been tested (many have not undergone *any* rigorous study), nearly all show positive efficacy while very little differential efficacy has been shown (Wampold et al., 1997). This finding that nearly all approaches show positive outcomes, but none seems to be better than any others—the lack of differential efficacy—has become known (after the Alice in Wonderland character) as the *Dodo Bird Verdict (all have won and all deserve prizes!)* (Luborsky, Singer, & Luborsky, 1975).

Common Factors

Efforts to explain this curious paradox of no differences have focused on possible reasons why different therapy approaches with clearly identified different techniques do not result in different outcomes. One of the best explanations has emphasized the commonality in therapy approaches, rather than their differences (Hubble, Duncan, Miller, & Wampold, 2010). The *common factors* explanation—what therapists do in sessions seem to be more alike than different—has generated decades of interest and controversy. It seems that common factors are the more curative factors, and yet they are not the factors most frequently emphasized in most theoretical approaches where the emphasis is usually on specific treatment methods and techniques. Although there is no agreed-upon set of ideal common factors, some include variables such as *therapist attitudes and behaviors* like empathy, positive regard, genuineness, encouragement, and reassurance, while others include *patient variables* such as hope, social support, and expectancy of positive outcome. Attempts to identify common factors have emphasized the interaction between therapist and patient and the acknowledgment that this interaction constitutes the *therapeutic relationship*. The interaction between a warm, empathic, reassuring therapist and a motivated, hopeful, and engaged patient may be as, or even more, important than any single, isolated common factor or any specific treatment method or technique. The explanation for the lack of differential efficacy despite different techniques may be that a therapeutic relationship is common to all approaches and this relationship may be the common factor most responsible for positive outcomes.

Empirically Supported Relationships

This interest in common factors and the importance of the psychotherapy relationship led to the empirically supported relationships (ESRs) movement, another effort of divisions of the American Psychological Association, with the goal of accumulating the evidence demonstrating the importance of ESRs in psychotherapy outcome (Norcross, 2002, 2011). Two volumes of meta-analytic research on ESRs have documented both the *general elements* of effective therapy relationships, such the alliance in individual therapy, and *particular elements* that work when adapting an approach to the needs of a particular patient. Thus, two important movements within the psychotherapy outcome research literature are the empirically supported treatments (EST) approach and the empirically supported relationship (ESR) approach.

These two approaches to psychotherapy outcome research are closely related, but they have a number of important differences. The EST approach places emphasis on specific techniques for specific diagnosed mental disorders; uses therapy manuals to direct the intervention; randomly assigns patients to different groups, one of which is a control group; and holds the randomized controlled trial (RCT) as the "gold standard" for outcome research. The ESR approach places emphasis on common factors and general elements of effective therapy relationships; does not use therapy manuals; and, given that relationships/common factors cannot be randomly assigned to groups, relies on correlational research designs.

These two perspectives spurred two groups—the EST group and the ESR group—each working to identify the evidence base for their side of the argument. Those supportive of specific intervention techniques (the EST movement) argued in favor of *specificity*, while those supportive of the common factors and

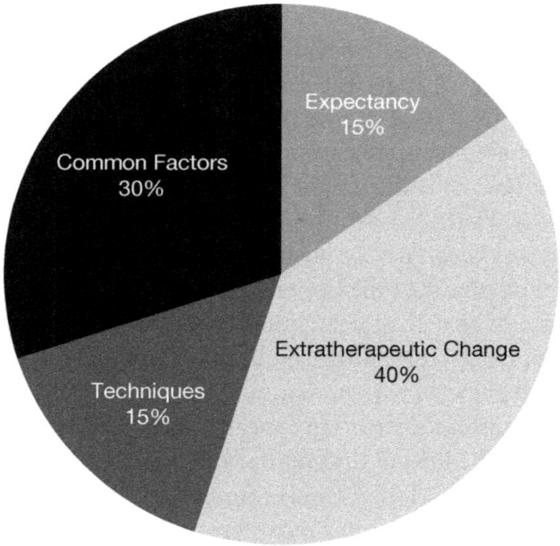

Figure 3.1 Percent of improvement in psychotherapy patients as a function of therapeutic factors.
SOURCE: Norcross, J. C., & Lambert, M. J. (2011). Evidence-based therapy relationships. In J. C. Norcross (Ed.), *Psychotherapy relationships that work* (2nd ed., Fig. 1.2, p. 13). New York: Oxford University Press. By permission of Oxford University Press, USA.

the importance of the therapeutic relationship (the ESR movement) argued in favor of *commonality*. More recent cooperative efforts (Norcross, 2011) have focused on a more comprehensive understanding of all relevant *therapeutic factors*. Broad-based efforts have been made to quantify the relative contribution of all possible therapeutic factors as illustrated in Figures 3.1 and 3.2 (Norcross & Lambert, 2011). Both illustrated models are *estimates* based upon decades of psychotherapy outcome research across thousands of studies and hundreds of meta-analyses. Figure 3.1 separates the already known explained variability in outcome among four categories: extratherapeutic change (40%), common factors (30%), techniques (15%), and patient expectancy/placebo (15%). *Extratherapeutic change* includes events such as spontaneous remission, social support, and patient self-change. As illustrated in Figure 3.1, nearly 40% of improvement in psychotherapy is accounted for by extratherapeutic change, with another 15% considered placebo in the form of a positive expectancy for change. The remaining 45% of the variance is split between the relative importance of specific treatment methods/techniques, accounting for 15%, and the common factors to all effective psychotherapy relationships, accounting for 30%.

Figure 3.2 illustrates a broader perspective by focusing on all possible variability in psychotherapy outcome and thus includes both *the already known and the unknown variability*. Because even the best research will continue to have flaws and psychotherapy research will always be limited by the complexity of human behavior change and researchers' efforts to measure it, this model estimates that 40% of the variance remains unexplained. This model separates and divides the

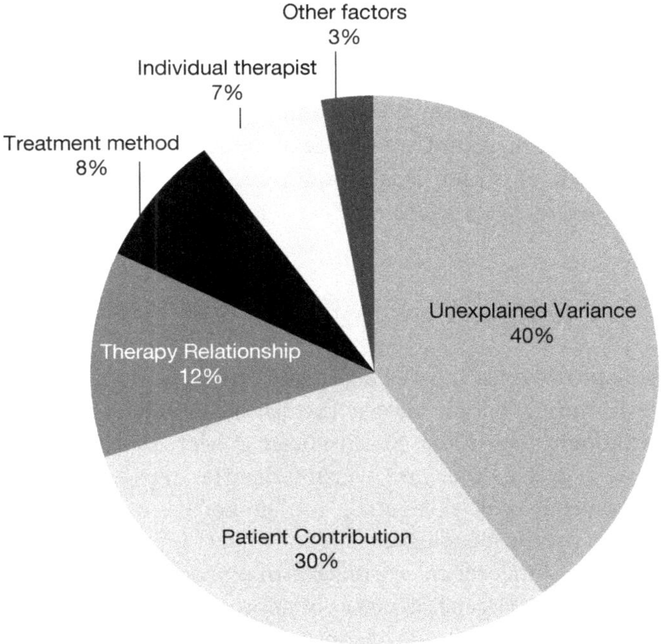

Figure 3.2 Percent of total psychotherapy outcome variance attributable to therapeutic factors.
SOURCE: From Norcross, J. C., & Lambert, M. J. (2011). Evidence-based therapy relationships. In J. C. Norcross (Ed.), *Psychotherapy relationships that work* (2nd ed., Fig. 1.1 p. 13). New York: Oxford University Press. By permission of Oxford University Press, USA.

factors common to all effective relationships, spreading them around among patient, therapy method, therapeutic relationship, and therapist variables, and it concludes with estimates that approximately 40%–43% of the variance is currently unaccounted for, while the remaining 57%–60% is accounted for by four other categories of variables: the therapist (7%), treatment method/techniques (8%), the therapy relationship (12%), and the patient's contribution (30%).

The two models present some consistent conclusions (Norcross & Lambert, 2011).

1. Much of the success or failure of psychotherapy is due to characteristics of the patient such as expectancy for improvement, motivation for change, and, of course, the severity of the presenting problem.
2. Both the therapeutic relationship and the treatment techniques or method are important to successful outcome.
3. Certain specific treatment techniques are particularly important for presenting problems, such as exposure-based techniques for anxiety symptoms/disorders.
4. It is important to adapt, tailor, or modify interventions to the specific needs of the patient, as this enhances the therapy relationship and improves outcomes.

In summary, psychotherapy research shows a number of impressive achievements, and background knowledge of this history is important to the EBP of psycho-oncology. When the psycho-oncologist is accessing and appraising the strength of the evidence, there will be significant gaps where no evidence exists. In such situations, background knowledge of the general psychotherapy research literature is needed, as is knowledge about those theories of psychotherapy that have been adapted for specific use with cancer patients.

THEORIES OF PSYCHOTHERAPY IN CANCER CARE

Psycho-oncologists typically have significant training in specific psychotherapy theories. Many function almost exclusively within a specific theoretical approach, although when asked, most indicate they are eclectic (Lambert, 2004). Estimates have suggested there are over 100 theories of psychotherapy; however, only cognitive-behavioral, existential, and supportive psychotherapy have an evidence base in psycho-oncology.

The application of theoretical approaches of psychotherapy to cancer care has evolved in two ways: (1) generalization of approaches from the general mental health literature, and (2) evolution of approaches in response to oncology-specific needs. In the first, approaches to psychotherapy with well-established empirical support (e.g., CBT, EFT, marital behavioral therapy) have been adapted for use with cancer patients, couples, and families. These approaches first established their efficacy and effectiveness in general mental health settings and were modified to apply to cancer care. In a second process, psychotherapies evolved exclusively within the oncology context in response to identified needs such as the concerns of specific cancer types (such as breast or prostate) or stages (early vs. late), the needs of specific persons (such as couples, family members, or caregivers), or some unique end-of-life issues (such as a hastened desire for death or the desire for a dignified death). In these approaches, interventions were developed—many guided by philosophical approaches to psychotherapy, such as existentialism—with goals specific to these unique needs and have been first tested in small pilot studies within the busy oncology setting to determine feasibility. If they were found to be feasible, they were later tested in larger randomized trials in an effort to determine absolute and, eventually, relative efficacy. Cognitive-behavioral therapy (CBT) is the most common approach generalized from the general mental health setting, and existential psychotherapies are representative of the second approach that evolved within the oncology setting.

Cognitive-Behavioral Therapies in Psycho-Oncology

Cognitive-behavioral theory (CBT) refers to a variety of therapeutic approaches that have in common the basic notion that a patient's thoughts and behaviors are instrumental in the etiology of psychological distress. Many CBT approaches claim their origin in Bandura's social learning and social cognitive theories (Bandura, 1986). Bandura proposed that all behaviors (this includes thoughts as covert behaviors) are learned behaviors. Behaviors are initially acquired by both doing/performing and by observing others/modeling and are subsequently maintained by two categories of variables, the antecedent stimuli, "cues," or "triggers" that signal when to perform a behavior, and the consequences that follow behaviors. Both of these categories of variables influence the likelihood of a behavior occurring or not occurring again in the future. With this basic foundation, others (Barlow, 2008; Beck, Rush, & Shaw, 1979; Lazarus & Folkman, 1984) expanded Bandura's ideas to the development of interventions designed to alter problematic thoughts and behaviors. CBT interventions for cancer patients include problem-solving therapy (Nezu, Nezu, Felgoise, McClure, & Houts, 2003), cognitive-behavioral stress management and coping skills training (Andersen et al., 2004; Antoni, 2003), cognitive therapy (Savard et al., 2006), Lazarus and Folkman's cognitive model of stress (Kayser, Feldman, Borstelmann, & Daniels, 2010), and behavioral marital therapy (Baucom et al., 2009). CBT is the most widely developed and tested theory for cancer patients.

A common CBT formulation of the etiology of unwanted symptoms, such as depression or anxiety, includes the identification of *automatic thoughts*, typically the result of one's *cognitive appraisal* of a particular life event or situation. With symptoms of anxiety, for example, a common appraisal is the *overestimation of harm/danger* in life situations. CBT identifies the connections between these automatic or distorted thoughts to maladaptive coping behaviors (e.g., isolation) and develops intervention strategies targeted at both cognitions and behaviors. In future chapters, CBT approaches with individuals, groups, couples, and families will be highlighted.

Specific CBT intervention *techniques* have also been widely used in psycho-oncology. These techniques include various relaxation procedures and guided imagery (Lewis & Sharp, 2011). Most relaxation procedures originate from Jacobson's (1938) formulation of progressive muscle relaxation (PMR), an intervention in which patients are taught to tense and relax muscle groups and encouraged to practice regularly to be able to voluntarily let go of excess muscle tension and generate the relaxation response (Benson, 1975). PMR is based upon the behavioral principle of *reciprocal inhibition,* (Wolpe, 1958) which posits that two opposing or incompatible states (e.g., tension and relaxation) cannot be present at the same time.

Existential Psychotherapies in Psycho-Oncology

Existential psychotherapy has its roots in the existential movement of 19th-century philosophers such as Kierkegaard, Nietzsche, and Sartre. It is an approach guided by existential philosophy that considers the ultimate concerns of life: the inevitability of death, freedom and its responsibilities, existential aloneness/isolation, and the importance of meaning in life (Yalom, 1980). Existential psychotherapy has been influential in the development of a variety of psychotherapy approaches in cancer care focused on issues of meaning, isolation, suffering, death, and end-of-life care (LeMay & Wilson, 2008).

Supportive-Expressive Group Therapy

Supportive-expressive group therapy (SEGT) is a group psychotherapy initially developed and tested mostly on women with metastatic breast cancer by Spiegel and colleagues in the 1970s (Spiegel, Bloom, Kraemer, & Gottheil, 1989). Its goals are to enhance mutual support, to encourage openness and emotional expression, to improve coping skills and doctor–patient relationships, to reorder priorities, and to detoxify death and the dying process (Classen & Spiegel, 2011). In its initial trial, in addition to a number of psychosocial benefits (such as improved mood, decreased depression, enhanced emotional control, improved coping, and improved overall quality of life), it was also found that SEGT improved survival of participants in the intervention group by about 16 months (Spiegel et al., 1989). A number of replications have found similarly positive psychosocial outcomes, but none have replicated the survival benefit (Classen et al., 2001; Goodwin et al., 2001; Kissane et al., 2007).

Meaning-Centered Psychotherapy

Meaning-centered psychotherapy (MCP) has also been influenced by existential psychotherapy, as well as the closely related work of Viktor Frankl's logotherapy and his emphasis on the importance of meaning in life, and spirituality as a construct of faith (Breitbart & Applebaum, 2011). MCP originated as an 8-week group psychotherapy for patients with advanced cancer and poor prognoses (Breitbart et al., 2010) and has also been modified in an individual format (Breitbart et al., 2012). The goals of MCP are to diminish despair, hopelessness, demoralization, and the desire for a hastened death, by unfolding an enhanced sense of meaning and purpose in life, even in the face of death. It strives to "reconnect with meaning in the midst of suffering" (Breitbart & Applebaum, 2011, p. 137). An RCT of the group intervention showed improved spiritual well-being; enhanced sense of meaning; and decreases (Breitbart et al., 2010) in anxiety, hopelessness, and desire for death.

Dignity Therapy

Dignity therapy (DT) is another psychotherapy influenced by existentialism, particularly existential despair and its relationship to a sense of dignity. Dignity, defined as "the quality or state of being worthy, honored or esteemed" (Chochinov & McKeen, 2011, p. 79), and generativity—Erik Erikson's developmental task encountered in middle adulthood that involves a sense of accomplishment in life and caring about and contributing to future generations—are emphasized. In this approach, a three- to four-session individual intervention was designed to affirm and maintain the dignity of terminally ill patients, by reflecting on past, memorable and meaningful life events while constructing a generativity or legacy document. The intervention consisted of contacts during which the therapist first introduced the concept and provided a set of possible questions to use to structure a more extensive audiotaped interview during session two. Session two involved patients answering relevant questions, designed to enhance a sense of meaning, purpose, and generativity. This interview was then transcribed, edited, and read back to the patient for changes/corrections. Its final version was then given to a designated person (typically family member) as a legacy document. In an RCT of 441 patients, no pre- to postdifferences in distress levels were noted between groups, but significant group differences were noted in improved quality of life, a higher sense of dignity, and that the intervention had been helpful to both patients and their families.

Other Relevant Theoretical Approaches

Emotionally focused couples therapy (EFT) is a well-established treatment for couples (Johnson, 2004), grounded in attachment theory (Levy, Ellison, Scott, & Bernecker, 2011). *Attachment theory* emphasizes the importance of early relationships with primary caregivers and the impact that these earliest relationships have on lifelong relationship patterns. As applied to couples, long-term relationships involve emotional bonds that can be threatened by a variety of life events. EFT addresses the security of these bonds as key ingredients in healthy relationships, particularly during times of distress and change. When applied to cancer, particularly advanced cancer, threats due to anticipated separation and loss can impact the relationship. EFT focuses on patients' and partners' experiences of the illness and the resulting relationship dynamics. Interventions attempt to maintain and strengthen the emotional bonds, to increase engagement within the relationship, and to encourage increased flexibility in responding to new demands, all with a goal of mitigating/managing grief and loss (McLean, Walton, Rodin, Esplen, & Jones, 2011). In the general mental health population, EFT has shown good efficacy with large effect sizes (Johnson, Hunsley, Greenberg, & Schindler, 1999). A manualized RCT of EFT for couples with advanced cancer, consisting of eight sessions, showed positive changes in overall marital functioning and patient-perceived caregiver (partner) empathy (McLean et al., 2011).

Mindfulness-based stress reduction (MBSR), originally developed by Jon Kabat-Zinn (1990), is typically a group intervention for a variety of chronic illnesses, anxiety, and depression. This approach involves the development, practice, and gradual acquisition of a state of nonjudgmental awareness. MBSR is a skills-based, educational approach where participants are taught a body scan, mindfulness meditation, a breathing break, and informal mindfulness. These skills are designed to help attain mindfulness, while alleviating a variety of symptoms and reducing overall suffering. Its format is typically an eight-session, manualized group intervention that meets 2.0–2.5 hours per week for 8 weeks, as well as for one all-day "mindfulness" experience following week six. A meta-analysis of nine studies of MBSR with breast cancer patients showed a moderate to large effect size in reducing stress, depression, and anxiety (Zainal, Booth, & Hubbert, 2013).

THE ROLE OF SUPPORTIVE PSYCHOTHERAPY IN CANCER CARE

One last, but important, theoretical approach to cancer care is *supportive psychotherapy* (SP). In the *Handbook of Psychotherapy in Cancer Care* (Watson & Kissane, 2011)—an excellent source of current psychotherapy approaches to the care of the cancer patient—the opening chapter by two premier leaders in the field of psycho-oncology declares:

> Supportive psychotherapy for patients with cancer and their families is the single most important tool of the psycho-oncologist (Lederberg & Holland, 2011, p. 3).

Despite this strong endorsement of the importance of SP, there is little consensus on what it is, how it is implemented, or what is its evidence base (Markowitz, Manber, & Rosen, 2008). Initially defined in the 1950s, within the then prevalent context of psychoanalysis, SP was viewed as a simpler form of therapy where the therapist used a direct conversational style, offered suggestions, and was supportive and encouraging in an effort to enhance self-esteem (Sjoqvist, 2007).

As the scientific study of psychotherapy evolved during the 1970s through the 1990s and into the 21st century, research focused on identifying the active ingredients in various forms of psychotherapy. Many specific forms of therapy—such as cognitive-behavioral—were tested in randomized trials. SP was often used as the control condition on which to test the hypothesized active ingredients of other therapies. As a control condition in these trials, there was little consensus or agreement on what SP was; rather it was designed to include the nonspecific, common ingredients of all therapies while controlling for the therapist's time and attention (Moorey, Greer, Bliss, & Law, 1998). Although books (Novalis, Rojcewicz, & Peele, 1993; Pinsker, 1997) and manuals (McMillan et al., 2006) were developed describing SP, components differed, and there was no agreement about the essential components of SP.

As previously explained, one of the most significant findings in the general psychotherapy outcome literature is the lack of differential efficacy. As more studies failed to show differential efficacy—often when being compared to SP—SP came to be a nonspecific approach to psychotherapy representative of a common factors approach, with its associated emphasis on the importance of the therapeutic relationship. Interestingly, when SP has been investigated as a control condition—representing the nonspecific, common factors approach—it has shown efficacy (Hellerstein et al., 1998; Markowitz, Kocsis, Bleiberg, Christos, & Sacks, 2005). For example, in a study of 353 women with gynecological cancer (Manne et al., 2007), those receiving SP reported fewer symptoms of depression than the usual care group at 6- and 9-month follow-ups, doing as well as the experimental condition (a coping and communication enhancement intervention), and some have called for supportive therapy as the treatment model of choice in many therapy contexts (Hellerstein, Pinsker, Rosenthal, & Klee, 1994).

However, despite these positive developments, a manualized form of SP has rarely been directly tested in any controlled trials as an experimental condition (Conte, 1994; Conte & Plutchik, 1986).

To summarize, SP has often been defined by exclusion, best known for what it did not include, rather than for what it did, as a control condition for other experimental interventions. As a control condition, it has shown efficacy. It has a mixed and poorly defined evidence base, particularly as a defined psychotherapy with agreed-upon essential components. Its evidence base will be examined in the next section.

An Evidence Base for Supportive Psychotherapy: Does One Exist?

At present, there is no agreed-upon evidence base for supportive psychotherapy in psycho-oncology. An evidence base for SP has not been developed in the usual manner. No essential ingredients or components have been defined. No universal treatment manual has been developed and tested. Most conclude, therefore, that there is no evidence base.

However, two lines of research suggest an emerging evidence base for SP: (a) the general elements of ESRs (Norcross, 2011) and (b) investigations of the generic process model of psychotherapy (GMP) (Orlinsky & Howard, 1987) with gynecological cancer patients (Manne, Kashy, Rubin, Hernandez, & Bergman, 2012; Manne et al., 2010).

Empirically Supported Relationship Research

The Task Force on ESRs completed meta-analytic reviews with estimated effect sizes (use of correlational coefficient r) and from the strength of this evidence identified six relationship elements as generally important in most psychotherapy relationships. Five of these general elements are relevant to SP in psycho-oncology. They are (a) alliance in adult individual psychotherapy (aggregate effect size of $r = .27$), (b) alliance in family therapy (weighted average effect size of $r = .26$), (c) cohesion in group therapy (weighted aggregate effect size of $r = .25$), (d) empathy (weighted effect size of $r = .30$), and (e) collecting client feedback (various effect sizes ranging from $r = .33$ to $.23$). These are considered moderate effect sizes, suggesting that patients who experience these elements are better off than about 60% of those who do not. To the extent that SP consists of any or all of these general elements of effective psychotherapy relationships, these findings may provide some empirical evidence for SP. However, none of these studies have included cancer patients.

Generic Model of Psychotherapy Research

Two investigations of the GMP with cancer patients have investigated nonspecific therapeutic processes hypothesized to occur in effective psychotherapy (GMP) (Manne et al., 2010, 2012). In the original RCT, 353 women with gynecological cancer were randomly assigned to a seven-session coping and communication-enhancing intervention (CCI), a seven-session supportive counseling intervention (SC), or usual care (Manne et al, 2007). Multiple outcome and process variables were collected. Results found that both interventions decreased symptoms of depression over usual care, but there were no differences between CCI or SC. Subsequent analyses were interested in learning more about what universal change processes might explain the benefits from both approaches, and thus, data from the two treatment conditions (CCI and SC) were combined and process variables from the GMP were investigated (Manne et al., 2010, 2012). The GMP variables of (a) therapeutic alliance, (b) therapeutic realizations (in-session benefits such as insight), (c) therapeutic openness/involvement in treatment, and (d) session progress were investigated. Results indicated that the therapeutic bond (a component of the therapeutic alliance) predicted openness, which predicted more therapeutic realizations. Therapeutic realizations predicted, in turn, greater session progress, and session progress predicted lower symptoms of depression at 3-month follow-up. These variables were found to be predictive of a sequence of processes leading to improved outcome in patients who received both CCI and SC. Such results are relevant to the question of an evidence base for SP.

To the extent that the SC condition in this study is representative of SP in psycho-oncology, these results provide some evidence of efficacy. Thus, at present, an evidence base for SP has not developed in the usual manner by developing a detailed treatment manual and testing its efficacy against control conditions in a well-designed RCT. Until or if this occurs, SP, as a theoretical approach in psycho-oncology, has no evidence base. However, the lines of research reviewed, using correlational designs and structural equation modeling (SEM), have found (a) moderately strong effect sizes for essential elements of effective therapy relationships, elements most likely to be present in SP and (b) many of the hypothesized relationships in the GMP were supported by SEM in the study of SP as an effective intervention for women with gynecological cancer.

At present, minimal research has investigated these variables in psycho-oncology and much more is needed (Schnur & Montgomery, 2010) to develop an evidence base for SP, but these studies provide interesting results from which to build.

CHAPTER SUMMARY

This chapter—along with Chapter 2—adds to the background knowledge of the psycho-oncologist. It begins with an overview of the general psychotherapy outcome research with adults—important knowledge in the face of gaps in the psycho-oncology evidence base. Key findings include (a) psychotherapy, in general, works and results in positive outcomes for many people; (b) these positive results are generalizable to real-world settings; (c) there is little support for the idea that some theoretical approaches, in general, are better than other approaches, and thus researchers have investigated those factors thought to be common across many approaches; (d) patient-focused research has shown that routine collection of feedback from patients improves outcomes and addresses many practical questions; (e) researchers have been divided on which factors are more important to positive outcomes—*specific* treatment techniques/methods or *common* factors that contribute to strong therapy relationships; and (f) a helpful approach to move beyond these controversies has focused on identifying which therapeutic factors account for how much of the variability in outcome (see Figs. 3.1 and 3.2), regardless of whether these factors are specific or common.

A second section of this chapter summarizes those theoretical approaches to psychotherapy that have been adapted or modified for use with cancer patients. Cognitive-behavioral and existential psychotherapy have the longest and strongest evidence base in psycho-oncology. Lastly, despite the recognition of supportive psychotherapy as viable and important to psycho-oncology, there is no consensus on what it is, how it is implemented, or what is its evidence base. This chapter concludes with a review of SP and offers ideas about an emerging evidence base. With this chapter as a resource for general background knowledge, the evidence-based practitioner can proceed through the process of evidence-based practice—as explained in detail in Chapter 4.

4

The Evidence-Based Practice of Psycho-Oncology

The most immediately important task of psycho-oncology is to close the yawning gap between current knowledge and actual clinical care of patients.

—Greer (1994)

There is little evidence that evidence-based practices are yet effectively disseminated or implemented in the vast majority of real-world practice settings.

—Frueh et al. (2012)

Evidence-based practice (EBP) in psycho-oncology is part of a larger effort to improve health care. Poor-quality health care in the United States is thought to be—among other causes—the result of delays in translating science to clinical practice, contributing to a "quality chasm" (Institute of Medicine, 2001). Health care costs continue to rise and health care policy in the United States has focused on cost containment, quality improvement, and increased accountability. These events have increased the importance of clinical science as the foundation of practice, and EBP has become a central component of health care reform (Institute of Medicine, 2001).

EBP is needed in psycho-oncology (Carlson & Bultz, 2004; Jacobsen, 2009; Jacobsen & Jim, 2008). Systematic reviews have concluded that psychosocial interventions in oncology are effective (e.g., Jacobsen et al., 2006; Meyer & Mark, 1995; Redd et al., 2001). Interventions show efficacy for relieving emotional distress, anxiety, depression, and improving quality of life (Faller et al., 2013). Effect sizes are generally small to medium, but in studies where patients are selected as a result of increased distress, effect sizes are large and positive results seem to last (Faller et al., 2013). Despite recognized efficacy, few evidence-based interventions are used in routine practice. Dissemination and implementation strategies are needed. The development of clinical practice guidelines (see Chapter 1) is one strategy for disseminating and implementing interventions, and learning how to do EBP is another. Practice guidelines disseminate knowledge, and competent EBP improves implementation.

As detailed in this chapter, EBP involves more than knowledge of best available evidence; it also requires competence in the skills involved in a systematic process for implementing EBP. This skill-development approach aims to train the evidence-based practitioner in enhanced treatment planning and evaluation, to improve patient outcomes, by attending to the three pillars of EBP: best available research evidence; clinical expertise; and patient characteristics, culture, needs, and preferences.

Psycho-oncologists competent in EBP will be positioned to bring quality care as a result of the following EBP advantages:

- Three major components of effective health care—best evidence, clinical expertise, and patient needs—are considered and integrated.
- The EBP process develops specific skills in how to proceed with implementing effective treatment. These include the following:
    - Specific procedures for formulating clinical questions
    - Steps for converting clinical questions into workable literature search strategies
    - Knowledge of online databases and search engines for online literature search skills
    - Knowledge and skill in appraising the identified literature by use of available check sheets and/or journal reporting standards

In addition, EBP encourages ethical practice. The routine reflection on one's own competencies and clinical expertise encourages compliance to the ethical standard to practice within the boundaries of one's competence and, when needed, to seek training to maintain competence. EBP's emphasis on patient collaboration through consideration of patient needs, characteristics, culture, and preferences is consistent with the ethical mandate to do no harm and to safeguard the welfare and rights of others.

EBP has been defined as "the integration of best research evidence with clinical expertise and patient values" (Institute of Medicine, 2001, p. 147). EBP has been said to have "a long past, but a short history" (Norcross, Hogan, & Koocher, 2008, p. 1). Psycho-oncology has *both* a short past and an even shorter EBP history, but it also has a promising future with the use of EBP (Jacobsen, 2009). All health care professions have now endorsed EBP. Those most relevant to psycho-oncology are psychology, psychiatry, social work, and oncology nursing, as well as the interdisciplinary field of behavioral medicine (Davidson et al., 2003; Spring et al., 2005). Table 4.1 provides a sampling of a number of important references to the EBP process across relevant disciplines.

Table 4.1. A Sampling of Evidence-Based Practice References Across Multiple Disciplines

Discipline	Reference and Description
Medicine	Straus, Richardson, Glasziou, & Haynes (2005). Third edition of the classic, pocket-size handbook that comes from the original working group who formulated basic principles of evidence-based medicine.
	Institute of Medicine (2001). An influential, broad-based report addressing the "chasm" between medical science and quality health care. Endorsed principles of evidence-based medicine.
Oncology	Devoto & Kramer (2006). Traces the development of research through the first use of comparison groups, the development of statistical methods, and the adoption by the FDA of the randomized controlled trial as the "gold standard." Notes the impact of the Flexner Report on medical education.
Psychology	American Psychological Association (2006). Official endorsement of evidence-based practice of psychology.
	Norcross, Hogan, & Koocher (2008). First handbook of evidence-based practice exclusively focused on mental health and the addictions. Modeled after Straus et al. (2005) for ease of access to relevant information—pocket size, includes a CD of entire contexts and additional information.
Psychiatry	American Psychiatric Association (2009). Development of practice guidelines for a wide variety of mental disorders.
Social work	National Association of Social Workers (2007). NASW report, in conjunction with NIMH, titled *Partnerships to integrate evidence-based mental health practices into social work education and research.*
	Gibbs (2003). Widely used textbook and practical guide. Has an accompanying Web site for ease of access to practical tools.
Oncology nursing	Oncology Nursing Society (2009). An online evidence-based resource. Putting Evidence Into Practice (PEP) (Fulcher et al., 2008) provides online access to evidence-based nursing interventions for specific patient problems.
Interprofessional	Society of Behavioral Medicine (SBM) has published relevant articles on evidence-based behavioral medicine (EBBM) by Davidson et al., (2003, 2004) and Spring et al. (2005).
	Council for Training in Evidence-Based Behavioral Practice (EBBP) (2009) has developed an excellent online resource funded by NIH's Office of Behavioral and Social Science Research (OBSSR).

THE BASICS OF EVIDENCE-BASED PRACTICE

Definitions and Core Components

Separate and discipline-specific definitions have been developed, but the most relevant to psycho-oncology are

- medicine,
- psychology, and
- interdisciplinary behavioral practice.

All originate from the Evidence-Based Medicine (EBM) Working Group (Sackett, Straus, Richardson, Rosenberg, & Haynes, 2000) and were adopted by the Institute of Medicine (2001, p. 147): "Evidence–based practice is the integration of best research evidence with clinical expertise and patient values." In psychology, the evidence-based practice of psychology is defined as "the integration of the best available research with clinical expertise in the context of patient characteristics, culture, and preference" (American Psychological Association, 2006, p. 273). From the National Institutes of Health–funded Evidence-Based Behavioral Practice project comes a broader, ecological definition of EBP as "making decisions about how to promote healthful behaviors by integrating the best available evidence with practitioner expertise *and other resources* [italics added], and with the characteristics, state, needs, values and preferences of those who will be affected" (Council for Training in Evidence-Based Behavioral Practice, 2009, p. 3). Although wording differs slightly, all of these definitions emphasize *the integration* of three components:

- best available *research evidence*,
- practitioner *expertise*, and
- *patient values.*

Best Available Research Evidence

In evidence-based *medicine*, Sackett and colleagues define best research evidence as emanating from basic medical sciences but coming particularly from clinical research focused on (a) the accuracy of diagnostic procedures (e.g., clinical examination); (b) the influence of prognosis; and (c) the efficacy and safety of a range of medical interventions, including prevention, treatment, and rehabilitation (Sackett, Rosenberg, Gray, Haynes, & Richardson, 1996). In the evidence-based practice of *psychology*, best available research is defined as scientific results related primarily to assessment and intervention strategies for relevant clinical problems, and also from basic psychological research. Evidence from a range of research designs and methodologies is acknowledged, but priority is given to clinically relevant research based on systematic reviews and notable effect sizes, demonstrating statistical and clinical significance (American Psychological Association, 2006). In interdisciplinary evidence-based *behavioral* practice, evidence is derived from research that is systematic, observational, experimental, and formulated from specific testable research questions and hypotheses (Council for Training in Evidence-Based Behavioral Practice, 2009).

Clinical Expertise

In the evidence-based practice of *psychology*, clinical expertise is the use of clinical competencies such as assessment, diagnosis, case formulation, treatment planning, intervention, and outcome measurement. Related skills include forming strong therapeutic relationships while attending to the influence of individual differences on treatment decisions. EBP of psychology also emphasizes practitioner self-reflective knowledge of how his or her own characteristics, values, and culture can interact with patient care (American Psychological Association, 2006). In interdisciplinary evidence-based *behavioral* practice, expertise is one important resource, considered along with others such as physical, technological, and financial assets that are necessary to successfully implement behavioral interventions. This approach to expertise reflects the ecological model (McLeroy, Bibeau, Steckler, & Glanz, 1988) upon which evidence-based behavioral practice is based, recognizing the importance of addressing health problems at multiple levels of intervention (e.g., individual, interpersonal, family, organizational, community, public policy). Specific categories of practitioner expertise include assessment, communication and collaboration, engagement and intervention and process skills (formulate questions, seek evidence, evaluate evidence, implement results and evaluate outcome) necessary to competently do evidence-based behavioral practice (Council for Training in Evidence-Based Behavioral Practice [EBBP], 2009).

Patient Characteristics, Values, Culture, and Preferences

In the EBP of *psychology*, the emphasis is on patient characteristics, culture, and context (American Psychological Association, 2006). The emphasis on individual differences, the impact of human development across the life span, and the role of human diversity (e.g., culture, race, ethnicity, and socioeconomic status) are just a few examples of a long history of research in psychology focused upon the uniqueness of each individual and its relevance to psychological interventions. In interdisciplinary evidence-based *behavioral* practice, patient values are expressed as client or population characteristics, needs, values, and preferences (Council for Training in Evidence-Based Behavioral Practice [EBBP], 2009) and collaborative decision making with health care providers is emphasized. With its ecological focus, the populations affected by the intervention will differ depending on the level at which the intervention occurs. Individuals, families, organizations, communities, or entire populations could all be the focus of the intervention as they represent those served.

Integration of the Three Components

All approaches emphasize the active integration of the three components. Figure 4.1 illustrates this integration and emphasizes the clinical decision-making process.

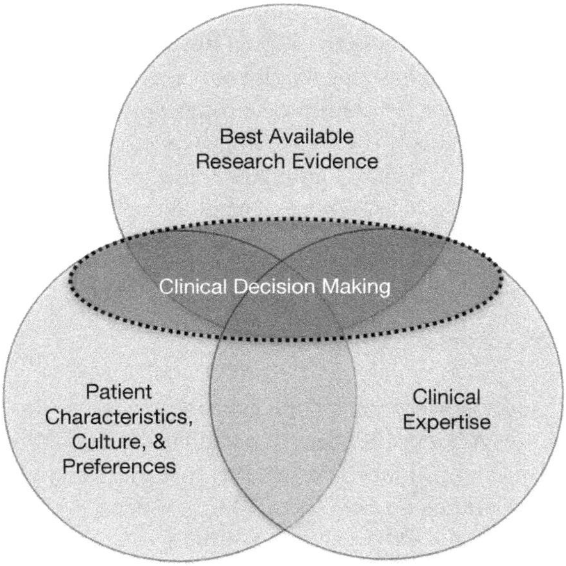

Figure 4.1 The three circles of evidence-based practice and the clinical decision-making process.
SOURCE: From Spring, B. (January, 2007). Evidence-based practice in clinical psychology: What is it: Why it matters: What you need to know. Invited address to Council of University Directors of Clinical Psychology, Savannah, GA. Reprinted with permission.

In Figure 4.1 the equal size and shape of each component is a hypothetical illustration in which all three components have an equal degree of importance in decisions to be made. In actual clinical examples, there will be varying degrees of emphasis or weight given to combinations of the three components. In addition, the relative weight given to each of the three components varies by discipline. In psycho-oncology the total amount of clinical research evidence is limited, the types of clinical questions for which research is needed are more complex given the recognition of vast differences between individual patients, and very little synthesizing and contextualizing of information has occurred (Jacobsen, 2009). The mental health professions, with roots in the social sciences, also have a stronger emphasis on individual patient differences and the impact of diversity on patient care. Consequently, EBP in mental health is likely to be asking questions of greater complexity, with more variability in potential answers, and yet, levels of evidence (e.g., effect sizes) comparable to medicine (2007). All of these differences combined suggest it is important to consider the relative weight of the three components in any clinical decision-making process (Norcross et al., 2008).

THE CORE COMPETENCIES OF EVIDENCE-BASED PRACTICE

The core competencies of EBP involve a series of repetitive, iterative steps (Council for Training in Evidence-Based Behavioral Practice [EBBP], 2009; Norcross et al.,

2008). The "5 A's" of *A*sk, *A*cquire, *A*ppraise, *A*pply, and *A*nalyze/Adjust summarize a traditional model. To these traditional five steps, Norcross and colleagues (2008) add a sixth step, emphasizing the importance of *translating* research to the needs of a particular patient, while also renaming *apply* to *integrating* and *analyze* to *evaluating*. This addition of the translating step and the renaming of *apply* to *integration*, and *analyze* to *evaluate*, emphasizes the "relentless complexity of people" (Norcross et al., 2008, p. 232) that is central to the mental health disciplines.

Step 1: Asking Questions: Formulating Specific and Answerable Clinical Questions

The start of any successful search for best available evidence is a well-formulated clinical question. As experienced practitioners come to ask specific, well-formulated questions, it becomes evident that these questions tend to arise from similar informational needs (Gibbs, 2003; J. C. Norcross et al., 2008; Straus et al., 2005). Although not exhaustive or mutually exclusive, Table 4.2 provides some sample questions by category.

In EBP, there is an important distinction between background and foreground questions (Norcross et al., 2008; Straus et al., 2005). Each functions to provide different types of information. *Background questions* look for already known and available general knowledge, while *foreground questions* look for highly specific knowledge most applicable to a specific patient or patient group. In psycho-oncology, background questions can be biomedical, psychosocial, or biopsychosocial.

Biomedical Background Questions

- What are some differences between early- and late-stage breast cancer?
- What side effects are expected when receiving combination chemotherapy and radiation therapy?
- For Stage II (cancer type) what are the 5-year survival rates?

Psychosocial Background Questions

- What psychotherapy approaches have the best evidence for treatment of advanced cancers?
- Are there any specific emotional or social issues unique to (cancer type)?
- Within families, who is most likely to become the primary caregiver?
- How does a diagnosis of early-stage cancer affect the relationship between recently married couples?

Biopsychosocial Background Questions

- Are certain chemotherapy or hormonal therapies associated with increased depression/anxiety?

Table 4.2. Type of Questions Asked in Evidence-Based Practice of Psycho-Oncology

Category	**Sample Question**
Diagnosis	Do this patient's symptoms meet diagnostic criteria for a mental disorder?
Intervention	Is supportive-expressive psychotherapy an effective intervention for a patient with symptoms of depression?
Etiology	What causes a patient to experience anticipatory nausea/ vomiting prior to a chemotherapy treatment?
Personal description	What is the phenomenological experience of a particular cancer-related life event (e.g., terminal illness) like?
Comorbidity	Which types of mental disorders are most likely to be experienced by the same person ("which go together"?)
Screening and assessment	Which self-report questionnaires are most valid and reliable for determining the presence of distress?
Therapeutic relationship	How important is the therapeutic relationship between a therapist and a cancer patient when providing supportive psychotherapy?
Progress monitoring	Is the patient improving as a result of the treatment intervention provided?
Harm	What potential for harm is there in a selected intervention?
Cost	How much does a specific intervention cost?

- During bone marrow transplant and periods of isolation do most patients experience increased anxiety/depression reactive to the isolation?
- What are the best psychological treatments for anticipatory nausea and vomiting?

Background questions in EBP do not ask about the particular details of a patient's history or the patient's particular prior experiences—often referred to as *the patient's background*—but rather about prior obtained knowledge. In contrast, foreground questions function to provide more specific answers to particular patient-focused, clinically relevant questions. The acronym PICO is recommended to guide the formulation of both background and foreground questions.

- *P—patient* (client, individual, couple, family, group, organization, community), problem, population
- *I—intervention* (broadly defined to include any planned interaction with a patient)
- *C—comparison* with another alternative intervention
- *O—outcomes* desired (reduced symptoms, quality of life)

PICO-formulated questions are specific in that they ask for information about *interventions* targeted to specific *outcomes*, as relevant to specific *patient* characteristics (e.g., age, diagnosis, stage). For example:

- P—for a 37-year-old single woman with early-stage breast cancer and self-reported symptoms of depression, who finished active treatment,
- I—is individual cognitive-behavioral therapy better than
- C—group cognitive-behavioral therapy for
- O—improving overall quality of life?

It is also important to note that in psycho-oncology, the comparison is often to no intervention. For example:

- P—for a 64-year-old, widowed (6 months) male, who recently began external beam radiation treatment for Stage II prostate cancer,
- I—will individual supportive psychotherapy—with a focus on the expression of grief-related sadness and loneliness—be better
- C—than no treatment, or treatment as usual, for
- O—frequency of crying episodes during which he avoids contact with friends.

The PICO format can prove helpful, but it is primarily focused on questions comparing specific interventions (Huang, Lin, & Demner-Fishmen, 2006). Psycho-oncology practitioners have a variety of important questions (see Table 4.2), many of which may not be best formulated via PICO.

Another useful format captured in the acronym COPES—*Client-Oriented Practical Evidence Search* questions—has been recommended for use in social work and other helping professions (Gibbs, 2003). COPES questions are *client-oriented* (CO) because they come from daily practice, are posed by busy practitioners, and oriented toward client needs. They are of *practical* (P) significance focused on real-world concerns, and a COPES question ultimately guides an *evidence search* (ES).

Step 2: Accessing the Best Available Research Evidence

Once a clinical question is formulated, the process of accessing available research begins. Many clinical questions will begin as background questions, seeking general knowledge (particularly if the questions are about a relatively new clinical issue or one new to the practitioner). For example, the previously formulated foreground question is as follows:

> For a 37-year-old single woman with early-stage breast cancer and self-reported symptoms of depression who recently finished active treatment, is individual cognitive-behavioral therapy better than group cognitive-behavioral therapy for improving overall quality of life?

becomes reformulated into broader, general-background-knowledge questions:

- Is cognitive-behavioral therapy effective in enhancing quality of life?
- In a cancer population, what constitutes quality of life, and how is it measured?
- Are there any potential harmful consequences in cognitive-behavioral therapy?

and the process of finding the evidence begins. It is necessary, however, to first review where available evidence comes from and what types of evidence are available to address the formulated questions.

Creation, Distillation, and Dissemination of Best Available Evidence

Best available evidence is first *created* and then *distilled* or summarized in order to facilitate its *dissemination* to practitioners. Three key roles are involved in this overall process: researcher, synthesizer, and practitioner (see Fig. 4.2).

The initial discovery of evidence begins with the input of the clinical researcher who designs, conducts, analyzes, and reports results. This has been called *knowledge creation* (Spring et al., 2005; Straus, Tetroe, & Graham, 2009). In this process, all of the knowledge (e.g., research design, methodology, statistics, and data analysis) of the competent clinical scientist is paramount. Knowledge creation

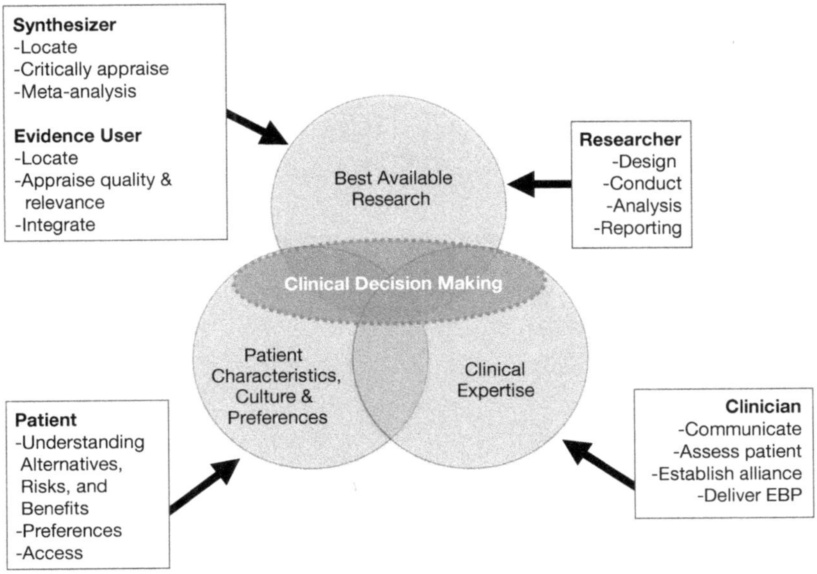

Figure 4.2 Creation, distillation, and dissemination in evidence-based practice.
SOURCE: From Spring, B. (2007). Evidence-based practice in clinical psychology: What it is: Why it matters: What you need to know. *Journal of Clinical Psychology, 63*(7), 611–631. Reprinted with permission.

occurs and relevant findings accumulate. As relevant findings grow, the output process begins. Next, the research synthesizers locate, appraise, and summarize the evidence. Systematic reviews, meta-analyses, and traditional reviews are examples of synthesized research summaries. This process has been called *knowledge distillation* (Spring et al., 2005; Straus et al., 2009). Here the expertise of reviewers is critical. (1) Reviewers must appraise the research on a wide variety of relevant criterion (e.g., internal and external validity as influenced by design, methodology, and data analyses). (2) Then they must also synthesize and summarize the evidence in the form of summaries or synopses that attempt to answer specific clinically relevant questions. With accessible synopses, the EBP practitioner or evidence user can then locate the evidence as it relates to her or his clinical question. Making this evidence accessible has been called *knowledge dissemination* (Spring et al., 2005; Straus et al., 2009). Knowledge dissemination involves the process of facilitating access of the information to the evidence-based practitioner through use of technology (e.g., online portals).

Types of Evidence-Based Practice Resources

Created and distilled evidence is then disseminated via a variety of EBP resources. Such resources are often illustrated by use of the EBP Evidence Resource Triangle (see Fig. 4.3).

The triangle is a conceptual scheme for organizing a wide variety of EBP resources, where categories of information begin with individual studies and

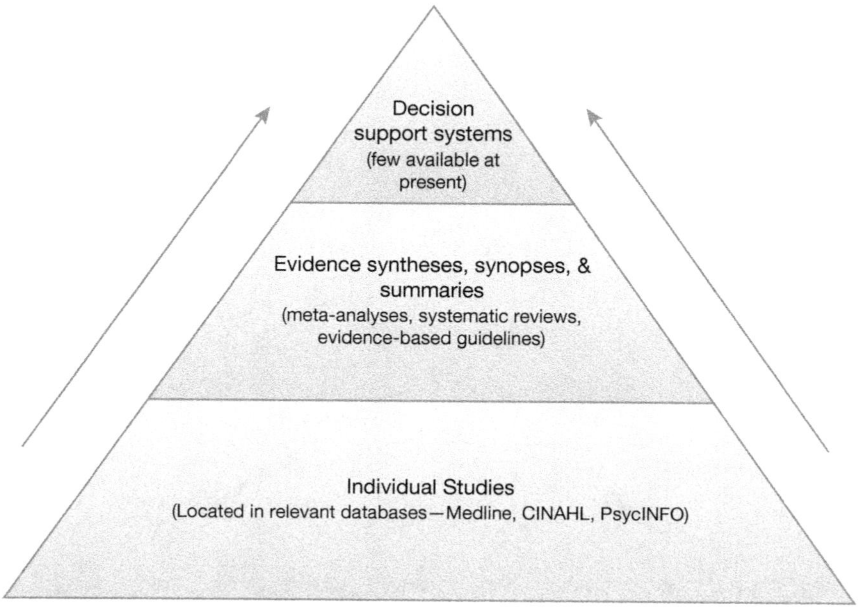

Figure 4.3 Evidence resource triangle.
SOURCE: Adapted from Haynes, R. B. (2006). Of studies, syntheses, synopses, summaries, and systems: The "5S" evolution of information services for evidence-based healthcare decisions, *Evidence Based Medicine, 11*(6), 162–164, with permission from BMJ Publishing Group Ltd.

become increasingly synthesized and contextualized to specific practice settings. At the lowest level of the hierarchy are individual studies such as original journal articles, often labeled *primary literature*. At this level, the literature is considered "unfiltered." Moving up the triangle, synthesized synopses and summaries include systematic reviews, meta-analyses, clinical guidelines, and online evidence-based textbooks, often called *secondary literature* or "filtered." At the highest level of synthesis and integration, decision support systems are computerized systems integrated into electronic medical records, making immediate access to evidence-based information readily accessible. Few decision support systems are available in psycho-oncology, yet there are an increasing number of synopses, syntheses, and summaries—secondary literature. Accessing best available evidence requires knowing how to sort through available resources. Table 4.3 presents definitions of categories of online resources, the types of evidence typically found, and a few examples.

Familiarity and practice in using these resources are essential to a successful search. However, for busy practitioners it is important to acknowledge the need (at least when faced with unfamiliar or infrequent clinical questions) for the help of medical librarians who typically use these resources daily (McKibbon, 1999). In addition to the general resources summarized in Table 4.3, Table 4.4 provides psycho-oncology-specific EBP resources relevant to answering many background questions.

With this understanding of knowledge creation, distillation, and dissemination, as well as some general and oncology-specific EBP resources, we now return to the EBP process of accessing best available research.

Designing a Search Strategy

Before quickly running to access the evidence resources, it is important to first devise a search strategy. Gibbs and colleagues (2003) provide a helpful process for designing a search strategy, which involves a series of sequential steps. *Step one* is to answer specific questions that correspond to each of the four components of the PICO (or COPES) format.

- P—*Patient or problem or population*—how would you describe the patient or problem or population in detail (demographics, medical status, etc.)? *A 37-year-old single woman, with early-stage breast cancer, who recently finished the active phase of treatment.*
- I—*Intervention* planned—what is the planned intervention?—["that which is to be implemented (e.g., screening/assessment procedure, therapy, treatment, program, consultation)"]—*Is individual cognitive-behavioral therapy*
- C—*Comparison*—what is the current or another alternative planned intervention? (e.g., standard care, current "gold standard" or "best practice," no treatment)—*better than group cognitive-behavioral therapy*
- O—*outcome* to be measured—what is the desired outcome or endpoint to the intervention?—*for improved overall quality of life?*

Table 4.3. General Evidence-Based Practice Online Resources and Types of Evidence

Online Resource	Type(s) of Evidence	Examples[a]
Clinical Decision Support Tools	*Multiple Types*	
These are computerized systems integrated into electronic health records, designed to make access to evidence-based information immediately accessible		UpToDate DynaMed
Metasearch Engines	*Multiple Types*	
These sites search multiple high-quality Web sites simultaneously and organize information into type of evidence accessed		TRIP Database SUMSearch
Filtered Information	*Secondary Literature*	
Information that has already undergone some summarizing and synthesizing	Systematic reviews Meta-analyses Practice guidelines Structured abstracts Electronic textbooks General public online	Cochrane Database (CDSR) Campbell Collaboration NICE, AHRQ(NGC) EB Mental Health MEDSCAPE (eMedicine) ACS, NCI, SAMHSAs NREPP
Unfiltered Information[b]	*Primary Literature*	
Information that has not undergone any summarizing or synthesizing	Individual studies	APA's PsycINFO PubMed (MEDLINE) CINAHL Elsevier's EMBASE

NOTES: This process is an ever-evolving one such that any table can only represent basic information available at a specific point in time.

[a]This is a list of accessible online resources at the time of the writing of this book (2010–2014), but it is anticipated that additional resources will be developed. Given the uncertainty of the sustainability of such resources, practitioners are advised to use the skills of medical librarians.

[b]Some unfiltered information databases can access secondary literature such as systematic reviews and meta-analyses with use of specific search strategies.

Table 4.4. Selected Psycho-Oncology Resources and Types of Evidence and Questions Addressed

Resource	Description	Type Evidence/ Questions
IOM (2008), *Cancer Care for the Whole Patient*	Report highlighting inadequate availability despite evidence base of psychosocial care	Evidence-based consensus report Background quest
Holland et al. (2010), *Psycho-Oncology*	The classic textbook of psycho-oncology	Secondary literature Background quest
APOS (2006), *Psycho-Oncology Quick Reference for Oncology Clinicians*	Small guide for psychiatric and psychological dimensions of cancer symptom management	Secondary literature Background quest
Watson & Kissane (2011), *Handbook of Psychotherapy in Cancer Care*	Edited book providing introductions to psychological therapies being developed for cancer patients, families, and caregivers	Background and foreground quest Secondary literature
Cancer Control P.L.A.N.E.T.	Portal to online resources for implementing and evaluating evidence-based programs	Multiple types Background and foreground quest
NCI's PDQ (Physician's Data Query)	Peer-reviewed, evidence-based summaries on adult and pediatric treatment, supportive and palliative care, screening and prevention, genetics, complementary and alternative medicine	Secondary literature Background quest
NCCN Guidelines for Screening for Distress	US consensus-based recommendations about how to identify psychosocial distress	Clinical practice guideline
Standards of psychosocial health services for persons with cancer and their families (Canadian Association of Psycho-social Oncology [CAPO], 2010)	Canadian consensus-based recommendations. Revision of original 1999 standards.	Consensus statement Background quest

(*Continued*)

Table 4.4. CONTINUED

Resource	Description	Type Evidence/ Questions
A Pan-Canadian Clinical Practice Guideline: Assessment of psychosocial health care needs of the adult cancer patient (Howell, et al., 2009)	Canadian recommendations for providing routine, standardized, and systematic assessment of the psychosocial needs of adult cancer patients	Clinical practice guideline
NBCC-NCCI (2003). *Clinical Practice Guidelines for the Psychosocial Care of Adults With Cancer*	Australian recommendations for optimal evidence-based psychosocial care for adults	Clinical practice guideline
IOM & NRC (2006). *From Cancer Patient to Cancer Survivor*	Report focused on transition of adult survivors during period of care after treatment has concluded. Emphasizes survivorship care planning.	Evidence-based consensus report Background quest
NICE (2004). *Improving Supportive and Palliative Care for Adults With Cancer*	Guidance for implementing supportive, palliative care services for adult patients and caregivers in the United Kingdom	Evidence-based consensus report Background quest

Step two involves listing keywords or specific search terms that correspond with each of the four PICO components. Online databases (e.g., Medline, PsycINFO, and CINAHL) organize their accessible knowledge in various ways, each using some form of a controlled vocabulary. *Controlled vocabularies* are systems for organizing information by use of specific search terms that can be found in databases. Some examples and their database include *subject terms* (academic search premier), *thesaurus* (PsycINFO), and *medical subject headings* (MeSh in Medline). A search strategy can be developed using either keywords or search terms from a controlled vocabulary. Search skills and knowledge of keywords or search terms develops with practice and familiarity.

For example, from the earlier question, keywords are likely to include the following:

- P—breast cancer
- I—individual cognitive-behavioral therapy
- C—group cognitive-behavioral therapy
- O—health-related quality of life

Step three involves listing possible synonyms or known terms from various controlled vocabulary databases (e.g., PsycINFO, CINAHL, and Medline):

- P—neoplasm; oncology
- I—psychotherapy, individual
- C—psychotherapy, group
- O—quality of life, well-being

The Gibbs and colleagues (2003) worksheet then guides the remainder of the search process.

Step four involves beginning the actual literature search. Ideally, the search will access syntheses or summaries such as systematic reviews or meta-analyses. The intent is to look first for information that is highest on the evidence resource triangle (see Fig. 4.3). A reasonable starting point could be a metasearch engine such as SUMSearch, or going directly to known secondary literature databases such as the Cochrane Collaboration or the National Guidelines Clearinghouse (NGC). This secondary filtered literature may directly answer the question, but if the formulated question is not answered with secondary literature, the search continues by accessing primary, unfiltered literature (see Table 4.3).

In the present example, the TRIP metasearch engine was used and the terms "breast cancer AND cognitive-behavioral therapy" found 20 systematic reviews. A quick review of abstracts from these 20 reviews resulted in the discovery of one from the Database of Abstracts of Reviews of Effects (DARE) titled *Psychosocial interventions for depression, anxiety, and quality of life in cancer survivors: meta-analyses* (Osborn, Demoncada, & Feuerstein, 2006). DARE is a well-known, structured abstracting service that is updated monthly and available online. It provides a concise and succinct abstract of systematic reviews. It is an example of filtered, secondary literature, and it provides a direct answer to the PICO question, in the summary:

> Cognitive-behavioral therapy was an effective short-term treatment for depression and anxiety, and had both short- and long-term effects on quality of life in adult cancer survivors. Individual interventions were more effective than group interventions.

Step five. Had our PICO question not been answered at this level of the evidence hierarchy, step five would then involve a search of unfiltered primary literature. Here the use of the controlled vocabulary terms and synonyms becomes important when searching databases such as PsycINFO, CINAHL, or PubMed. Referring back to the original worksheet becomes essential to identify potential terms. General knowledge of how to use these evidence-based resources is essential, but the prospect of a busy practitioner keeping up with the latest changes and innovations makes it difficult. Expert knowledge of the use of thesauri, keyword searching, Boolean operators, shortcuts, truncation, specialized filters, and the many other skills of the medical librarian are beyond the scope of most evidence-based practitioners. Therefore, training and periodic consultation with a skilled medical librarian becomes essential. Also, archiving these well-formulated clinical questions will help for future searches.

Once the best, most up-to-date evidence is accessed—whether primary unfiltered original studies or secondary filtered reviews or synopses—it needs to be appraised, by asking, "How do we know that this is best available evidence?"

Step 3: Appraising the Research Evidence

Learning how to evaluate the best available research evidence requires an understanding of research design, methodology, statistical analyses, and the reliability and validity of reported results and conclusions.[1] A detailed discussion of these topics is beyond the scope of this book, as most psycho-oncology practitioners already have some familiarity with these concepts. For those who do not, many excellent resources exist to help in this process (Council for Training in Evidence-Based Behavioral Practice [EBBP], 2009; Gibbs, 2003; Heneghan & Badenoch, 2006; Norcross et al., 2008; Rubin & Bellamy, 2012). For those with little background in research or for those looking for an online source for updating knowledge, a helpful starting point is the EBBP Web site, specifically, its critical appraisal training module (http://www.ebbp.org/training.html) and its critical appraisal resource page (http://www.ebbp.org/appraisal.html). The training module is designed to introduce some of the details of understanding basic terms, such as internal and external validity, and various forms of bias as they apply to the most common research designs relevant to EBP. Detailed examples are provided for key issues to appraise in randomized controlled trials (RCTs) and time series designs, as well as how to appraise the validity and reliability of the evidence provided in systematic reviews and clinical practice guidelines. The critical appraisal resource page has a number of links to other helpful online sources that provide checklists to use to appraise various types of research studies. Another helpful resource is Gibb's textbook *Evidence based practice for the helping professions* (Gibbs, 2003). Whichever sources are used, the starting point in understanding the appraisal process is to recognize the relationship between the types of questions asked and the research designs used to answer such questions. Only certain research designs can answer certain types of questions. Thus, the types of questions asked (intervention, assessment, cost, harm, etc.) influence which research designs to look to for answers. Table 4.5 provides an overview of

1. At the present time, it is not realistic to expect that the busy practitioner can do the detailed appraisal process as described here. Future electronic health records (EHRs) are to include decision support systems designed to facilitate this process. This detailed description of Step 3 is provided as an initial step in the development of competency in appraising research evidence. See Appendix C for an abbreviated time-saving approach.

Table 4.5. Types of Research Questions Asked and Best Study Type

Question Type	**Research Type/Designs**
Diagnosis/comorbidity/screening and assessment	Cohort study (with use of current "gold standard" for diagnosing)
Intervention (treatment, therapy)	True experimental, randomized controlled trial
Etiology/harm	Randomized controlled trial, cohort study, case control, case series
Therapeutic relationship	Psychotherapy process
Cost	Economic analysis
Description/meaning/purpose	Observational, qualitative research (small sample, detailed information)

SOURCE: Adapted from the Council for Training in Evidence-Based Behavioral Practice (EBBP) training module, *Searching for Evidence,* http://www.ebbp.org, copyright © Bonnie Spring, PhD, Northwestern University.

some common types of questions asked and the study design(s) best equipped to answer them.

Once the type of question has been determined and the appropriate design(s) are identified, accessed literature can then be appraised. Various checklists and journal reporting standards have been developed to help in the appraisal process.

Helpful Appraisal Resources

Identifying a variety of helpful appraisal resources begins at the EBBP critical appraisal resource page (http://www.ebbp.org/appraisal.html), where links to a number of online sources are provided. The psycho-oncologist is most likely to be appraising the literature to answer a question about the effectiveness of an intervention, sometimes comparing the relative effectiveness of one type of psychotherapy to another. This type of question is best answered by use of true experimental designs such as RCTs. Thus, one helpful resource is a *checklist for critically appraising* the internal and external validity of a single RCT from the Centre for Evidence-Based Medicine (CEBM) in Toronto (http://www.cebm.net/index.aspx?o=1157). The CEBM site also has critical appraisal worksheets for use with systematic reviews and studies answering diagnostic and prognostic questions. Gibbs's textbook (Gibbs, 2003) includes a widely used rating form—Quality of Study Rating Form (QSRF)—designed to evaluate the quality of the evidence, and this form is used in future chapters to appraise the accessed literature. A modified version of the QSRF and scoring instructions are provided in Appendix B.

Journal reporting standards provide another helpful appraisal tool. In recent years, researchers, journal editors, methodologists/design/statistics specialists, along with specific content experts, formed working groups to address concerns about the lack of transparency in many published, peer-reviewed articles. There were concerns about the difficulties in knowing exactly how a study or a systematic review/meta-analysis was carried out. Too many specific decisions—made by researchers and reviewers during the execution of the study—were left out of the published articles, and the adequacy of the methodology and overall conclusions were being questioned. Increased transparency of the process was needed. To address these concerns, a number of detailed reporting standards with very useful checklists have been developed, and today many journals require that all submitted manuscripts follow these standards. Table 4.6 provides a brief explanation of a variety of reporting standards, along with an indication of which standards apply to which methodology or design, and whether the standards apply to primary or secondary literature.

Table 4.6. RESEARCH REPORTING STANDARDS AND APPLICABLE DESIGNS

Guidelines or Standards[a]	**Applicable Methodology/Design**
PRIMARY LITERATURE	
CONSORT[b]	*Randomized Controlled Trials (RCTs)*
Standards developed by medical researchers for studies in which participants are randomly assigned to different groups (RCT). A 25-item checklist guides evaluation of methodology and reporting. A flow diagram illustrates details of participants' enrollment, allocation, follow-up, and analysis.	
CONSORT extension[c]	*RCTs of Nonpharmacologic Trials*
Extension and elaboration of CONSORT standards as applied to nonpharmacologic trials. Elaborates on 22-item checklist and modifies flow diagram.	
TREND[d]	*Quasi-experimental Designs*
Developed via CDC initiative to establish standards for quasi-experimental (nonrandomized) designs. A 22-item checklist emphasizes description of theory, intervention, procedures for comparing groups, and methods of adjusting for possible bias due to nonrandomization.	
STROBE[e]	*Observational studies in epidemiology: Cohort, case-control, and cross-sectional*
Initiative to identify accurate and complete reporting in observational studies. A 22-item checklist with 18 items relevant to all observational studies and 4 items related to cohort, case-control, and cross-sectional designs.	
STARD[f]	*Studies of Accuracy of Diagnostic Procedure*
International group of scientists and editors developed reporting standards for studies of diagnostic accuracy (e.g., specificity, sensitivity). A 25-item checklist emphasizes use and reporting of reference standards (i.e., "gold standard").	

(*Continued*)

Table 4.6. Continued

Guidelines or Standards[a]	**Applicable Methodology/Design**
AERA[g]	*Multiple Designs*
Applies to reports of education research grounded in the empirical traditions of the social sciences. Can apply to both quantitative and qualitative research.	
Secondary Literature	
PRISMA[h]	*Systematic Reviews and Meta-Analyses*
International group of review authors and methodologists updated previous standards (QUORUM). A 27-item checklist and a four-phase (identification, screening, eligibility, included) flow diagram	
MOOSE[i]	*Meta-Analyses of Observational Studies*
A CDC-funded project focused on observational studies in epidemiology. A checklist proposes guidelines for background, search strategy, methods, results, discussion, and conclusion.	
Primary and Secondary Literature	
JARS[j]	*Multiple Designs*
Standards that consolidate many of the above for use in American Psychological Association (APA) journals. Three lists of standards: (1) new data collection (regardless of design); (2) experimental manipulation or intervention (with two separate modules for random and nonrandom assignment); and (3) meta-analyses.	

NOTES: See NLM Research and Reporting Guidelines and Initiatives for a more comprehensive list (National Library of Medicine, 2014).

[a]It is important to note that terms such as guidelines, standards, or recommendations are sometimes used interchangeably and sometimes have specific definitions for each context.

[b]Schulz, Altman, and Moher (2010).

[c]Boutron, Moher, Altman, Schulz, and Ravaud (2008).

[d]Des Jarlais, Lyles, and Crepaz (2004).

[e]von Elm et al. (2007).

[f]Bossuyt et al. (2003).

[g]American Educational Research Association (AERA) (2006).

[h](Moher, Liberati, Tetzlaff, and Altman (2009).

[i]Stroup et al. (2000).

[j]American Psychological Association (APA) JARS Working Group (2008).

Along with previously mentioned worksheets and checklists, journal reporting standards provide a helpful roadmap for working through the critical appraisal of the research evidence. Knowledge of the scientific process, close attention to specific reporting standards and the use of a variety of worksheets and checklists are essential to an effective appraisal of accessed best available evidence.

Appraising the Research Evidence: Basic Concepts and Steps

Because a detailed and comprehensive explanation of how to appraise the research evidence is beyond the scope of this book, what follows are definitions of key terms and some psycho-oncology-specific considerations when appraising the evidence.

Key Terms and Basic Concepts

- *Internal validity* is the extent to which the results of a study are true. For example, is it the actual planned treatment intervention that caused the change in behavior, or is the behavior change the result of some other source of error?
- *External validity* is a property of a scientific study that reflects how well the study results can be generalized to other people or situations, such as those in your particular oncology setting.
- *Bias* or *experimental error* is any systematic distortion of the real effects of a study that results from how the study was carried out. Bias can therefore lead to invalid conclusions about the effectiveness of an intervention.
- The *goal of appraising the evidence* is to determine if a study's results are valid and reliable.
- The *goal of well-designed applied research* is to consider internal and external validity so that, as much as possible, they are well balanced and study results/outcomes can be both inferred to be caused by the intervention (rather than from experimental error that biased results) and generalized to other situations/people.
- There are many *sources of potential bias*, but for intervention studies, most bias comes from the study's procedures, such as how the participants were selected (e.g., do all potential participants have an equal chance of being selected?), how participants were assigned to the study's groups (e.g., random or nonrandom), how well and by whom the intervention was provided (e.g., followed a well-written, easy-to-follow manual), how the study outcomes were measured (e.g., by use of standardized, reliable questionnaires), and how the data were analyzed (e.g., appropriate statistics used).

Psycho-Oncology-Specific Considerations When Appraising the Evidence

Given the current psycho-oncology evidence base, the following sources of potential bias are of particular importance to consider.

Recruitment and Selection

- Were all possible consecutively screened patients eligible? If not, how were they chosen (e.g., referred only, convenience sample)?

- Were they selected due to "high" or "low" scores on certain screening measures (e.g., anxiety, fatigue)?

Randomization

- How were patients allocated and randomized to treatment groups?
- Who did the randomization? Were random assignments done by persons not involved in providing the intervention?
- Did the randomization procedure result in groups that were comparable on important variables (e.g., age, gender, stage)?

Demographic and Disease Status

- Who participated in this study (e.g., age, race, ethnicity, disease type)?

Intervention

- Is the intervention described in sufficient detail (i.e., a manual) to know how to implement it?
- Does the description fit other similarly defined and described interventions?
- Was adherence to (i.e., integrity checks) its implementation measured in some way (e.g., use of a treatment manual, close supervision by experts, sessions videotaped and reviewed)?

Lost to Follow-Up and Intent-to-Treat Analysis

- Can you easily track (i.e., is there a CONSORT style flow chart) how many patients were assessed for eligibility, enrolled, randomized, and lost to follow-up and why they were lost?
- How were those lost to follow-up handled in the data analysis (e.g., separate results presented for "completers" and "noncompleters")?

Outcome Measures

- Are they adequately described?
- Are they reliable and valid?
- Have they been used in other studies?
- Were raters used, and if so, were they blind to treatment conditions?

Steps for Appraising the Best Available Research Evidence

With an understanding of key terms and concepts and consideration of these psycho-oncology specifics, the process of appraising the best available research evidence involves a series of steps:

- Determine the type of question(s) being asked and consider whether such a question is adequately addressed by the research design of the accessed study (see Table 4.5).

- Use available worksheets, checklists, and journal reporting standards to evaluate the evidence. Be certain to use the appraisal resource developed for the particular type of evidence (primary or secondary literature) or research design (RCT, quasi-experimental, economic analysis, etc.).
- After using these appraisal resources, consider whether they provide conclusive evidence of valid and reliable results. If so, continue on to consider external validity (i.e., generalization to your particular patient or setting) in the next EBP step—translating the research to a particular patient. In this next step, the focus shifts to the practical questions of how applicable these results are to your particular patient.

Step 4: Translating the Research to a Particular Patient: A Component of Clinical Expertise

Complex questions and gaps in the evidence base (Glasgow, Davidson, Dobkin, Ockene, & Spring, 2006; Jacobsen, 2006) make translating research to the needs of an individual patient challenging. Translation requires balance between an appreciation for the rigors of science and clinical relevance. It is the evidence-based practitioner's responsibility to determine the best fit between the available evidence and the needs of a particular patient. The end result is a treatment plan that is implemented skillfully and flexibly while being evaluated and modified, as needed, as a result of patient feedback as needed. Successful translation of best available evidence requires specific competencies, supported by the use of practice models designed to bridge the science-to-practice gap. Self-reflective practice is an important competency for EBP, and the local clinical scientist is a model of practice that encourages EBP.

Self-Reflective Practice

Reflective practice is "practice conducted with personal and professional self-awareness and reflection" (Fouad et al., 2009), particularly "reflection on action" in which the EBP practitioner is aware of the variety of influences on clinical judgment and has "the ability to reflect on one's own experience, knowledge, hypotheses, inferences, emotional reactions, and behaviors and to use that reflection to modify one's practices accordingly" (American Psychological Association, 2006, p. 277).

The Local Clinical Scientist

The local clinical scientist (LCS) is a model of practice, applicable to psycho-oncology, that integrates science and practice, with hopes of bridging the science-to-practice gap. The LCS model acknowledges the challenges in integrating science and practice (Trierweiler & Stricker, 1998). Science is interested in *knowledge for knowledge sake* and values its academic freedom to investigate and expand an ever-growing base of knowledge. Practice, in contrast, is interested in *knowledge for what it can accomplish* and places public service as its highest value. When viewed as daily *activities*, science and practice seem incompatible. However, when viewed as *attitudes and values*, science and practice can be compatible; they can be well integrated. The fundamental similarity in attitude is the belief and value placed upon the importance of observation, whether that is the objective observation and measurement of empirical science or the subjective self-reflective observation of the practitioner. Science and practice can be integrated when the evidence-based practitioner shares, with the scientist, the value of and belief in skilled observation. Stricker and Trierweiler (1995) note that the LCS is "an approach that recognizes the contributions of science and the scientific attitude as well as the realities of daily clinical practice" (p. 996).

The local clinical scientist needs to understand various meanings of the term "local" (Stricker & Trierweiler, 1995) to best implement EBP. First, *local* can mean the application of a general finding (e.g., cognitive-behavioral therapy for depression) to a particular case (e.g., 34-year-old, single female reporting depressive symptoms soon after being diagnosed with early-stage breast cancer). Here the concept of local focuses on generalization of the universal to the specific. Second, *local* can mean attention to and appreciation of local knowledge—the specifics of a particular ethnic, racial, geographic, or other cultural group. It is particularly relevant to the process of integrating patient characteristics, culture, and preferences. Finally, *local* can mean idiosyncratic and refer to the particulars of the unique history (e.g., delay in seeking care after a self-discovered breast lump), family (e.g., daughter of a mother who died from breast cancer), individual experiences (e.g., recent death of a close coworker), or comorbidities (e.g., other noncancerous diseases or other disabilities) of a specific patient.

Questions of Local Context to Consider When Translating Research to a Particular Patient

When translating best available evidence to the needs of a clinical situation, the following questions arise, as organized by patient derived, cancer derived, and life context.

- *Patient Derived.* How closely does the research match your clinical situation on biological sex, age, ethnicity, minority status, and other demographic variables? If the answer to this question suggests a poor fit, is there reason to believe that the efficacy of the intervention will not be effective with your particular patient?
- *Cancer Derived.* How closely does the research match your clinical situation on disease-related variables, such as cancer type, stage, prognosis, and treatment status? If not, is there reason to believe that the efficacy of the intervention will not be effective with your particular patient?
- *Life Context.* Are there any other important issues of life context such as significantly different health-related beliefs, life span development issues, or other cultural or religious variables that might interfere with the ability to generalize research to your particular patient?

Use of Reporting Standards

When translating best available evidence to a particular patient, the use of checklists from relevant journal reporting standards can be helpful (see Table 4.6). For example, if the research to be translated is an RCT, use of the CONSORT checklist (Schulz, Altman, & Moher, 2010) or the CONSORT extension on non-pharmacological research (Boutron, Moher, Altman, Schulz, & Ravaud, 2008a) can be very helpful. If translating research focused on a diagnostic question, the STARD checklist (Bossuyt et al., 2003a) can be helpful. These checklists provide a framework for investigating the transportability of the evidence to the local clinical situation. When using checklists from reporting standards, it is helpful to imagine how the needs of your patient compare to the details of a particular study. The checklist items from the Methods and Results sections are most helpful.

Relevant questions include the following:

- *Participants.* What are the eligibility or inclusion and exclusion criteria for participants in the study, and how do these compare with your patients?
- *Intervention.* What is the intervention provided? Are its specific components adequately explained, with sufficient detail, to be implemented? If not, can you get access to a manual or another more detailed description? Are you competent to provide the intervention? Do you need to modify the intervention for the particular needs of your patient? If so, how?
- *Outcome.* Are the study outcomes, as measured, the same or similar to the agreed-upon (in collaboration with your patient) goals and outcomes for your particular patient? Do you have access to the instruments (e.g. self-report questionnaires) to measure the outcome?

Step 5: Integration—Pulling It All Together

The next step in the EBP process is integrating the accessed and appraised (1) research evidence with (2) clinical expertise and (3) patient characteristics, culture, and preferences. This process of integration is the least researched and developed of the core *AAA TIE* competencies, and it has been suggested that the clinical questions asked in mental health practice are more varied and complex (Norcross et al., 2008) than in the EBP of medicine. Therefore, the specific competencies that make up an evidence-based practitioner's clinical expertise needs to be considered.

Clinical Expertise and Its Competencies

The professional practice of mental health services involves the use of specific competencies. Clinical expertise can be viewed as the sum total of specific competencies in combination with clinical experience. Experience alone does not equal expertise (Collins, Leffingwell, & Belar, 2007) nor does simple knowledge of specific competencies. It is the combination of experience in using specific competencies that results in clinical expertise.

In the professional practice of psychology, competency domains have been organized into two broad categories: foundational and functional (Rodolfa et al., 2005).

Foundational competencies include attitudinal, intellectual, and interpersonal skills, along with scientific knowledge, an appreciation of issues of diversity, and awareness of ethical and legal standards. An attitude of intellectual curiosity, appreciation for science, knowledge of the limitations and potential errors in clinical judgment, and a commitment to continued education and training are all important foundational competencies. As previously mentioned, self-reflective practice and the role it plays in clinical decision making is another important component of clinical expertise. These foundational competencies lay the groundwork for effective use of functional competencies. The *functional competencies* most relevant to psycho-oncology include skills such as assessment, treatment planning, case formulation, interpersonal expertise, and clinical decision making, all resulting in a cogent rationale for clinical strategies. Clinical expertise in psycho-oncology involves the combination of both foundational and functional competencies. Table 4.7 provides a list of specific components of clinical expertise (American Psychological Association, 2006) as identified in the evidence-based practice of psychology and directly relevant to the practice of psycho-oncology. Many of them converge in the central integrating process of clinical decision making.

Clinical Decision Making

Clinical decision making is central to the integration process and occurs at the intersection of the three major components of EBP (see Fig. 4.1). *Clinical decision making* is both a process and an outcome. As a process, clinical decision making is an iterative, recurrent process that involves attention to patient feedback, practitioner self-reflection, flexibility, and skill in adapting and modifying an initial treatment plan to the unique and changing needs of a patient. As an outcome, it is the conclusion of a process that involves research knowledge, theoretical conceptualization, expertise in assessment and diagnostic judgment, the development of a systematic case formulation, and a resulting treatment plan. Throughout this process, clinical decisions are guided by cogent rationales for specific intervention techniques and strategies (American Psychological Association, 2006).

Cognitive Errors and Heuristic Bias

Clinical decision making is complex and prone to cognitive errors and bias. It is an impossible task to consistently and accurately process all of the relevant verbal and nonverbal stimuli that a clinical encounter elicits. Consequently, human beings use strategies or shortcuts to organize this vast amount of information in hopes of reducing the complexity of decision making. These cognitive shortcuts or *heuristics*, although sometimes accurate and helpful in making sense of a complex world, can also be problematic. Because they are often used without

Table 4.7. Key Components of Clinical Expertise and Patient Characteristics in Evidence-Based Practice of Psycho-Oncology

Clinical Expertise	**Patient Characteristics**
Assessment, diagnostic judgment, systematic case formulation, and treatment planning	Variations in presenting problems or disorders, etiology, concurrent symptoms, or syndromes and behavior
Clinical decision making, treatment implementation, and monitoring of patient progress	Chronological age, developmental status, history, and life stage
Interpersonal expertise	Sociocultural and familial factors (e.g., gender, gender identity, race, ethnicity, social class, religion, disability status, family structure, sexual orientation)
Continual self-reflection and acquisition of skills	
Evaluation and use of research evidence	
Understanding the influence of individual, cultural, and contextual differences on treatment	Current environmental context, stressors (e.g., unemployment, recent life events) and social factors (e.g., institutional racism, health care disparities)
Seeking available resources as needed (e.g., consultation, adjunctive or alternative services)	Personal preferences, values, and preferences related to treatment (e.g., goals, beliefs, worldviews, treatment expectations)
A cogent rationale for clinical strategies	

awareness, they become a problem when they interfere with an otherwise more accurate clinical judgment by "short-circuiting" the process and causing practitioners to conclude and make judgments too quickly, with unwarranted certainty. They interfere with the self-correcting process of the self-reflective practitioner.

Theory and research in clinical judgment (e.g., Spengler, Strohmer, Dixon, & Shivy, 1995) has identified a number of common errors that can occur when heuristic biases are unknowingly used and strategies to correct them are not. Box 4.1 provides a list and brief definition of some common heuristic biases (Norcross et al., 2008) and related debiasing strategies. To avoid errors in clinical judgment, it is important to use debiasing strategies.

Box 4.1

Common Heuristic Biases and Debiasing Strategies

Common Heuristic Biases

Availability

Making judgments based upon the ease with which information comes to mind; to assume that a salient or easily remembered example is an accurate representation of a larger population. *Concluding that the prostate patient you are interviewing is significantly worried and in distress about erectile dysfunction after recently attending a continuing education workshop on this topic.*

Anchoring

Focusing on and giving greater importance to information obtained first or earliest in a clinical encounter or failure to adjust initial judgments based upon additional information, obtained later. *Concluding that a patient with Stage IV cancer will have weeks to months to live before learning about what type of cancer.*

Representativeness

Forming probability estimates based upon one's perception that events co-occur, whether they actually do or do not. Sometimes also referred to as illusory correlation; ignores base rates. *A diagnosis of cancer results in depression.*

Confirmatory Bias

The tendency to pay closer attention to information that "fits" already existing hypotheses, while ignoring or deemphasizing information that does not. Holding to the hypothesis that *women who undergo surgery for breast cancer will suffer from body image problems*, despite research to the contrary.

Fundamental Attribution Error

An error in concluding the cause of an event by attributing causes of events occurring to others as due to internal factors (personality, disposition), while attributing causes of events occurring to self as external (situation, environment). *This patient is experiencing significant anxiety not due to her recent diagnosis of cancer (situation), but because she has always been very anxious (disposition).*

Diagnostic Overshadowing

The tendency to underestimate the importance of, or ignore, an issue (patient characteristic, problem, diagnosis, symptom, event) due to attention being diverted to a perceived more important or more salient issue. *A hostile and combative lung cancer patient, recently informed of new metastatic disease (bad news), is angry at his doctor because of the bad news, not because his doctor informed him casually (told him while on the elevator) and without any empathy (quickly turned away and moved on).*

Debiasing Strategies

Consider Alternative Outcomes

Get in the habit of questioning initial conclusions or hypotheses and actively seek out and search information for alternative explanations to events. Decide not to be particularly enamored by your first impressions, nor to be overly confident of conclusions.

Increase Attention to Usually Ignored Data

The core of EBP is to attend closely to research findings—all relevant findings. Pay close attention to those findings that might contradict or be in opposition to your favored theory, hypothesis, or treatment techniques.

Minimize the Role of Memory

Memory is fallible and prone to errors. Note how some heuristics emphasize salient or recently obtained information over a more considered and thorough recall of a wide variety of information. Use technology to help store and retrieve information.

Use a Disconfirmation Strategy

Throughout the clinical decision-making process, remember to look for information contrary to your hypotheses—seek out disconfirmatory evidence. This needs to be an active and intentional process to be effective.

Rely on Actuarial Judgment When Available

Ever since Meehl's book on clinical versus statistical prediction (Meehl, 1954), it has been known that despite clinicians' beliefs to the contrary, they are not particular good at predicting patient outcomes. Thus, whenever feasible, rely on judgments that come from data over clinical impression.

NOTE: See Norcross, Hogan, and Koocher (2008) for additional examples as they relate to evidence-based practice.

Use of these and related debiasing strategies is a critical component of self-reflective practitioners who continuously question their own clinical decision-making process. Making good clinical decisions also involves collaboration with patients.

Patient–Provider Collaboration: Psychosocial Health Services Compared to Biomedical Health Services

In psychosocial interventions, certain assumptions, roles, and relationships are different than in traditional biomedicine. The traditional biomedical model assumes the curative factors to be the *specific ingredients* of a particular biomedical treatment (e.g., chemotherapy drug, surgical removal of diseased tissue, radiation to malignant cells), and this assumption dictates certain defined patient–provider roles. Successful outcome results from expert understanding of treatment options, selection of the most effective treatment and the provision of best available evidence by the provider, and compliance with the treatment by the patient. For the effective ingredient to result in the desired outcome, the provider's role is to be the expert in selecting and administering the treatment, and the patient's role is to be educated and informed, *but mostly compliant.*

In psychosocial interventions, these roles are different and collaboration between patient and provider is crucial to successful outcome. The assumption that the curative factors come exclusively from specific ingredients of treatment techniques is not warranted. In fact, as previously discussed in the review of psychotherapy research in Chapter 3, there is controversy about which ingredients (e.g., techniques, common factors, the therapeutic relationship, patient characteristics, or provider characteristics) contribute the most to positive outcomes. Thus, psychosocial interventions rely on patient–provider collaboration. A unique patient, presenting with specific problems, concerns, and symptoms, collaborates with an expert provider capable of using a range of competencies to affect a positive outcome. This enlarges the decision-making process and makes it essential to consider patient characteristics, culture, and preferences.

Integrating Patient Characteristics, Culture, and Preference

The importance of integration of patient characteristics, culture, and preferences comes from the underlying question of how well does the available research evidence generalize to patients whose characteristics (age, gender, cancer type and stage), culture, and preferences may differ from those of the persons who make up the samples researched. First, what are some of the relevant patient characteristics to consider? Table 4.7 provides a broad list that suggests a number of important clinical questions to consider in the clinical decision-making process:

- Are there certain patient characteristics that might alter how a particular treatment is provided?
- Are there cultural and social characteristics that necessitate adapting or modifying a particular intervention?
- Does the provision of an intervention to a 35- or 40-year-old patient require modification from that provided to a 70- or 75-year-old patient?
- Are there certain variables to always consider, regardless of type or severity of presenting problem, such as readiness to change, level of resistance, or perceived social support, that may impact treatment?
- How important are client expectations to treatment outcome?
- How does one consider these characteristics?
- Is there a systematic way to do the integration?

A growing literature on shared decision making (Adams & Drake, 2006; Barratt, 2008; Charles, Gafni, & Whelan, 1997, 1999) is beginning to address these questions.

Shared Decision Making

In the process of integrating research evidence and clinical expertise with patient characteristics, culture, and preferences, models of shared decision making (SDM) highlight the specific process of indicating, negotiating, and eventually choosing one's treatment preferences—one component of patient–provider collaboration and a critical step in the EBP process of integration. "In shared decision-making, the practitioner becomes a consultant to the client, helping to provide information, to discuss options, to clarify values and preferences, and to support the client's autonomy" (Adams & Drake, 2006, p. 90).

The process of SDM has been given little attention in psycho-oncology. In the biomedical literature, a few conclusions can be drawn. Most patients say that they want health and medical information. Most patients want to select their health care provider and want a close relationship with him or her. Lastly, patients vary considerably regarding how much they want to participate in treatment decisions (Adams & Drake, 2006). Some patients prefer to make the choice to delegate to their physician (the role of decision maker), whereas others want to be directly involved in weighing the risks and benefits of treatment options and communicating their personal values to their practitioner(s). Efforts to improve the SDM process have focused on enhancing patient–practitioner communication skills and the development of decision aids. Enhancing communication skills is a strategy designed to improve the patient–provider relationship and thus has been compared to a similar construct in psychotherapy research: the working alliance, particularly the component of "mutuality"—the notion of patient–provider agreement on goals and tasks, all within the context of a close emotional bond (Fischer, 2006). Thus, as SDM continues to focus on enhancing communication within the context of the patient–practitioner relationship, attending to research on working alliance is important.

Decision aids are tools that provide information about treatment options to patients to help them actively participate in decision making. Decision aids are not designed to advise one option over the other, but rather to provide information about treatment options that will help patients clarify their own values and to communicate to their practitioner those characteristics of the options of most importance to them. Few, if any, decision aids have been developed in psycho-oncology.

Adopt, Adapt, or Abandon

Ultimately, the clinical decision-making process in step 5 (Integration) leads to one of three options: adopt, adapt, or abandon (Norcross et al., 2008). (1) If the available research evidence suggests that a particular treatment is a good fit for specific patient characteristics, (2) if the provider has the necessary clinical expertise, and (3) if it is the patient's preference to accept the available treatment, then (4) the decision to adopt the intervention is warranted. Here, the EBP process of integration results in a clinical decision to provide the treatment with the best available evidence. However, if the best available evidence, in combination with clinical expertise and patient characteristics and/or preferences, determines that the treatment is not a good fit, the clinical decision may be to adapt or modify the intervention. The clinical expertise of the practitioner will be needed to balance issues of treatment fidelity and fit. *Fidelity* is concerned with the degree to which a treatment is provided in a manner consistent with how it was provided in the studies from which research evidence comes. *Fit* is concerned with patient characteristics, culture, and preferences. As Norcross and colleagues (2008) explain,

> Dynamic tension occurs in resolving the conflict between fidelity and fit, both essential elements of EBP. We seek fidelity of implementation in the delivery of the manualized intervention as found effective in controlled research. At the same time, we seek fit in adapting the service to accommodate the needs of the specific patient. (p. 234)

Finally, if it is determined that (1) the best available evidence is a poor fit, or (2) if there is no relevant evidence, or (3) if a patient declines/refuses the recommended treatment, or (4) if the practitioner is not competent to provide the intervention, then (5) a decision to abandon the research evidence is warranted.

Decisions about two of these options—when to *adopt* or *abandon*—are comparatively straightforward once the literature is identified, accessed, and appraised. In contrast, the process of *adapting* best available evidence is much more complicated and, in different contexts, has been called *treatment selection, prescriptive matching,* and *evidence-based responsiveness* or *adaptation* (Norcross & Lambert, 2011). Much less has been written about the processes involved in adapting best available evidence to fit patient characteristics, given practitioner expertise. Such literature will become a crucial next step in the evolution of EBP.

Adaptation of Best Available Research Evidence

The idea that the options of adopting, adapting, or abandoning the evidence are three separate categories is mistaken and oversimplifies the decision-making process. Rather than discrete categories, they are better conceptualized as existing along a continuum, where one end represents the decision to adopt the evidence and the other end to abandon it. The middle of the continuum then comes to represent varying degrees of adaptation of the evidence.

Shifting the notion of a decision-making process from categorical to continuous expands the options on how to most effectively use the best available research.

This middle of the continuum represents the broad and varied forms of adaptation, modification, and integration of the evidence, as influenced by the previously described tension between fit and fidelity. EBP calls for clinicians to strive for fidelity (i.e., close adherence to treatment procedures), while attending closely to fit with the ultimate goal to "make it work." Figure 4.4 presents fit and fidelity as continuous variables along a continuum from low to high. Fit and fidelity vary together. As fit declines from high to low, so too does the concern for fidelity. Where both fit and fidelity are high, the best decision is to adopt; when both are low, the decision is to abandon. However, when either or both are intermediate,

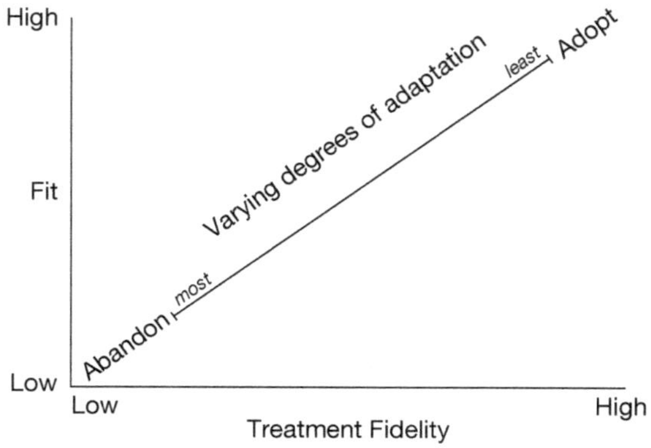

Figure 4.4 Evidence-based adaptation.
Fit is the degree to which patient characteristics and clinical expertise (i.e., provider competence) are comparable to the patient characteristics and the clinical expertise in the best available evidence. Treatment fidelity is the degree to which the treatment provided is like that in the best available research—typically by use of a treatment manual.

the decision-making process becomes more complex and questions of when, how, and how much to adapt become paramount.

Step 1: Decide When to Adapt.

Determining when it is time to adapt the best available evidence is not easy. The first occasion for considering adaptation is during the *development of an initial treatment plan.* Adaptation is considered when there is evidence that a particular intervention might be beneficial, but there is poor fit. Poor fit can exist between the studied sample (nomothetic data) and the individual patient characteristics, preferences, and/or culture (the idiographic). Poor fit can be seen in many forms, but some include significant differences in demographics or presenting problems. A second occasion for considering when to adapt is anytime *during ongoing treatment*, when there is evidence of poor progress or treatment failure. In such situations, adaptation needs to be considered (Lambert, 2010), such as any increase in symptoms suggestive of deterioration/decline, or any possibility of dropping out and/or any evidence of harm. The regular and routine collection of outcome data to measure, monitor, and manage patient progress—patient-focused research—in the general psychotherapy literature (Harmon et al., 2007; Howard et al., 1996) can facilitate decision making about when to adapt an ongoing treatment.

Step 2: Decide How and How Much to Adapt.

There is no single method for how best to adapt available research evidence. Rather, a few authors have described methods of adaptation that vary in terms of the degree of difference from the original evidence-based treatment. A variety of suggested forms of adaptation have been proposed that include varying methods of modification, such as supplementation, augmentation, and sequential presentation of treatment components. Three authors offer methods of adaptation that vary in degree from the primary evidence-based intervention.

First, Persons (2005) describes a mix-and-match method based upon the development of a case formulation, ongoing hypothesis testing, and frequent monitoring of patient progress. She describes how it can be used when various barriers to the direct application of complete treatment protocols do not allow for sufficient flexibility to meet patient needs. She emphasizes the importance of understanding theorized mechanisms of pathology and change, noting how clinical expertise includes knowledge of such mechanisms to guide the development of working hypotheses, organized within a case formulation that incorporates these mechanisms of both etiology and change. For example, Persons presents an idiographic case formulation developed for a patient experiencing anxiety, depression, problems at work, and alcohol abuse, triggered by negative events of a new job and move to a new city. Using theorized mechanisms of pathology and change from both Beck's cognitive theory of depression (i.e., role of schema reactive to negative life events) and principles of behavioral activation (i.e., withdrawal/isolation results in low levels of positive reinforcement), the skilled therapist can *mix and match* which interventions best fit the hypothesized causes of distress. This allows for adaptation and more flexibility than in the original treatment protocol. This approach to adaptation is relatively minimal in the *how much* adaptation, as it remains pretty close to adopting the original protocol and is at the high end of fit and fidelity on Figure 4.4.

Second, Ruscio and Hollohan (2006) suggest a variety of ways to adapt evidence-based interventions with complex cases. They begin by providing a list of characteristics of complex cases and then offer ways to adapt interventions. On the least end of the adaptation continuum, they suggest combinations of interventions in which the primary intervention is *augmented* by providing supplementary additional interventions to address patient complexity, a type of "adjuvant" therapy. A primary intervention could be augmented by either a *sequential* administration of multiple evidence-based interventions in a sort of *back-to-back* format, or *offered concurrently* in which multiple interventions are offered in alternating sessions or even within portions of individual sessions. For example, the cancer patient with a past history of obsessive-compulsive disorder, for whom symptoms of obsessions and compulsions intensify during a course of chemotherapy, may respond best to a concurrent offerings of both exposure and response prevention (Steketee, 1996) to some increased obsessions and compulsive rituals of fears of germs/contamination, while also being provided an evidence-based, stress management intervention for coping with chemotherapy (Jacobsen et al., 2002) that includes a realistic understanding of increased risk for infection. In the moderate range of the adaptation continuum (see Fig. 4.4), Ruscio and colleagues suggest a *tiered approach* in which a clinician may decide that the preferred or *first-line* treatment is not an option because it may not be acceptable or appropriate for a particular patient. If faced with this tiered approach, the clinician would then use a *second-line* intervention that may have less empirical support but be more acceptable to the patient. For example, for a cancer patient experiencing generalized anxiety disorder, but for whom cognitive restructuring is very difficult due to some chemotherapy-related neurocognitive deficits, the second-line intervention of applied relaxation (Ost, 1987) may be more effective. Lastly, Ruscio and Hollohan (2006) describe *accommodation* of the evidence-based intervention in which the intervention is modified to fit patient characteristics, such as a limitation (e.g., highly concrete thinking style) or conversely a strength (e.g., familiarity with and daily practice of meditation). The research on empirically supported psychotherapy relationships (see Chapter 3) is a similar form of adaptation. This research supports the adaptation of the general elements of an effective therapy relationship, to respond to the particular needs of an individual patient. A number of particular elements of effective psychotherapy relationships that have an empirical evidence include culture, individual preferences, and stage of change.

A third way to adapt (Shapiro, 2009) involves a synthesis of clinical judgment with evidence-based interventions, relying on an understanding of theories of psychotherapy and their connections between etiology and intervention techniques. This method of adaptation falls closest to the low end of the fit and fidelity continuum on Figure 4.4. Shapiro's (2009) is an eclectic approach, using major theories of psychotherapy and, like Persons, it focuses on the connections between theorized causal factors and specified intervention techniques. "The major theories of psychotherapy—behavioral, cognitive, psychodynamic, and family systems—posit connections between etiologic factors that cause and/or maintain disturbances and therapeutic strategies that address these factors" (Shapiro, 2009, p. 50). Shapiro (2009) considers the connection between a theory's stated etiology and how that translates to empirically supported intervention techniques. Shapiro suggests adaptation of the evidence base can occur throughout an intervention, when a skilled therapist listening closely to his or her patient hears information that connects theorized etiology with intervention techniques, suggesting a matching of etiology and intervention, as guided by theoretical principles. Such a method of adaptation relies more heavily on components of clinical expertise such as case formulation, clinical decision making, and skill in implementing specific intervention techniques, along with a familiarity of multiple theories of psychotherapy.

Integration of the Three Evidence-Based Practice Components: Relative Weights Will Vary by Case

The process of EBP, with its integration of (a) best available research evidence; (b) clinical expertise; and (c) patient characteristics, culture, and preferences implies an equal weighting of all three components. In the provision of psychosocial health services in psycho-oncology, however, an equal weighting of all three components is rarely the case. In some cases, where the evidence base is strong, research will be dominant and clinical expertise and patient characteristics may be much less important. In other cases, the converse may be true; particularly in situations where there is very little evidence base, clinical expertise will become important and more heavily weighted. There will also be clinical situations in which the evidence base is strong and clinical expertise is important, but given issues of patient characteristics (e.g., cultural diversity or terminal illness, or religious preferences) and preferences, this third component will be most heavily weighted (Norcross et al., 2008).

Step 6: Evaluation of Evidence-Based Practice

In the final step, the evidence-based practitioner evaluates the effectiveness of the entire EBP process. Although evaluation can occur at various levels (institution, profession, etc.), the emphasis here is on the individual practitioner. Evaluation of the individual evidence-based practitioner is focused mostly on evaluating patient outcomes but also on adherence and quality of all of the EBP steps (Straus et al., 2005). In addition, of course, psycho-oncology practitioners are guided by discipline-specific ethical standards (e.g., American Psychological Association, 2002), available clinical guidelines, and the variety of previously reviewed calls to action to bring high-quality psychosocial interventions to cancer patients.

Effectiveness of Service Provision: Tracking Patient Outcomes

Evaluation of individual evidence-based practitioners involves a process of evaluating the effectiveness of service provision. Because most services are offered to individual patients in individual, small group, family, or couples formats, the evaluation of the individual evidence-based practitioner is a process of "tracking patient outcomes" (Norcross et al., 2008, p. 247). The provision of services by an individual practitioner should thus include measures of treatment outcome. Much can be learned by modeling this evaluation on the principles of outcome assessment in psychotherapy (Ogles, Lambert, & Fields, 2002).

Measuring Outcome

The process of measuring outcome—a component of patient-focused research—involves the selection of valid and reliable outcome measures, setting up the data collection procedures, and scoring results. Selecting outcomes begins by considering what types of information are most important to collect. Some conceptual organizing schemes exist (Ogles et al., 2002) that can be helpful in considering the range of information possible, and it is important to consider from whom the information is collected (i.e., patient self-report, therapist rating, others' observation, physiological data). Some standards have been recommended that include patient symptoms, interpersonal relationships, and overall functioning, as measured by multiple sources. In psycho-oncology it is also essential to measure self-reported quality of life (e.g., Cella et al., 1993).

Setting up the data collection procedures and scoring results comes next. This involves decisions about the frequency and the process. How frequent to collect data is influenced by resources, staff availability, patient cooperation, and overall how time consuming or cumbersome the collection process can be. The question, at what intervals to measure, can range from every session to pre-post a course of treatment. Although some recommend every session (Lambert et al., 2010; Miler & Duncan, 2004), the feasibility of doing so is influenced by the availability of technology to help with the process. In psycho-oncology, even if outcome is measured at every session, it is also important to be certain to measure outcome at critical transition points, such as the start and end of a course of chemotherapy or radiation therapy, at times of transition between treatments, periodically during ongoing survivorship, and at times of recurrence. Systems currently exist that make the administration, scoring, and utilization of data much more feasible in the context of a busy practice (Miller & Duncan, 2004; OQ Measures, 2004), although adaptation or modification of these systems to use in an oncology setting has not occurred and thus requires consideration of how best to use and modify.

Monitoring Outcome

Monitoring outcome involves using the data collected to track patient progress during the treatment process with the intent of informing the practitioner. During the late 1990s and 2000s, patient-focused research addressed the question, Is treatment working for this particular patient? (Howard et al., 1996). With the advent of new, more sophisticated statistical procedures that allowed for the measurement of individual patient change over time, it became feasible to chart the course of change and develop expected treatment response curves. Individual patient responses were then compared to the expected response curve most appropriate to that particular patient (Lambert et al., 2010). This comparative response information is then used to manage outcome.

Managing Outcome

Managing outcome involves using the data collected to alter and modify treatment as needed (Ogles et al., 2002). This involves the use of outcome data to trigger various types of comparative feedback that informs the practitioner how the patient is doing. The system quickly and effectively alerts whether the patient's rate of change is as expected and treatment is progressing well (green signal as a dot on patient chart), whether change is less than adequate and the practitioner should consider altering the intervention (yellow signal), or whether the patient's rate of change is such that he or she is not making adequate change (red signal) and a significant alteration is needed (e.g. referral, completely new treatment plan). These latter signal alarm cases have been the focus of a number of RCTs, in which various types of feedback have been provided, with the goal of altering treatment for patients not making change as expected (Lambert et al., 2010). Types of feedback have included the rate of change, patient perception of the therapeutic relationship, degree of social support or motivation, and clinical support tools to help therapists decide how to alter their treatment intervention. These RCTs have shown that providing practitioners with feedback about patient change improves outcomes; particularly of red-signal alarm cases (Lambert et al., 2010). These studies have not included patients diagnosed with cancer, and thus it is not clear how, or if, this system would work in psycho-oncology, but it provides an excellent model from which to guide future psycho-oncology research.

Adherence to Evidenced-Based Practice Steps and Quality of Critically Appraised Topics

Individual practitioner evaluation can also include informal self-reflection on adherence and quality of one's EBP. Self-reflection on each of the EBP basic competencies results in a series of questions a practitioner can use to evaluate her or his practice. Straus and colleagues (Straus et al., 2005) have suggested a number of questions for each of the five core competencies. Box 4.2 summarizes these and related questions as they relate to the EBP steps.

One particularly important question from Box 4.2 asks, *Do I have a method for saving my questions for similar circumstances?* This is the question about archiving well-conducted evidence searches and appraisals. Although there is no single way to do so, keeping brief summaries of previously completed question

---

Box 4.2

Evaluation—Questions for the *AAA TIE* Evidence-Based Practice Steps

Asking Questions

- *How frequently am I asking clinical questions?*
- *Have they been answerable and well formulated?*
- *What types of questions (intervention, screening/assessment/diagnosis, etiology, comorbidity, purpose/meaning, quality of life, cost, qualitative/descriptive, harm) have I been asking?*
- *Have they been both foreground and background questions?*
- *If related to treatment interventions, have I used the PICO format?*
- *Do I have a method for saving my questions for future, in similar circumstances?*

Accessing Best Available Evidence

- *How frequently am I searching?*
- *Do I have knowledge of the best sources for my discipline?*
- *Which sources (secondary/filtered, primary/unfiltered) am I using the most?*
- *Am I searching all relevant databases (PsycLit, CINAHL, Medline)?*
- *Have metasearch engines (TRIP, SUMsearch) proved helpful?*
- *Am I finding relevant information for both background and foreground questions?*
- *Am I becoming more efficient in the process of finding evidence?*

- *Do I know how, and am I regularly using truncations, Boolean operators, MeSH headings, and other controlled language aids?*
- *How well do my searches compare to those of the experts like medical librarians?*

Appraising the Evidence

- *Am I actually critically appraising the evidence myself, or am I just accepting the conclusions of the synthesized evidence?*
- *Am I using specific worksheets, checklists, and journal reporting guides?*
- *Am I noticing that the types of questions asked are often addressed in specific types of research designs?*
- *Is it becoming easier to appraise the evidence?*
- *Am I becoming more efficient and accurate in using some of the appraisal measures such as effect sizes, confidence intervals, and odds ratios?*
- *Do I consider the current state of research (design types, methodological limitations in prior studies) in psycho-oncology when appraising new evidence?*

Translating the Evidence

- *How honestly and genuinely do I reflect on my own practice?*
- *Do self-reflections and self-awareness result in changes in clinical decisions?*
- *Do I have an approach (e.g., local clinical scientist) to the science-to-practice gap?*
- *As a local clinical scientist, do I understand the various meanings of the term "local" and can I translate the evidence in light of the specific "local" clinical situation?*
- *Do I closely consider questions of local context when translating the evidence?*
- *Can I review the appraised evidence and determine its relevance to my particular clinical situation?*

Integrating Research Evidence, Clinical Expertise, and Patient Characteristics

- *How well am I pulling it all together?*
- *Do I possess the requisite clinical assessment and intervention skills?*
- *Am I aware of potential biases and flaws in clinical decision making?*
- *Am I knowledgeable about my patients' particular unique characteristics, culture, and preferences?*
- *How well do I collaborate with my patients?*
- *Can I explain treatment options to my patients?*
- *Do I regularly present a potential treatment plan and its options to my patients to get their preferences?*
- *Do I know what to do if my patient does not prefer my preferred and recommended treatment?*
- *Am I prepared to acknowledge that for many clinical decisions, evidence may not exist, and I will need to rely on clinical decision making and expertise?*

SOURCE: Sackett, D. L., Straus, S. E., Richardson, W. S., Rosenberg, W. M., & Haynes, R. B. (2000). *Evidence based medicine: How to practice and teach EBM.* London: Elsevier Churchill Livingstone. Adapted with permission from Elsevier.

searches and appraisals that have resulted in useful "bottom-line" conclusions would save time when similar clinical questions arise in the future. Over time, the evidence-based practitioner can contribute to a growing list of critically appraised topics (CATs). For personal use, a psycho-oncologist might simply store his or her CATs in a Dropbox file or in some other accessible online format in order to easily share with others. However, a good example of this archiving procedure can be found at the Centre for Evidence Based Medicine (CEBM) Web site and their software tool CATmaker (http://.cebm.net/index.aspx?o=1216). This downloadable software tool is designed to help the archiving process be done more efficiently and routinely. A completed CAT includes a well-organized summary of the entire EBP process, including the clinical bottom-line results, the citation, clinical question, search terms, study description, evidence summary as appraised, and a prompt for when a future updated search and appraisal may be needed to keep the CAT up to date. Thus, a final step in evaluating the individual practitioner within Step 6 is to complete and archive the current critically appraised topic.

CHAPTER SUMMARY

This chapter provided an introduction to the relatively short history of EBP in medicine, oncology, psychology, and other related disciplines. Most of this chapter was devoted to the detailed elaboration and explanation of the six core competencies of EBP, summarized by the acronym AAA TIE (asking, accessing, appraising, translating, integrating, and evaluating). This series of iterative steps guides the evidence-based practitioner in the challenging process of integrating evidence, patient characteristics, and clinical expertise toward the aspirational goal of improved patient outcomes. Chapter 5 begins Part II of the book where more specific and detailed descriptions of particular psychosocial health services are described. In Chapter 5, *screening* and *assessment* of the cancer patient/family, as the initial step in identifying those in need of services, is described.

PART II

Psychosocial Health Services in Psycho-Oncology

5

Screening and Assessment

This chapter is organized into two sections: screening for psychosocial distress and the assessment of psychosocial adaptation. Identifying the psychosocial distress of the adult cancer patient involves these two separate, yet related processes:

- *Screening* is defined as a rapid process of determining who needs referral for more extensive assessment by the use of brief self-report questionnaires administered by office staff, the core oncology team, and/or available technology.
- *Assessment* is the in-depth clinical interview focused on factors relevant to coping and adaptation, done by a qualified health care professional, using a semistructured interview.

This chapter is about both screening and assessment and provides an exemplar for how to screen for distress and how to assess for psychosocial adaptation. It also provides background knowledge for the evidence-based practitioner looking for answers to some of the following background questions:

- Screening—*How many patients need psychosocial care?*
- Screening—*Do patients who indicate high levels of distress seek psychosocial care? Do those patients who indicate distress desire psychosocial care?*
- Screening—*How is distress defined, and is it the same thing as anxiety and depression?*
- Screening—*Are there valid and reliable screening instruments?*
- Screening—*Is there a best way to do screening for psychosocial distress?*
- Screening—*When should patients be screened?*
- Assessment—*What is the best way to do an assessment of psychosocial adaptation?*
- Diagnosis—*What are the typical rates of distress, anxiety, and depression in cancer patients?*
- Diagnosis—*Does the type or stage of cancer influence how many patients experience distress?*
- Diagnosis—*Which screening method is the best for my local situation? How should screening be done in my setting?*

- Progress monitoring—*Does screening result in decreased anxiety or depression?*

BACKGROUND KNOWLEDGE IN SCREENING FOR PSYCHOSOCIAL DISTRESS

As is well documented in the Institute of Medicine's 2008 report, cancer patients experience an increased prevalence of a variety of psychosocial problems that often go unrecognized by health care providers, and they are associated with a number of adverse health effects. Consequently, guidelines have been developed for the routine screening for psychosocial distress, and these guidelines are soon to be required for all accredited cancer care programs in the United States. In this context, distress is viewed as existing along a continuum ranging from

a. normal emotional reactions,
b. to problematic symptoms that are below the threshold of an official mental disorder,
c. to diagnosable mental disorders, such as the adjustment disorders, major depressive disorder, generalized anxiety disorder, and posttraumatic stress disorder.

Prevalence of Distress

The prevalence of psychosocial distress has been investigated in various ways. The earliest attempts were focused on diagnosable mental disorders (e.g., Derogatis et al., 1983) and used structured clinical interviews, following specific *DSM* criteria, and found prevalence rates for specific *DSM* mental disorders ranging from 20% to 40% of newly diagnosed patients, with adjustment disorders being the most prevalent. This was beneficial to note both (a) higher prevalence rates of mental disorders in cancer patients than in the general population, and (b) that the majority of cancer patients *do not* experience a mental disorder. Most patients cope well. These earliest studies also noted that many patients report significant distress that does not rise to the level of severity of a fully diagnosable mental disorder. These problematic levels of distress were important to identify, refer, and treat. Thus, more recent investigations have used brief, standardized, self-report questionnaires such as the Brief Symptom Inventory (BSI) or the Hospital Anxiety and Depression Scale (HADS). For example, results from a large sample (N = 4,496) of patients completing the BSI showed overall prevalence of *distress* of 35.1% with 24% for *anxiety* and 19% for *depression* (Zabora, BrintzenhofeSzoc, Curbow, Hooker, & Piantadosi, 2001). The HADS is one of the most frequently studied self-report questionnaires (Mitchell, 2010a). For example, a study in England using the HADS found 22% reported distress, 23% anxiety, and 16% depression (Strong et al., 2007).

Correlates of distress, such as cancer type or stage, have also been investigated and found to vary somewhat, but not dramatically. Two studies (Carlson et al., 2004; Zabora et al., 2001) using the BSI found patients with lung, brain, and pancreatic cancers to experience the most distress, yet others have concluded that one's age (<65 years), being female, and having active disease may be better predictors of distress than cancer type (Strong et al., 2007). A helpful overview of prevalence of various forms of distress (Mitchell, 2010b) is illustrated in Figure 5.1, which summarizes the prevalence rates for distress, anxiety, and depression as determined by either self-report or clinical interview.

As summarized by Mitchell (2010b), whether the identification process is by a more formal clinical interview or by a briefer screening method that uses a self-report questionnaire, *distress/adjustment disorders* are most prevalent at 48% via a clinical interview or 57% via self-report screening. *Anxiety* is next highest at 18% (clinical interview) and 38% (self-report screening), and *depression* shows the least prevalence at 13% (clinical interview) or 20% (self-report screening) (Mitchell, 2010a). These data come from studies representative of a variety of cancer patients, diagnosed with varying types and stages of disease, collected from a variety of cancer care settings, in patients currently receiving or having recently received some form of active cancer treatment. In addition, data on distress in longer term cancer survivors are also available.

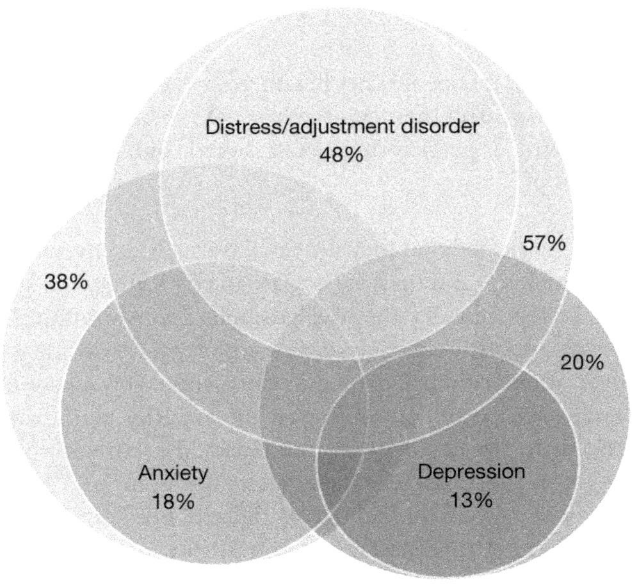

Figure 5.1 Meta-analytic rates of distress, anxiety, and depression by interview (inner circle) and self-report (outer circle).

SOURCE: MITCHELL, A. J. (2010B). SCREENING PROCEDURES FOR PSYCHOSOCAL DISTRESS. IN J. C. HOLLAND, W. BREITBART, P. B. JACOBSEN, M. LEDERBERG, M. LOSCALZO, & R. MCCORKLE (EDS.), *PSYCHO-ONCOLOGY* (2ND ED., FIG. 52.2, P. 390). NEW YORK: OXFORD UNIVERSITY PRESS. BY PERMISSION OF OXFORD UNIVERSITY PRESS, USA.

The prevalence of distress in long-term cancer survivors was the focus of a study by Hoffman and colleagues (2009), noting the increasing numbers of cancer survivors in the United States and the importance of understanding the longer term psychological effects of the cancer experience. This study of a nationally representative sample of 4,636 self-identified cancer patients, who responded to the 2002–2006 National Health Interview Survey, compared those reporting serious psychological distress (e.g., felt hopeless, felt so sad nothing could cheer them up, felt nervous, felt restless/fidgety, felt worthless) from those not reporting such distress. Results showed that cancer survivors experienced a significantly higher prevalence of serious psychological distress (5.6%) than those who were never diagnosed with cancer (3.0%). Those survivors who were younger, unmarried, had less than a high school education, were uninsured, had multiple comorbidities, or had difficulties with routine activities of daily life were more likely to report psychological distress.

Receipt of Psychosocial Care as Reported by Cancer Survivors

Given these prevalence rates, it might be expected that most individuals who experience distress receive psychosocial care. This is not the case (Institute of Medicine, 2008), and estimates suggest that a relatively low percent of patients in need of care actually receive it. Forsythe and colleagues (2013) studied a representative sample of US adults diagnosed with cancer and asked two questions:

- Did their doctor, nurse, or other health professional talk to them about how cancer may affect their emotions or their relationships?
- Did they receive or participate in professional counseling or a support group?

Over half (55.1%) indicated that they did not have such a conversation with their health care provider, nor did they participate in counseling or a support group. Conversely, 31.4% reported that they did have such a conversation, 4.4% reported that they received professional counseling/support groups, while 8.9% reported both the conversation and participation in counseling. Fewer patients report the receipt of psychosocial care than do report the experience of distress, anxiety, or depression. This disparity between the reported prevalence of distress and the participation in psychosocial care suggests the need for a more systematic and clearly planned method for identifying those in need of psychosocial health services. This is the goal of screening and assessment.

Clinical Practice Guidelines and Their Implementation

The NCCN Clinical Practice Guidelines in Oncology (NCCN Guidelines®) for Distress Management (National Comprehensive Cancer Network, 2014) are consensus-based, clinical practice guidelines designed to identify, refer, and provide treatment for patients experiencing psychosocial distress. The guidelines, first adopted by the National Comprehensive Cancer Network® (NCCN®) in 1997, provide guidance for both the primary oncology team (e.g., oncologist, nurse, social worker) as well as key referral sources (e.g., mental health, social work, and chaplaincy services) on how to define "distress," how to do a brief screening procedure, when and to whom to refer, and how further, discipline-specific assessment should proceed. For distress screening to become well established and sustainable, NCCN® has also adopted standards of care for distress management, as listed in Box 5.1.

Given the potential for stigma associated with terms such as *psychiatric, psychological, maladjustment, emotional,* or *mental* the term *distress* was intentionally chosen, in hopes of lessening any stigma or embarrassment and increasing patient willingness to report. The NCCN Guidelines® specifically define distress as

> a multifactorial unpleasant emotional experience of a psychological (cognitive, behavioral, emotional), social, and/or spiritual nature that may interfere with the ability to cope effectively with cancer, its physical symptoms and its treatment. Distress extends along a continuum, ranging from common normal feelings of vulnerability, sadness, and fears to problems that can become disabling, such as depression, anxiety, panic, social isolation, and existential and spiritual crisis. (National Comprehensive Cancer Network, 2014, DIS-2)

Advocating for increased attention to psychosocial distress, distress has been promoted as the *sixth vital sign* along with pulse, temperature, respiration, blood pressure, and pain (Bultz & Carlson, 2006), in hopes of routine initiation of conversations about psychosocial needs and concerns. The American Society of Clinical Oncology (ASCO) has recommended an adaptation of a Pan-Canadian Practice Guideline (Howell et al., 2010) on screening, assessment and care of patients with symptoms of depression and anxiety (i.e., distress) for use in the United States (Andersen et al., 2014).

A number of self-report questionnaires have been used for identifying distress, anxiety, and depression. Some are conventional mood severity scales, such as the Profile of Mood States (POMS) and the Hospital Anxiety and Depression Scale (HADS), while others follow the briefer, NCCN Distress Thermometer (DT) format. Table 5.1 lists some examples.

Short screening instruments (<15 items) have included valid and reliable self-report questionnaires that take 5–15 minutes to complete and can screen for single disorders such as depression, or a broader array of concerns such as quality of life, mood states, or symptoms of other mental disorders. The goal is for the screening instruments to be accurate in identifying the presence or absence of distress. In addition, given the time constraints in a busy oncology practice, cost-effectiveness, efficiency, and local acceptability have become important in selecting a specific screening procedure. Finding a valid, reliable, efficient, and locally acceptable procedure is an ongoing goal for many community cancer centers, particularly in light of newly defined accreditation standards

Box 5.1

NCCN Standards of Care for Distress Management

- Distress should be recognized, monitored, documented, and treated promptly at all stages of disease and in all settings.
- Screening should identify the level and nature of the distress.
- All patients should be screened for distress at their initial visit, at appropriate intervals, and as clinically indicated, especially with changes in disease status (i.e., remission, recurrence, progression, treatment-related complications).
- Distress should be assessed and managed according to clinical practice guidelines.
- Interdisciplinary institutional committees should be formed to implement standards for distress management.
- Educational and training programs should be developed to ensure that health care professionals and certified chaplains have knowledge and skills in the assessment and management of distress.
- Licensed mental health professionals and certified chaplains experienced in psychosocial aspects of cancer should be readily available as staff members or through referral.
- Medical care contracts should include reimbursement for services provided by mental health professionals.
- Clinical health outcomes measurement should include assessment of the psychosocial domain (e.g., quality of life, patient and family satisfaction).
- Patients, families, and treatment teams should be informed that management of distress is an integral part of total medical care and provided with appropriate information about psychosocial services in the treatment center and the community.
- Quality of distress management programs/services should be included in institutional continuous quality improvement (CQI) projects.

SOURCE: Adapted with permission from the NCCN Clinical Practice Guidelines in Oncology (NCCN Guidelines®) for Distress Management V.1.2014. © 2014 National Comprehensive Cancer Network, Inc. All rights reserved. The NCCN Guidelines® and illustrations herein may not be reproduced in any form for any purpose without the express written permission of the NCCN. To view the most recent and complete version of the NCCN Guidelines, go online to NCCN.org. NATIONAL COMPREHENSIVE CANCER NETWORK®, NCCN®, NCCN GUIDELINES®, and all other NCCN Content are trademarks owned by the National Comprehensive Cancer Network, Inc. (National Comprehensive Cancer Network, 2014).

calling for the implementation of routine documented distress-screening procedures (American College of Surgeons & Commission on Cancer, 2012). The use of online and other technology-based distress screening procedures (Cancer Support Community, 2012; Clark, Bardwell, Arsenault, DeTeresa, & Loscalzo, 2009) has increased as the need for readily available, efficient, and cost-effective procedures has increased.

Table 5.1. SAMPLE SELF-REPORT QUESTIONNAIRES FOR SCREENING FOR DEPRESSION, ANXIETY, AND DISTRESS

Title	Items	Time (min)	Constructs Measured
Distress Thermometer	1	2	Severity of distress
+ Problem List[a]	36	5–7	Practical, emotional, physical, spiritual/ religious problems related to the distress
Brief Symptom Inventory (BSI)[b,c]	53 (18)	7–10 (3–5)	Somatization, anxiety, interpersonal sensitivity, depression, hostility, phobic anxiety, paranoid ideation, psychoticism, obsessions-compulsions
Hospital Anxiety and Depression Scale (HADS)[d]	14	5–10	Symptoms of anxiety and depression
PRIME-MD Patient Health Questionaire (PHQ)[e]	9 (depression), 22 (anxiety)	5–10	*DSM-IV* diagnostic criteria for depression and anxiety
Profile of Mood States (POMS)[f]	65	5–10	Six mood states: anxiety, fatigue, confusion, depression, anger, vigor
Functional Assessment of Chronic Illness Therapy[g]	27	5–10	Four dimensions of quality of life: physical, functional, social, emotional
Psychological Distress Inventory (PDI)[h]	13	3–7	Distress
Zung Self-Rating Depression Scale[i]	20	5–10	Symptoms of depression

[a]National Comprehensive Cancer Network (2014).
[b]Both a 53- and an 18-item version.
[c]King, Heisel, and Lyness (2005).
[d]American Cancer Society (2009).
[e]Spitzer, Kroenke, and Williams (1999).
[f]Porter, Spates, and Smitham (2004).
[g]Cella et al. (1993).
[h]Feuerstein (2007).
[i]Weir et al. (2003).

The most widely promoted and investigated method is the Distress Thermometer and its accompanying Problem List (Fig. 5.2), as shown in the NCCN Guidelines (National Comprehensive Cancer Network, 2014). The overriding goal is that no patient experiencing distress should go unrecognized or untreated. The NCCN Guidelines call for distress to be screened by the primary oncology team (oncologist, oncology nurse, and social worker) at all stages of disease, at a variety of times along the clinical course of the disease, in all relevant settings. Figure 5.3 illustrates the clinical course of the disease for most cancer patients. Along this continuum, note key periods when distress screening could occur: diagnosis, start of treatment, completion of treatment, recurrence/metastases, periodic follow-up, and so on.

The Distress Thermometer and Problem List are administered in the waiting room prior to an appointment, either via pen and paper or technology such as a touchscreen computer. The primary oncology team then reviews the completed Distress Thermometer and Problem List. Various cutoff scores have been investigated with most considering a score of 4 or 5 as indicating clinically significant distress warranting further follow-up. It has been recommended that scores of 0–3 (none to mild) be managed by the primary oncology team by providing information that answers patient questions or concerns, while scores of 4–6 (mild to moderate) result in providing educational information about available support resources and a referral to appropriate specialists as *potentially helpful, but optional*, and scores of 7–10 resulting in a *strongly recommended referral* to appropriate health care professionals (Hoffman, Zevon, D'Arrigo, & Cecchini, 2004).

The 2014 NCCN Guidelines recommend using a cutoff of 4. Typically the oncology team would respond to scores of 4 or greater with an evaluation of the Problem List to see which types of problems have been endorsed and which referral sources to consider. In collaboration with the patient, a referral would then be made for any patients scoring a 4 or higher on the Distress Thermometer.

Accuracy and Efficiency of Screening Procedures

Since the late 1990s, a significant body of research has developed investigating the accuracy of distress screening procedures. Two reviews (Meijer et al., 2011; Mitchell, 2007, 2010a) have summarized results. The first review was focused on the ability of screening procedures to identify accurately both those who are experiencing distress and those who are not. The ability of a screening procedure to identify accurately those *who are* experiencing distress ("rule in") is defined as the *sensitivity* of the procedure or the procedure's ability to accurately identify *true positives*. Conversely, the ability of a screening procedure to accurately identify those *who are not* experiencing distress ("rule out") is defined as the *specificity* of the procedure or the procedure's ability to accurately identify *true negatives*. Overall, this review found that many screening procedures incorrectly identified a number of patients as depressed, when in reality they were not. These instruments had a large number of false positives because a large number were incorrectly "ruled in" as depressed. Given a large number of false positives, the combination of those accurately identified as depressed with those

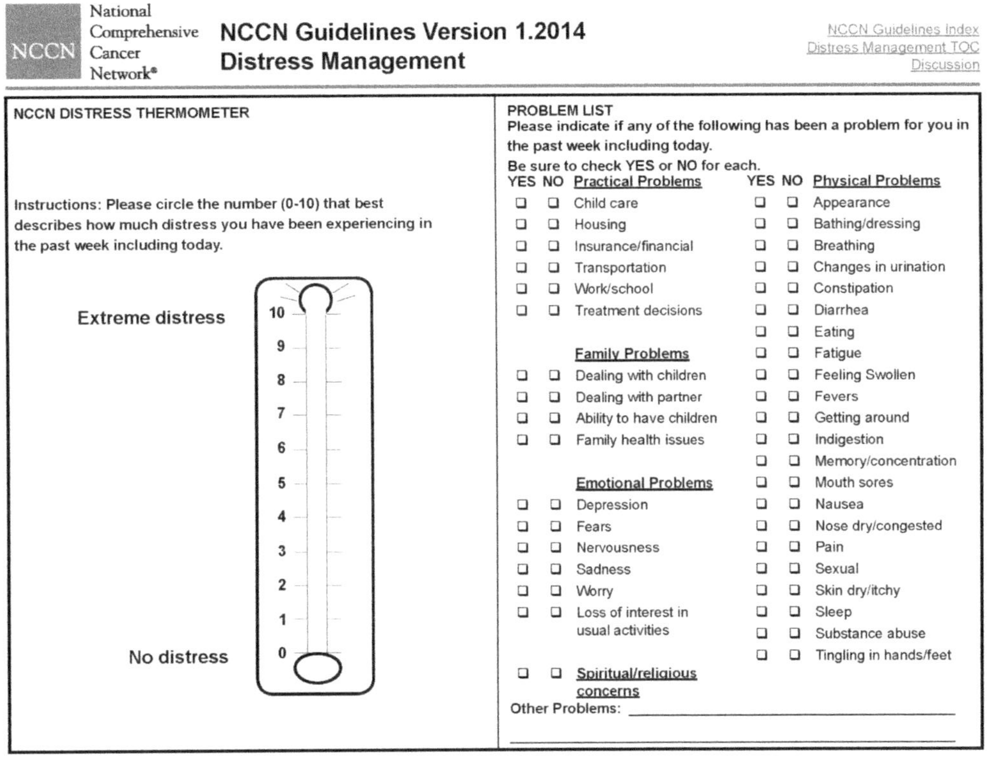

NCCN National Comprehensive Cancer Network®

NCCN Guidelines Version 1.2014
Distress Management

NCCN Guidelines Index
Distress Management TOC
Discussion

NCCN DISTRESS THERMOMETER

Instructions: Please circle the number (0-10) that best describes how much distress you have been experiencing in the past week including today.

PROBLEM LIST

Please indicate if any of the following has been a problem for you in the past week including today.

Be sure to check YES or NO for each.

YES	NO	Practical Problems	YES	NO	Physical Problems
❑	❑	Child care	❑	❑	Appearance
❑	❑	Housing	❑	❑	Bathing/dressing
❑	❑	Insurance/financial	❑	❑	Breathing
❑	❑	Transportation	❑	❑	Changes in urination
❑	❑	Work/school	❑	❑	Constipation
❑	❑	Treatment decisions	❑	❑	Diarrhea
			❑	❑	Eating
		Family Problems	❑	❑	Fatigue
❑	❑	Dealing with children	❑	❑	Feeling Swollen
❑	❑	Dealing with partner	❑	❑	Fevers
❑	❑	Ability to have children	❑	❑	Getting around
❑	❑	Family health issues	❑	❑	Indigestion
			❑	❑	Memory/concentration
		Emotional Problems	❑	❑	Mouth sores
❑	❑	Depression	❑	❑	Nausea
❑	❑	Fears	❑	❑	Nose dry/congested
❑	❑	Nervousness	❑	❑	Pain
❑	❑	Sadness	❑	❑	Sexual
❑	❑	Worry	❑	❑	Skin dry/itchy
❑	❑	Loss of interest in usual activities	❑	❑	Sleep
			❑	❑	Substance abuse
			❑	❑	Tingling in hands/feet
❑	❑	**Spiritual/religious concerns**			

Other Problems: ______________________

Figure 5.2 The distress thermometer and problem list.

SOURCE: Reproduced with permission from the NCCN Clinical Practice Guidelines in Oncology (NCCN Guidelines®) for Distress Management V.1.2014. To view the most recent and complete version of the NCCN Guidelines, go online to NCCN.org. NATIONAL COMPREHENSIVE CANCER NETWORK®, NCCN®, NCCN GUIDELINES®, and all other NCCN Content are trademarks owned by the National Comprehensive Cancer Network, Inc.

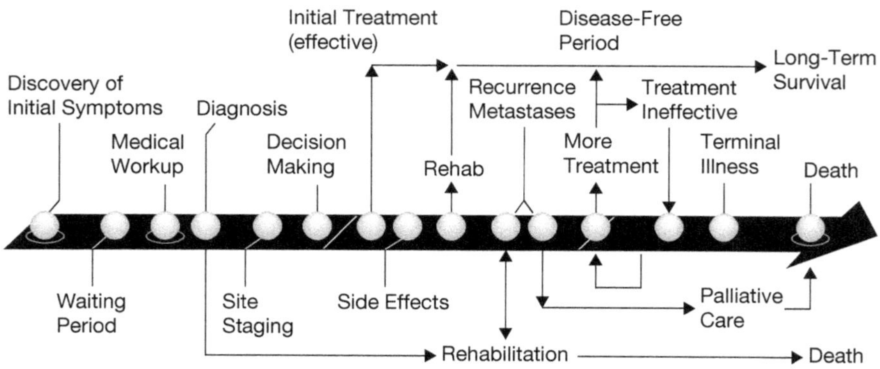

Figure 5.3 The clinical course of the disease.
SOURCE: From Nicholas, D. R., & Veach, T. A. (2000). The psychosocial assessment of the adult cancer patient. *Professional Psychology: Research and Practice, 31*(2), 206–215. Copyright 2000 by the American Psychological Association. Reproduced with permission. The use of APA information does not imply endorsement by APA.

inaccurately identified as depressed—known as the positive predictive value (PPV) of the procedure—was only 32.4%. Conversely, screening procedures did a better job at correctly identifying those who were not depressed (true negatives). They were correctly "ruled out" as not depressed. The combination of those accurately identified as not depressed with those inaccurately identified as not depressed—known as the negative predictive value (NPV)—was 93.4%.

In studies of screening procedures for anxiety and distress, a similar pattern was found, where more patients were correctly identified as not experiencing anxiety or distress (true negatives) than were those correctly identified as experiencing anxiety or distress (true positives). With anxiety, the PPV was 55.2% and the NPV was 80.25%. For distress, the PPV was 59.7% and the NPV was 82.8%. Thus, as a result of incorrectly identifying a number of patients as distressed, depressed, or anxious, these very brief screening procedures are better at correctly ruling out those not in distress than ruling in those who are.

In an update to the 2007 review, Mitchell and colleagues (2010a) evaluated the accuracy and efficiency of six methods for identifying psychosocial distress. These six were chosen from a total of 45 short (5 to 14 items, taking a total of 2 to 5 minutes to complete) and ultra-short (1 to 4 items, taking less than a total of 2 minutes to complete) methods identified in a comprehensive search. The six methods were chosen because their accuracy was tested against a semistructured clinical interview as the "gold standard" for comparison. The six were

- the NCCN Distress Thermometer,
- the HADS (total score),
- the Psychological Distress Inventory (PDI),
- the Distress Thermometer and the Impact Thermometer used together,
- a single-verbal questionnaire (e.g., "Are you depressed?"), and
- a two-question procedure ("Have you lost interest or pleasure?" or "Are you depressed?").

All six methods showed comparable accuracy to one another with their ability to identify those who are experiencing distress (i.e., sensitivity) ranging from 67% to 81%, and their ability to accurately identify those who are not (i.e., specificity) ranging from 67% to 93%. All showed moderate accuracy and thus there was no clear basis upon which to recommend any one procedure over the other.

Efficiency (the time to administer, complete, and score the instrument and patient acceptability) and patient willingness to cooperate with the screening procedures are additional important considerations when developing a screening procedure. The choice of which procedure to use is best made by considering the accuracy of the instrument as well as the overall efficiency and patient acceptability of the procedure. Recognizing the heterogeneity of local cancer care settings, and the evidence-based practice of acknowledging patient characteristics, culture, and preferences, the EBP of distress screening suggests that local patient acceptability be considered, along with the procedure's accuracy and efficiency, as the basis on which to select a screening procedure.

In summary, ongoing investigations of the accuracy of screening procedures have found that most of these methods are better at ruling out the presence of distress than at ruling in distress. Thus, if a systematic, planned psychosocial screening program is to be implemented, it is likely that a number of screening procedures could be used that will correctly identify patients in distress. To enhance the accuracy of these procedures, some have suggested that the short (e.g., Psychological distress inventory) and ultra-short (e.g., Distress Thermometer) methods can be improved in a variety of ways (Mitchell, 2010b). These include (a) combining procedures such as using the Distress Thermometer and the impact thermometer together, (b) repeating the procedure multiple times across the course of the illness, and (c) adding questions that directly inquire about patient interest or perceived need for professional help.

Efficacy of Screening Programs on Patient Outcomes

Even with the NCCN Guidelines and the development of valid, reliable, and accurate brief screening instruments, continued research is needed to investigate whether these screening procedures, when combined with a comprehensive referral and treatment program, result in improved patient outcomes, such as decreased anxiety or depression. At present there is no convincing evidence that screening results in improved outcomes in cancer patients (Carlson, Clifford, Groff, Maciejewski, & Bultz, 2010; Meijer et al., 2011). What has yet to be determined is whether screening is the start of an effective process that (a) identifies patients in need who (b) can be successfully referred to a competent care provider (c) capable of providing effective interventions that can then (d) be demonstrated to have resulted in improved outcomes. A very limited number of studies have attempted to answer such questions. Carlson and colleagues (2010) reviewed seven longitudinal studies testing the efficacy of screening programs in oncology and concluded that such programs appear to result in more discussions between patients and oncology staff about psychosocial issues, but not necessarily in any improved outcomes. A systematic review by Meijer and colleagues (2011) identified only one randomized trial of a *treatment* for depression in cancer care (Strong et al., 2008), and unfortunately this study—although it did find moderately reduced depression—was not a randomized trial of *screening*. In this study the identification of eligible patients occurred via a structured clinical interview, not a brief screening procedure. Thus, it remains unknown if screening programs do, in fact, result in improved patient outcomes. One suggestion is that improved outcomes via a screening program might first need to consider a patient's interest in, perceived need, or unmet needs for psychosocial services. That is, do patients who report distress perceive any unmet needs and want to participate in psychosocial services?

Screening for Distress and Unmet Needs/Desire for Psychosocial Services

The NCCN Guidelines and most of the research on screening for distress have assumed a relationship between the identification of distress and the desire for receiving psychosocial services. When a patient is identified as in distress, it has been assumed that that same patient is interested in receiving psychosocial services. This is not always the case (Merckaert et al., 2010; van Scheppingen et al., 2011). Some patients who report significant amounts of distress are not interested. One study of lung cancer patients (Graves et al., 2007) found that only 30% of those reporting distress wanted any help, while another found only 43% wanted help (Tuinman, Gazendam-Donofrio, & Hoekstra-Weebers, 2008).

Which patients are most likely to express interest in psychosocial services? Although no definitive answer is yet known, some studies (Merckaert et al., 2010; van Scheppingen et al., 2011) have identified characteristics of those reporting a perceived need and expressing interested in psychosocial services. One study of 381 patients with varied types of cancer (Merckaert et al., 2010), noting significant gender differences, reported that about one in four (26%) women and one in ten (11%) men reported a desire for psychological support services. Other studies have found those most likely to report unmet needs or interest in psychosocial services as being female, single, younger, and having a support-seeking coping style. Conversely, males with prostate cancer have been identified as those reporting less need or interest in psychosocial services.

Considering these findings, a different approach to screening seems to be needed. In addition to attempts to screen for distress, it seems also necessary to identify patient-identified interest, desire, or perceived need for psychosocial services. From this perspective, screening becomes a process of identifying distress and also *meeting unmet needs*, that is, identifying those patients who score either high or low on a distress screening instrument, and who report an interest in or a perceived need for psychosocial services (van Scheppingen et al., 2011).

In addition to this ongoing research regarding screening, there are also consensus-based guidelines by the NCCN suggesting risk factors and patient characteristics to consider. These include both *who* is at risk, as well as *when*

Box 5.2

Risk Factors for Psychosocial Distress: Patient Characteristics

- History of psychiatric disorder/substance abuse
- History of depression/suicide attempt
- Cognitive impairment
- Communication barriers (language, literacy, physical barriers)
- Severe comorbid illnesses
- Social problems
  - Family/caregiver conflicts
  - Inadequate social support
  - Living alone
  - Financial problems
  - Limited access to medical care
  - Young or dependent children
  - Younger age; woman
  - History of abuse (physical, sexual)
  - Other stressors
- Spiritual/religious concerns
- Uncontrolled symptoms

along the clinical course they may be more vulnerable to distress. These factors are listed in Boxes 5.2 and 5.3.

BEST AVAILABLE EVIDENCE: HOW TO SCREEN FOR PSYCHOSOCIAL DISTRESS

The evidence-based practitioner is now equipped with knowledge that addresses background questions regarding psychosocial distress screening. Next, the following PICO question is asked:

> For an outpatient, adult cancer care setting, what is the best procedure for implementing an accurate, efficient, and acceptable screening that is feasible to implement and reduces distress (anxiety, depression, patient-identified problems)?

Box 5.3

Risk Factors for Psychosocial Distress: Periods of Increased Vulnerability

- Finding a suspicious symptom
- During diagnostic workup
- Finding out the diagnosis
- Awaiting treatment
- Change in treatment modality
- Significant treatment-related complication(s)
- End of treatment
- Discharge from hospital after treatment
- Transition to survivorship
- Medical follow-up and surveillance
- Treatment failure
- Recurrence/progression
- Advanced cancer
- End of life

SOURCE: Adapted with permission from the NCCN Clinical Practice Guidelines in Oncology (NCCN Guidelines®) for Distress Management V.1.2014. © 2014 National Comprehensive Cancer Network, Inc. All rights reserved. The NCCN Guidelines® and illustrations herein may not be reproduced in any form for any purpose without the express written permission of the NCCN. To view the most recent and complete version of the NCCN Guidelines, go online to NCCN.org. NATIONAL COMPREHENSIVE CANCER NETWORK®, NCCN®, NCCN GUIDELINES®, and all other NCCN Content are trademarks owned by the National Comprehensive Cancer Network, Inc. (National Comprehensive Cancer Network, 2014).

The following is a review of accessed best available evidence and an exemplar for distress screening, designed to answer this question.

Given new accreditation standards by the Commission on Cancer (CoC) of the American College of Surgeons (ACOS) requiring a distress screening program, interest in dissemination and implementation research has grown, and funding resources for distress screening are likely to increase, paralleling recent increases in training on how to implement distress screening programs. As reviewed earlier, there is no single best way to screen for distress in cancer care. Rather, close attention to efficiency and patient acceptability are paramount in the local cancer care setting. What evidence is available?

Unfiltered, Primary Literature

A review of unfiltered, primary literature in PsycINFO, Medline, and CINAHL, searching for published articles on screening for psychosocial distress with the search terms "screening AND distress" in "cancer OR neoplasm" found a steady increase in numbers of published studies from 107 in 2009 to 208 in 2014. However, when a more limited search of randomized controlled trials was done for this same period, a total of only 20 unique randomized controlled trials were found, published between 2009 and 2014. Of these 20 studies, only 3 were randomized trials of psychosocial distress screening programs in outpatient settings. All three were from the same research group, with two describing different randomized trials (Carlson, Groff, Maciejewski, & Bultz, 2010), and the third being a secondary analysis of data on pain, fatigue, and common problems (Carlson, Waller, Groff, & Bultz, 2013). Of the other 17 randomized trials, nine were diagnostic screening studies for various cancers, four were psychosocial intervention studies, two were studies of distress related to genetic screening, two were studies of psychosocial distress screening in inpatient oncology settings, and three were abstracts of psychosocial distress screenings listed in the clinical trials registry. Thus, these last three are relevant as data become available.

A Psychosocial Distress Screening Exemplar

The two large-scale longitudinal studies by Carlson and colleagues (Carlson, Groff, Zhong, & Butz, 2012; Carlson, Groff, et al., 2010) investigated 3- and 12-month outcomes of structured programs designed to screen for psychosocial distress in outpatient settings. They are offered as exemplars of best available research investigating the efficacy of psychosocial screening programs as determined by their impact on longer term outcomes—as available via a limited search in November 2013.

These studies investigated different types of screening procedures on levels of distress, anxiety, depression, fatigue, and pain with very large samples. In the first study (2010), online screening for psychosocial distress was followed by random assignment to three levels of care. A large number (n = 1,134) of newly diagnosed breast and lung cancer patients were randomly assigned to one of three different conditions:

- *Minimal screening* during which they completed, in the presence of a screening team member, an online Distress Thermometer and a demographics form and were given educational information about psychosocial program availability and self-referral information but did not receive a feedback report nor was their screening information provided to other health care providers
- *Full screening* in which patients completed the online Distress Thermometer, a problem list, fatigue and pain thermometers, and a self-report measure of anxiety and depression, and received a printed personalized feedback report, a summary of which was also placed in the medical record for other providers to see
- *Personalized triage* in which they received all that was provided in the full screening group, plus an offer to speak by phone to a member of the psychosocial team about any concerns. When requested, a team member

> contacted the patient within 3 working days. The team member then closely followed an algorithm that guided suggested referral procedures.

All participants were contacted at 3 months and completed outcome measures that included the Distress Thermometer and measures of anxiety and depression. This first study (Carlson, Groff, et al., 2010) tested these three forms of screening for their relative efficacy in decreasing overall distress at 3 months follow-up. The primary results at 3 months showed (a) for lung cancer patients who received the personalized triage, 20% fewer remained in the highly distressed range of scores than those who received either of the other two conditions and (b) for breast cancer patients, their mean distress scores were significantly lower if they received either triage or the full screening compared to the minimal screening. On secondary outcome measures, the best predictor of decreases in anxiety and depression was if the patient received a referral to psychosocial services. This study also showed good patient acceptability and that it was feasible to do routine computerized screening in a large, busy oncology setting, as almost 90% of eligible participants completed the screenings.

In the second study (Carlson et al., 2012)—a larger and longer study of 3,133 patients who were newly diagnosed with a wide variety of types of cancer—patients were randomly assigned to one of two groups in which a computerized triage procedure was tested against a personalized triage. For both groups follow-ups were done at 3, 6, and 12 months. All patients completed the online screening procedure at touchscreen kiosks located in the waiting area, as directed by receptionists. After completing the screening they were randomly assigned to either a *computerized triage group*, in which they immediately received a printout with a summary of their expressed concerns and instructions on how to access appropriate services, or to a *personalized triage group* in which they also received a printout and were contacted by phone by a staff person within 3 days. During this phone contact, appropriate referral options were discussed based on the same distress-screening triage algorithm as in the computerized triage group. Specific services recommended could include psychosocial support, resource counseling, pain management, fatigue management, and nutrition management for both groups.

A number of interesting results were found. First, in both groups there was a significant decline in distress, anxiety, depression, pain, and fatigue from baseline to the 12-month follow-up. This result likely reflects the natural course of symptoms as they decline from time of diagnosis throughout the first year. There were no significant differences between groups in the amount of decline in symptoms—both screening procedures showed similar declines. Second, when gender and change over time were investigated, it was found that men in a computerized group improved more than men in a personalized group, and conversely, women in a personalized group improved more than women in a computerized group, and regardless of group, women showed a greater degree of improvement than did men. Third, it was found that patients who used the offered psychosocial services showed a significantly greater decrease in distress and depression than those who did not use available services, and finally, a higher percentage of patients accessed services if they received the personalized screening procedure. Thus, this study suggests that even though patients in both groups improved over time, those who showed greater improvement were those who used the available psychosocial services, and those in the personalized screening procedure accessed more available services. Decreasing unwanted symptoms of distress, anxiety, depression, pain, or fatigue seems feasible using either screening procedure; yet greater improvement came from the use of psychosocial services, and more patients used these services when they received the personalized screening. These relationships can be illustrated as follows:

online screening → personalized triage → psychosocial services → decreased symptoms

These two studies conclude that although screening for distress is feasible, important to do, and results in decreases in unwanted symptoms/problems, more improved outcomes occur *when patients accept and utilize referrals* to appropriate psychosocial services. Future research needs to focus on both optimal methods of screening and on identifying effective methods of increasing patients' acceptance of referrals that result in accessing and utilizing needed psychosocial services.

BEST AVAILABLE EVIDENCE: HOW TO DO AN ASSESSMENT OF PSYCHOSOCIAL ADAPTATION FOR THE ADULT CANCER PATIENT

In contrast to growing empirical evidence on screening for psychosocial distress, any comparable empirical evidence for the assessment of psychosocial adaptation does not exist. Extensive literature searches over multiple years since the early 1990s have failed to identify quantitative research on the development and testing of various psychosocial assessment procedures. In the primary professions of psychology, psychiatry, social work, oncology nursing, and chaplaincy, the clinical interview is the primary process for the assessment of psychosocial adaptation. Theoretical and conceptual models along with clinical practice guidelines for how to do the face-to-face clinical interview have guided this literature. Within the three components of evidence-based practice—best available research evidence; clinical expertise; and patient characteristics, preferences, culture—these professions consider the clinical interview a component of clinical expertise. The evidence-based practice of psychology, for instance, places "assessment, diagnostic judgment, systematic case formulation, and treatment planning" (American Psychological Association, 2006, p. 276) as components of clinical expertise. This may then explain the limited empirical evidence base. Thus, at present, clinical practice guidelines are the best source of evidence on how to do an assessment of psychosocial adaptation. Assessment occurs via a clinical interview, focused on factors relevant to coping and adaptation done by a qualified professional following a semistructured procedure. The NCCN Guidelines state that the supportive care professional who receives the referral for a patient's distress management should evaluate the patient using the clinical practice guidelines for that discipline (e.g., mental health, social work, or chaplaincy services) (National Comprehensive Cancer Network, 2014). Assessment by the specialty mental health professional will, of course, vary by the referral question, but the NCCN Guidelines call for routine evaluation of the following components of adaptation:

- Psychosocial distress
- Behavioral symptoms
- Psychiatric history and relevant medications
- Pain and other symptom (e.g., fatigue, nausea/vomiting) control
- Body image and sexuality concerns
- Impaired capacity
- Safety (e.g., suicidality)

In addition, common referral questions may warrant additional assessment of the following:

- Dementia
- Delirium
- Mood disorders
- Adjustment disorders
- Substance-related disorders
- Personality disorders

Detailed discussion of assessment of all of these disorders is beyond the scope of this book. (See *Psycho-Oncology* [Holland et al., 2010] for more information on assessment of each of these potential presenting problems.) However, the mental health professional will follow established standards of care for their discipline and quick reference guides such as the *Quick reference for oncology clinicians: The psychiatric and psychological dimensions of cancer symptom management* (McQuaid & Nassau, 1999). Clinical practice guidelines (e.g., NCCN) recommend that cancer patients identified as experiencing distress be evaluated further.

In a series of related conceptual models, psychosocial adaptation of the adult cancer patient appears to be influenced by three broad categories of variables: sociocultural context, medical context, and the psychological context (Rowland, 1989). These three categories of variables have been organized into a conceptual model for the assessment of the adult cancer patient (Nicholas & Veach, 2000) and offered as an exemplar of best available evidence in the next section.

A Conceptual Model of Psychosocial Adaptation: Person, Situation, and Life Context

In the assessment of the adult cancer patient, in addition to addressing the specific referral question, the outcome of primary interest is psychosocial adaptation. *Psychosocial adaptation* has been defined as the ongoing adjustment to cancer-related life stressors encountered by each patient along the clinical course (Spencer, Carver, & Price, 1998). Some broad markers of successful adaptation include the following:

- Continued, active involvement in daily life
- The ability to minimize excessive disruptions to life roles
- Skill at regulating emotional distress (Spencer et al., 1998)

Figure 5.4 illustrates an integrative conceptual model for the psychosocial adaptation of the adult cancer patient. This is a transactional model that recognizes the interaction between person, situation, and life context. The process of psychosocial adaptation to the unique illness experience of each patient occurs at the intersection of patient-derived variables (person), cancer-derived variables (situation), and cultural, development variables (life context). *Quality of life* is viewed as the outcome of the ongoing process of adaptation. This model has been used as a guiding framework for the development of a semistructured interview process of the adult cancer patient (Nicholas & Veach, 2000). Those variables tailored to the specific assessment of the adult cancer patient, and derived from the conceptual model in Figure 5.4, are reviewed next.

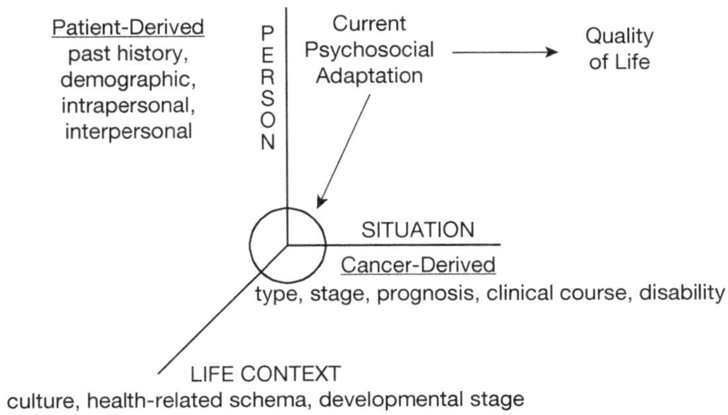

Figure 5.4 A model of psychosocial adaptation in cancer. Current psychosocial adaptation occurs at the intersection of patient-derived person variables, cancer-derived situation variables, and broader life context and largely determines ongoing quality of life.
SOURCE: Nicholas, D. R., & Veach, T. A. (2000). The psychosocial assessment of the adult cancer patient. *Professional Psychology: Research and Practice, 31*(2), 206–215. Copyright 2000 by the American Psychological Association. Reproduced with permission. The use of APA information does not imply endorsement by APA.

Person Variables

Person variables can be organized into four categories: past history, demographics, intrapersonal, and interpersonal. Table 5.2 presents the relevant variables along with a theoretical and/or empirical rationale for their importance in assessing overall psychosocial adaptation. In addition to considering a range of person variables, it is also important to have a clear understanding of closely related, but different constructs, as listed in Table 5.2.

The distinction between intrapersonal and interpersonal resources is the first to be examined. *Intrapersonal resources* consist of the intrapsychic or internal coping resources each patient brings to the task of coping with the varied stressors of cancer. Intrapersonal resources can be furthered divided into two closely-related components: coping style and coping strategies. *Coping style* is a patient's relatively stable and enduring pattern of coping, conceptualized as a trait-like disposition, such as optimism. In contrast, *coping strategies* are situation-specific techniques

Table 5.2. Person Variables Relevant to the Assessment of the Adult Cancer Patient

Variables	Theoretical and Empirical Rationale
Demographics	
Age	Younger age associated with increased risk of distress and prevalence of nausea/vomiting
Gender	Related to different patterns of social support and help seeking
Relational status	Related to availability of social support
Socioeconomic status	Related to incidence of certain types of cancer; lower socioeconomic associated with access to care, treatment patterns, survival rates, morbidity, and mortality
Prior history	
Mental disorders	Risk factor for increased distress, anxiety, depression; adjustment disorders most common; subthreshold posttraumatic stress disorder symptoms relevant to assess; dementia/delirium in older adults
Substance use/ abuse	Stress of cancer can result in increased/worsening of use/ abuse; continued use interferes with coping; risk factor for head and neck cancers
Mental health treatment	Proxy variable for prior mental health history
Illness experiences	Can influence expectations about treatment, prognosis, coping efforts; important to understand health-related schema (i.e., illness beliefs about cause, treatment, side effects, prognosis, stigma of cancer, culturally influenced)
Recent losses	Significant losses can influence coping

(*Continued*)

Table 5.2. Continued

Variables	Theoretical and Empirical Rationale
Intrapersonal resources (internal coping)	
Coping style (trait-like disposition)	Dispositional optimism associated with better coping
Coping strategies (situational responses)	Strategies that result in increased engagement and commitment to ongoing life goals facilitate adaptation. There are three types: *problem-focused* attempts to solve specific problems, *appraisal-focused* can alter purpose/meaning of events, and *emotion-focused* can help to regulate and control distressing emotions
Interpersonal resources (external resources that provide social support)	Receiving emotional support associated with better overall adaptation; broader social networks associated with increased survival; *gender* can influence patterns of support—perceived availability, support seeking and utilization; men more agentic (oriented toward self, individual autonomy/achievement, less relational), women more communal, oriented toward others and relationships); *structural* sources of support consist of family, friends, church, neighbors, etc.; *functional* uses of support as three types: emotional, informational, and instrumental (i.e., practical aid like transportation, financial)

SOURCE: Nicholas, D. R., & Veach, T. A. (2000). The psychosocial assessment of the adult cancer patient. *Professional Psychology: Research and Practice, 31*(2), 206–215. Copyright © (2000) by the American Psychological Association. Adapted with permission. The use of APA information does not imply endorsement by APA.

or responses designed to cope with specific (some very common—others unique) cancer-related situations that challenge one's ability to adapt. In contrast to these internal coping resources, *interpersonal resources* are the people and related social structures or networks of family, friends, neighbors, church, and community that provide the potential for social support.

Social support has been conceptualized in different ways, often summarized as consisting of two different forms: structural and functional (Helgeson & McUmber, 2010). *Structural support* describes the existence of various types of connections with other people such as marital status, the size of one's family or social network, or the frequency of contact with network members. Structural support does not take into consideration the quality, type, or depth of support; it is simply a measure of numbers of people available. Conversely, *functional support* considers how social support may function to effect adaptation, such as the type and amount of support received, as well as the perceived availability of support. Functional support is organized into three types: emotional (i.e., ability to express emotions with others), informational (i.e., receipt of accurate/helpful cancer-related information), and instrumental (i.e., practical aide like transportation or financial help). Thus, in the assessment of the adult cancer patient, the evaluation of social support is crucial, particularly the patient's perception of the availability of social support. It appears that even if not accessed, received, or utilized, it is important that a patient have the perception that social support is available when needed.

Finally, consideration of the concept of engagement is key to the assessment and evaluation of how an individual patient utilizes resources. *Engagement* is the degree to which a patient remains actively involved and interested in those things of importance in his or her life. In contrast, *disengagement* characterizes one who withdraws, becomes isolated, and/or "gives up" and does not remain involved in things of importance. Researchers in coping with cancer (Spencer et al., 1998) have summarized a wide variety of coping styles, strategies, and various outcomes and have suggested that one consistent core factor in the assessment of psychosocial adaptation is the concept of engagement. Thus, *engagement versus giving up* is one summary way to evaluate the relationship between intra- and interpersonal resources and their impact on psychosocial adaptation.

Life Context: Personal Identity as Formed via Culture and Family

Life contexts are the circumstances of time, place, culture, and personal identity that form the settings for events. Personal identity is the result of (a) shared, *universal* human experiences; (b) shared *group* experiences (racial and ethnic identity, cultural attitudes/values, religious beliefs); and (c) nonshared *individual* life experiences (Sue, 2001). Understanding how personal identity forms from universal, group, and individual experiences is crucial to competently consider how issues of culture, ethnicity, religion, family, race, gender, sexual orientation, and other life experiences influence adaptation.

Shared group experiences as a member of a particular *cultural group* can influence adaptation. Three areas of potential influence of culture on psychosocial adaptation to cancer include (a) one's health-related schema or explanatory model for cancer, (b) communication barriers with the health care team, and (c) expectations about the role of family in patient care. An *explanatory model* is a personal or commonsense representation of what causes an illness, influenced by cultural and family experiences, and can be quite disparate from health care providers' explanatory models (Landrine & Klonoff, 1992). Health care providers' explanatory models are embedded within a Western cultural view of disease as an intrapersonal (occurring within the person) event, often time-bound and caused by microlevel, natural agents such as genes, viruses, bacteria, and stress. Within this broader Western cultural view, cancer is viewed as a disease that occurs within an individual, caused by genetic alterations influenced by a wide variety of "hits" in the form of risk factors such as smoking, diet, lack of exercise, sun, and other environmental exposures. Patients' explanatory models, in contrast, can be quite different, particularly as influenced by non-Western cultural beliefs, and can include explanations of disease as more of a continuous, fluid, interpersonal event resulting from violations of moral, religious, or social role expectations, and/or caused by supernatural events such as fate, or punishment (Landrine & Klonoff, 1992). Expressions of these varied explanatory models can be seen in patients' statements that attribute cause to personal failures (e.g., "a few months before I was diagnosed, it was a very stressful time in my life") or beliefs about the connection between life stressors, altered immune functioning, and resulting disease onset.

It is important to identify and understand a patient's personal explanatory model for his or her cancer and to identify discrepancies between the patient's explanation and the provider's explanation, particularly as it influences adaptation. Other patient–provider communication barriers can include linguistic/language differences, varied expectations for sharing information (e.g., "If it's really important to know, my doctor will tell me" versus "I have a right to have all of my questions answered"), culturally influenced communication preferences (e.g., subtle, indirect communication), time constraints of busy practice settings, and provider stereotyping in the absence of clear, accurate communication (Nicholas, Aegisdottir, & Kruczek, 2006).

Shared group experiences as a member of a *family*, particularly recognizing that family is the primary organizing structure for the communication of cultural experiences, explains both how shared family experiences and the role of family in a patient's care are important variables to consider in assessing psychosocial adaptation. Individualistic (predominantly Western culture) versus collectivistic cultures (predominantly Eastern, Asian cultures) differ in regard to the relative importance of personal or group/family identity. The typical Western individualistic culture values personal identity, independence, and autonomy, while the typical Eastern, collectivistic culture values group/family identity, interdependence, and reliance on others (Nicholas et al., 2006). These differences can result in different expectations for the relative importance of family and the level of active participation of family in a patient's care. Even definitions of family are changing, and given current confidentiality and informed consent requirements, many patients and families face a health care system not receptive to their desires for shared communication and decision making within families. These "culture clashes" can affect psychosocial adaptation and need to be assessed.

Life Context: Age and Developmental Stage

Shared group experiences, as represented in one's *age cohort*, affect personal identity as related to cancer, as cultural and societal attitudes, beliefs, and fears of cancer have changed over time (Holland & Weiss, 2010). The stigma of a diagnosis of cancer has lessened in the United States, and dramatic changes about the "right to know" one's diagnosis and treatment options have developed in the United States since the 1940s–1950s. Despite change, many older adults may continue to consider cancer as a stigmatizing disease that should not be spoken about openly, with prognosis viewed as "a death sentence." Younger age cohorts exposed to a greater openness and less stigma about cancer are less likely to share many of these beliefs.

In addition to these shared group experiences, a patient's personal identity is influenced by *age* and its associated *developmental stage and tasks* (Rowland, 1989). A patient's age is significantly related to psychosocial adaptation. Age is often one of the strongest predictors of distress, as a diagnosis of cancer at a young age challenges our basic assumptions about how life is expected to unfold (Fawzy, 1994).

> Information about the time at which cancer occurs in the life cycle, and what tasks are threatened or interrupted as a consequence, provides insight into the psychological problems likely to result from the diagnosis and to arise during the treatment and course of the illness.
> (Rowland, 1989, p. 26)

A 32-year-old female diagnosed with breast cancer, during a time in life where focus is on parenting and child-rearing, faces very different challenges than a 58-year-old female who may be at the peak of her career, launching children into adulthood, and anticipating retirement. Table 5.3 provides some detail about potential developmental interruptions, challenges, or delays. The five categories of potential disruptions or delays are presented as prototypic examples and do not describe issues of relevance to many patients. However, having a general familiarity with these potential issues is important in each assessment of psychosocial adaptation.

Situational Variables: Clinical Course of the Disease

The clinical course of the disease is conceptualized as a time, place, or location along a disease continuum that is accompanied by common psychological and psychosocial issues. Figure 5.3—the clinical course of the disease—was introduced earlier in the explanation of implementing distress screening. It is also useful when assessing psychosocial adaptation because it illustrates the locations along the disease continuum that can be associated with common psychological and psychosocial concerns. It begins with the earliest signs or symptoms (e.g., lump, bleeding) of disease, progressing through

- seeking (or delay in seeking) medical care,
- the initial medical workup,
- the hearing of the diagnosis and treatment options,
- decision making,
- primary treatment(s),
- end of primary treatment(s),
- transition to survivorship,
- ongoing survivorship,
- recurrence or metastasis,

Table 5.3. Adult Development and Theoretical, Potential Disruptions to Life Tasks

	Altered Relationships	Dependence	Achievement	Body Image	Existential
Young Adult (19–30 years) *Intimacy vs. Isolation*	Fear/guilt about close relationships. May withdraw/ isolate self. May be rejected by others due to stigma of illness. Daily routine disrupted	Concern about increased dependence on others; overprotected by family. All occurring at time when normally independence would be increasing	"On hold" uncertain future. Worried about ability to meet achievement goals	Concerns about attractiveness to others (sexual partners). Lowered libido, self-esteem regarding sexuality. Physical symptoms trigger fears of return	Finality of death; threat to personal identity and future generations
Mature Adult (31–45 years) *Generativity vs. Stagnation*	Absence from family routine; fears of abandonment in both patient and family. Relationship strains from crises of illness, treatment regimen. Fears of or real isolation due to neutropenia, other treatment side effects. Worries about future ability to do roles	Overdependence due to illness and treatment. Role reversal strain. Overcompensation due to concerns about overdependence and too early return to physical activity, work, life roles	Job interruption. Anxiety about inability to return to work; life goals to be adjusted, unfulfilled. Worry about long-term financial commitments	Lowered libido. Any prior sexual problems exacerbated; premature loss of reproductive ability. Illness worsens normal body changes associated with aging	Disruption of developed identity. Spiritual crises (angry at God, concerns of afterlife, doubting faith)

(*Continued*)

Table 5.3. CONTINUED

	Altered Relationships	**Dependence**	**Achievement**	**Body Image**	**Existential**
Older Adult (46–65 years) *Ego Integrity vs. Despair*	Concern about inability to care for own parents; fears loss of chance to know/nurture grand-children. Unable to maintain social life. Long-term relational problems confronted. Conflict about changing nature of relationships	Guilt, feels a burden to others; fears of dependence on others, possible long-term disabilities. Loss of lifelong independence. Financial burden on others.	Anger, frustration with possible early retirement. Feels "cheated" out of healthy retirement. Disappointment with potential loss of future achievements, purposeful and meaningful work	Acceleration of aging process (real or imagined). Altered self-image reactive to treatment effects (e.g., hormonal treatments)	Depression reactive to inability to deny reality of death. Heightened reflection, life review could lead to despair and sense of meaninglessness
Aging Adult 66+ years	Increased isolation; fewer resources available; lowered adaptability to change; fears of abandonment; diminished ability to nurture others	Fears of being a burden to others, or opposite, overreliance and unnecessary dependence. Shameful about asking for help	Worry about financial security for self or others dissolving. Anger about loss of enjoyment in late life	Inability to carry out personal hygiene. Common diseases of aging compounded by cancer. Difficulty assimilating and integrating complex information. Greater susceptibility to complications of illness; greater risk of central nervous system dysfunction as related to treatment	Concerns of the dying process; grief from multiple losses; loss of own dignity; sudden need for life review to consider issues of life purpose, integrity.

SOURCE: Adapted from Rowland, J. H. (1989). *Handbook of psycho-oncology: Psychological care of the patient with cancer*, edited by Holland and Rowland (1989). Table in Appendix G, pp. 768–769. Adapted by permission of Oxford University Press, USA.

- secondary treatment(s),
- palliative care, and
- terminal illness.

The psychological and psychosocial issues of the illness experience are influenced by where an individual patient is along this continuum. The location on the clinical course represents the situational variables in the conceptual model (see Fig. 5.4). The mental health professional doing the psychosocial assessment interview should understand the common issues associated with particular locations along the clinical course. Table 5.4 provides details of common questions or concerns, emotional reactions, and signs of positive psychosocial adaptation.

The Semistructured Clinical Interview Procedure

Based upon the conceptual model explained earlier, the semistructured interview procedure includes seven steps.

Step 1: Preinterview Chart Review

An understanding of the medically derived situational variables is important to gather prior to beginning the interview. A chart review should precede the clinical interview. Medical information of importance to gather includes type of cancer, site, stage, time since diagnosis, location on the clinical course, current and planned cancer treatments, prior medical history (e.g., any prior cancer diagnoses), and current medications. Psychosocial variables of importance include relational status, family information, current living environment, and employment status. Discussion with the referral source is needed to get clarification of the referral question. Common reasons for referral include patient distress, family distress, prior mental health history, history of or current substance use, symptoms of depression or anxiety, additional concurrent psychosocial stressors, and cognitive deficits. However, this general psychosocial assessment interview is also relevant to the cancer patient experiencing the many normal, situational stressors inherent in a diagnosis and treatment of cancer.

Step 2: Introductions, Rationale, and Patient Expectations

Some patients and accompanying family members or friends may be unclear about who the interviewer is and why they are being interviewed. Thus, a brief rationale and explanation is usually warranted. After this explanation is provided, there should be some acknowledgment of understanding by the patient.

Step 3: The Human Experience of the Illness

After brief introductions and explanations, it is important to give the patient the opportunity to "tell her or his story." Here is where the distinction between the terms *illness* and *disease* becomes important (Lerner, 1994). Many view the *disease* as the biological and traditional biomedical aspects of a patient's

Table 5.4. Clinical Course of the Disease, Questions/Concerns, Emotional Reactions, and Positive Psychosocial Adaptation

Location	Common Questions/Concerns	Emotional Reactions	Positive Psychosocial Adaptation
Discovery of symptoms	*What could be wrong? It's probably nothing serious.* *This could be very serious!*	Surprise, confusion, vacillating fears, apprehensive anxiety	Maintain balanced perspective while initiating process of accessing medical care. Maintain involvement in daily life. Minimize role disruptions.
Seeking or delay in care	*I need to get this checked out right away? I can't deal with this right now; too much else going on right now; I am just going to wait.*	Denial and avoidance, fear, terror, apprehensive anxiety	Manage (i.e., self-regulate) expected emotional distress. Seek social support as needed. Access medical care appropriate to symptoms. Maintain involvement in daily life; minimize role disruptions.
Medical workup	*What will have to be done to find out what this is? I don't think I want to know! It is so hard to wait. I can't bear to wait!*	Impatience, vacillating fears, apprehensive anxiety, vulnerable	Manage expected emotional distress. Persist in completing full workup. Maintain involvement in daily life; minimize role disruptions.
Hearing diagnosis, stage, treatment options	*Why me? How did this happen? Did I do something wrong? Did they make a mistake? Are these results really about me? Could I die from this? What next?*	Shock, denial, disbelief, numb, confused or "foggy," anxiety, depression, fear	Manage expected emotional distress; accept limitations in processing info. Seek emotional and informational support. Ask questions as needed. Understand medical information (e.g., type, stage, prognosis, pros/cons of treatment options).

Decision making	*I don't know what to do? How can I ever make up my mind? These are major life decisions, so I have to get them right!* *Where can I find accurate information to help decide?* *I trust my doctor, so I will do what he/she recommends.*	Confused, terrified, "stuck," easily distracted, apprehensive anxiety, depression	Seek informational support as needed. Communicate, consult, and collaborate with physician and other health care staff. Make decisions.
Primary treatment(s) (surgery, chemotherapy radiation, hormonal therapies)	*How difficult will the treatment be? Will I survive this? What side effects will I get? I now have a chance to beat this!* *I need to remain positive (but I don't always feel positive)!* *Do they know what they are doing?*	Apprehensive anxiety, fear, avoidant, shock, numb, energized ("ready to get started"), focused clear purpose, hopeful, vulnerable	Manage expected emotional distress. Understand treatment plan (treatment types, schedule, side effects, etc.). Communicate, consult, and collaborate with health care team. Complete course of treatment and manage side effects. Seek and accept emotional, informational, and instrumental support as needed. Minimize disruptions to life roles while remaining as actively engaged in life as possible.
End of treatment(s)	*I survived this. I am so glad these are over. When will I begin to feel better/back to normal?*	Relieved, optimistic, apprehensive anxiety, lost focus.	Manage expected emotional distress. Manage any continued treatment effects (e.g., fatigue, anorexia, nausea).

(*Continued*)

Table 5.4. Continued

Location	**Common Questions/Concerns**	**Emotional Reactions**	**Positive Psychosocial Adaptation**
Transition to survivorship	*I am so glad treatments are over, but scared not to be seeing my doctors as regularly. So what do I do now? I feel sort of lost. Will it come back? How often will I see my cancer doctors?* *What signs should I be looking for? Not sure I can move on with my life.*	Ambivalent, relieved, frightened, scared, lost, uncertain future, grateful, vulnerable	Manage ambivalent emotions. Accept sense of loss and understand fears. Acknowledge relief and sense of accomplishment. Communicate, consult, and collaborate with health care team; set up survivorship care plan.
Ongoing survivorship (no evidence of disease)	*Will the cancer come back? When will I (can I) stop thinking about cancer? What does the future hold for me? Am I going to have to deal with these treatment effects forever? When I get sick now, which doctor do I go to? I am moving on with my life. My life now has clearer priorities. Life seems so uncertain. I worry about getting a second cancer.*	Intrusive worry, Apprehensive anxiety, uncertain future, reordered priorities, clear purpose/meaning, confused, frustrated with poorly coordinated care, fears of recurrence, hopeful	Return to active engagement with daily life and important life roles. Acknowledge and accept altered view of life goals and priorities. Manage fears of recurrence and other uncertainties. Maintain hope. Minimize disruptions to life roles while remaining as actively engaged in life as possible. Active participation in survivorship care plan.
Recurrence or metastasis	*My worst fears have been realized! What did I do wrong? Am I now going to die from this? What now? Do I want to go through more treatment(s)?* *I beat this last time, I can do it again! I don't know if I can do this again. I am going to die from this.*	Devastated, terrified, confused, fear of dying, shock, denial, disbelief, demoralized, numb, difficulty processing info, guilty	Manage expected emotional distress. Gradually accept reality of disease progression. Communicate, consult, and collaborate with health care team. Seek informational support as needed. Make decisions.

Secondary treatment(s) (surgery, chemotherapy radiation, hormonal therapies)	*Last time it wasn't so bad.* *I just can't do this again, last time it was terrible. Well, this time around I at least know more about what to expect.* *I hope it works this time.*	Ambivalent, hopeful, clear focus, fearful	Manage expected emotional distress. Understand new treatment plan (type schedule, side effects, etc.). Communicate, consult, and collaborate with health care team. Seek and accept emotional, informational, and instrumental support. Maintain hope—may alter what is hoped for (e.g., to be present for certain important life events). Complete course of treatment; manage side effects.
Palliative care	*Now what? I don't know what to expect. Will I be in pain? Who will take care of me? I feel like a burden. I don't want to suffer. This can't be happening.*	Confused, fearful, anxiety, depression, denial	Manage expected emotional distress. Communicate, consult, and collaborate with health care team. Communicate end-of-life decisions (e.g., advance directives) to family and health care team. Live dignified life. Maintain quality of life. Minimize suffering.
Terminal illness	*I am going to die from this. Why me? Why now? What happens after death? I don't want to die alone.*	Fear, depression, acceptance, withdrawal, isolation, desire to discuss afterlife	End life in desired way (e.g., at home, with family, pain-free). Health care team focuses on needs of family, significant others (grief, bereavement).

SOURCE: Adapted from Loscalzo, M. and Brintzenhofescoz, K. (1998). Brief crisis counseling. In J. C. Holland (Ed.), *Psycho-Oncology* (pp. 662–675). New York: Oxford University Press. Adapted by permission of Oxford University Press, USA.

experience: cancer type, tumor size, pathology, stage, surgical, radiation, or chemotherapy treatments, and so on; while the *illness* is the unique, individual, idiosyncratic, human experience of the disease. This distinction helps to account for the many patients who may have identical or highly similar diseases to other patients, but very different illness experiences. Here the interview is focused on the human experience of the illness—each patient's unique, idiographic experience. Encourage the patient to tell his or her story while you listen attentively, utilizing basic nondirective counseling skills (e.g., paraphrasing, reflection of feelings). For many patients, this is the first opportunity to tell their personal account of what they have been through; how they first did or did not notice symptoms, sought medical care, completed the diagnostic workup, reacted to the diagnosis, told others, made decisions about treatment, and so on. The mental health professional is often the only health care provider whose sole task is to attend, listen closely, and understand nonjudgmentally, while empathizing and developing a working alliance. Many patients find the simple process of telling their stories very helpful and cathartic.

While hearing the patient's "cancer story," it is important to guide the patient to focus on emotions

> *Throughout all that has been happening, how would you describe how you have felt emotionally? How has your mood been?*

as well as coping efforts

> *How would you say you have been coping with all that has happened? What types of things have you been doing to help cope?*

Each story will vary depending upon where the patient is along the clinical course. As the story unfolds, it is important to eventually direct it toward the present.

> *Tell me about your current situation and how things have been most recently.*

To assess accuracy of understanding the biomedical aspects of the disease, it is important to ask about cancer type, stage, prognosis, treatment plan, and so on.

Step 4: Life Context: Family and Social Support, Engagement Versus Giving Up, Developmental Disruptions, and Additional Psychosocial Stressors

As the story continues to unfold, it is important to evaluate the life contexts of social support, family reactions, developmental disruptions, and presence of other, concurrent psychosocial stressors. This usually begins by asking about family.

> *Tell me about your family. How have they reacted to your illness?*

Having a family genogram drawn by the interviewer, prior to the interview, can help guide the focus to key family members and the patient's perception of their emotional reactions, coping skills, and so on. When additional stressors are present, it is during this portion of the interview that the patient will often explain and elaborate. Listening with the conceptual framework of social support and its structural and functional components is important. Consider the size of the social network, the degree of social integration, the depth of social support, perception of availability of support, and willingness to seek and access support, in addition to failed efforts of support; these are all important to listen for in the assessment of emotional, informational, and instrumental support.

> *Do you feel that you are receiving good support from others? Who has been available for you as a source of support? In what ways have they provided support? Overall, how satisfied are you with your social support?*

With the construct of psychosocial adaptation defined as (a) continued, active involvement in daily life, (b) the ability to minimize excessive disruptions to life roles, and (c) skill at regulating emotional distress (Spencer et al., 1998), and with overall engagement versus giving up as a key component to adaptation, it is important to focus the interview on these issues. At opportune times it is important to ask:

> *Have you been able to remain involved in most of the things that are important to you? For example, in what ways has your illness changed or altered your usual routine or roles, such as being a spouse, a parent, or an employee? How do you feel about these changes? Have you tried to minimize these changes, and if so, how?*

These, or similar questions can also serve as a way to open up discussion about developmental disruptions. Often the answers to these questions suggest some delay, alteration, or disruption to what a patient (or family member) might otherwise be doing with her or his life had the patient not been diagnosed with cancer (e.g., *I would love to still be able to be working. I miss my work and didn't really want to have to retire so soon*).

Also, if the patient has not previously mentioned, it becomes important to listen for and directly ask about additional psychosocial stressors.

Step 5: Symptom Assessment and Presence of Mental Disorders

At this point, the interview becomes more structured. A potential transition might be:

> *During any serious illness, people can experience more serious difficulties with emotions such as anxiety and depression. I have a few questions to ask that focus specifically on these types of emotions.*

Ask questions to assess the presence of specific symptoms, indicative of specific diagnosable mental disorders. Use of a structured interview such as the Structured Clinical Interview for DSM (SCID) (Spitzer, Williams, Gibbon, & First, 1992) can provide the specific questions. Assessment of depression and anxiety, as potential indications of overall distress, are warranted with all patients, and other sections of the SCID can be used depending upon identified symptoms (e.g., posttraumatic stress disorder, specific phobia). In addition, the use of self-report questionnaires such as the HADS or PHQ with the intent of gaining information for presence or absence of a mental disorder can also be helpful (see Table 5.1). Most of these questionnaires can be completed by the patient in 5–10 minutes at the conclusion of the interview. It is important to note that many cancer patients will report symptoms of various disorders such as anxiety, depression, and/or posttraumatic stress disorder but will remain below the threshold for meeting the full criteria for a diagnosable disorder. During this portion of the interview, it is also important to gather information about prior history of mental health disorders and/or prior history of mental health treatments.

Step 6: Final Question and Closing

Before concluding the interview, it is important to check with the patient about any other topics of importance to her or him.

Step 7: Treatment Planning

Following the completion of the interview, begin the process of treatment planning. Throughout the interview, you have been developing your definition of the presenting problem(s); evaluating the presence of specific emotional, social, and physical symptoms, and related causal factors; while beginning the case formulation. Important components of the case formulation include the accuracy of understanding the disease, its treatment, potential side effects, prognosis, and so on, the patient perception of social support and its availability, the patient's willingness to access support, and types needed. Finally, a clinical judgment about overall psychosocial adaptation is needed, and it is based on the assessment of the patient's continued active engagement in daily life, attempts to minimize disruptions to life roles (such as spouse, parent, or employee) while being able to manage expected emotional distress. Your clinical judgments of patient understanding, social support, and psychosocial adaptation can be easily communicated to other oncology staff by use of a simple "poor, fair, good, very good, or excellent" rating scheme. When you rate adaptation as poor or fair, intervention is warranted and treatment planning begins at the conclusion of the interview.

Treatment planning is influenced by the severity of distress and the presence or absence of a diagnosable mental disorder. It is important to distinguish differences in severity between patients who may be experiencing normal adaptation to mild or moderate distress (as determined by their score on a Distress Thermometer) from those whose symptoms meet diagnostic criteria for an adjustment disorder or are either below or above the threshold for a diagnosable mental disorder.

CHAPTER SUMMARY

This chapter introduced the concepts of screening and assessment. Background knowledge about screening for psychosocial distress was provided, and best available evidence on the accuracy of screening procedures was reviewed. An exemplar that shows how a well-organized, structured distress-screening program has shown some long-term benefits was described, and summary thoughts about the psychosocial distress screening process and the importance of its efficiency and patient acceptability were provided. A conceptual model for doing a comprehensive psychosocial assessment focused on three broad categories of relevant variables: person, situation, and life context. The end result is to introduce you to the initial step in the process of identifying which cancer patients experiencing psychosocial distress are in need of further services.

6

Individual Psychosocial Health Service Interventions

This chapter focuses on individual interventions for adult cancer patients, experiencing varying levels of severity of distress, anxiety, and depression, often as the result of the lack of resources to address identified psychosocial needs. Some of the most comprehensive resources in psycho-oncology have included psychosocial health services offered via an individual modality. Before beginning a clinical encounter with a new patient, the evidence-based practitioner needs general background knowledge. Some background questions seeking general knowledge about *individual* psychosocial health service interventions include the following:

- What types of individual interventions have been successfully used with cancer patients?
- What theoretical approaches to psychotherapy are most commonly used with cancer patients?
- With whom have these interventions been effective?
- How do these interventions work and how strong are their effects?
- For which types of presenting problems are they most effective?
- What are the specific intervention techniques used; is there an accessible treatment manual?
- How many sessions have been needed?
- How long is each individual session?
- Who provides the interventions?
- How acceptable are these interventions to most patients?

The following summary of general background knowledge is designed to answer some of these background questions.

BACKGROUND KNOWLEDGE

In the three editions of Holland's *Psycho-Oncology* texts (Holland, 1998; Holland & Rowland, 1989; Holland et al., 2010), each has a major section on interventions.

In the earliest edition, individual interventions were emphasized in chapters on psychotherapy, psychopharmacology, and behavioral techniques (relaxation, self-regulatory therapies). In much expanded second and third editions (Holland, 1998; Holland et al., 2010), chapters on screening for distress, brief crisis counseling, psychotherapy, cognitive-behavioral interventions, problem-solving therapy, self-management support, art therapy, telephone counseling, meditation, religion and spiritual beliefs, bedside interventions, and rehabilitation have also emphasized predominantly individual interventions. In the *Handbook of psychotherapy in cancer care* (Watson & Kissane, 2011), a 21-chapter edited book, the first nine chapters present individual models of therapy. Thus, although significant gaps in the evidence base continue to exist, there is a large body of evidence from which to select, the majority of which are interventions provided individually to patients experiencing varying degrees of distress along various locations of the disease continuum.

Research Evidence: Individual Interventions

Summaries of reviews that include individual interventions have been published (Faller et al., 2013; Jacobsen & Jim, 2008) and clinical guidelines exist (see Table 1.2). Meta-analytic reviews of individual interventions have reported increasingly effective interventions as first noted in small to medium effect sizes (Mark & Meyer, 1995) that have grown to medium to large, particularly when patients are prescreened for the presence of elevated levels of emotional distress (Faller et al., 2013). Medium to large effect sizes have been interpreted to mean the patients receiving the intervention score between the 66th to 82nd percentiles on treatment outcomes compared to those not receiving the treatment. Those receiving the intervention are 16 to 32 percentage points above the average patient not receiving the treatment. In success rates, medium effect sizes indicate 60% to 64% success, and large effect sizes indicate 76% to 82% success.

However, to best understand the details of individual psychosocial interventions, reviewing unfiltered primary literature is necessary. A few selected primary studies are summarized in Table 6.1.

Unfiltered Primary Literature

The studies selected for Table 6.1 are exemplars of best available evidence for individual psychosocial health service interventions. They include randomized controlled trials (RCTs) provided along the clinical course from the first clinic visit, through active treatment, periods of recurrence, survivorship, and end-of-life care. Studies were selected that have medium to large sample sizes, positive outcomes—as determined by effect size estimates—and the potential to be disseminated to the local cancer setting.

Study Characteristics

Cancer Type, Stage, and Disease Continuum

The nine studies in Table 6.1 are interventions designed to affect psychosocial distress, anxiety, and/or depression. Of the nine studies, six are of patients with

Table 6.1. Exemplars of Best Available Evidence for Individual Interventions Along the Clinical Course: Study Characteristics and ease of Dissemination

	Study Characteristics		Ease of Dissemination[a]		
Citation/ Clinical Course	**N, Diagnosis, Stage/ No. of Groups**	**Results/Outcomes**	**Intervention Description, Theory, Accessibility[c]**	**Therapist Characteristics**	**Percent Acceptability/ Trainability[b]**
McQuellon et al. (1998) *At first appt.*	120 participants; Median of 40 days since diagnosis; any cancer type; 3 groups (clinic, tour, TAU)	Lower state anxiety/overall distress at 1 week; fewer patients report depressive symptoms greater satisfaction large effect ($d = 1.33$) for state anxiety	1, 15–20-minute orientation to clinic (tour, handout describes procedures, answered questions; L&F No manual No Accessibility	3 masters-level counselors, 1 doctoral student, 1 PhD psychologist	64% (180/279) of eligible agreed 83% (150/180) completed study High trainability[d]
Jacobsen et al. (2002) *At start of chemotherapy*	411 participants (58% breast cancer) at least 4 IV chemo cycles; 3 groups professionally administered, self-administered, TAU	Self- administered did better on physical functioning, role limitations, vitality, mental health than both groups; professionally administered no better than self-administered—less costly small effect ($d = .20$) for emotional adjustment	1, 60-min session professionally administered; 15-minute video, 35-minute audio of PMR, 12-page booklet in self-administered; CBT manualized-RTIP High accessibility	Doctoral-level psychologists, training provided	81% (411/507) of eligible agreed 87% (382/441) completed study Moderate trainability

Manne et al. (2007) *On active treatment*	353 participants; gynecological cancer 55% Stage III or IV, 3 groups (CBT, SC, TAU)	Both groups improved over usual care on depressive symptoms at 6, 9 months (small effects) SC better for those with more physical symptoms and more expressive of positive emotions	6, 60-min weekly sessions + 1 phone booster session CASPT Manualized Low accessibility	11 social workers 8 psychologists (5–15 years therapy experience), 6 hours of training, individual and group supervision	41% (353/852) of eligible agreed 81% (197/242) completed 1–6 sessions Moderate trainability
Enzo et al. (2003) *On active treatment*	132 participants; mixed types (44% breast), prescreened for significant distress; 3 groups (individual PST, PST with significant other, WL)	Both groups improved over waitlist on quality of life, distress, depression; very large effects ($d = 2.04$ to 4.49), clinically significant, long-term effects	10, 90-minute weekly sessions PST Manualized Medium accessibility	15 psychology graduate students, 3 social workers, 15 hours training + weekly supervision	57% (150/262) of eligible agreed 88% (132/150) completed study High trainability
Pitceathly et al. (2009) *On active treatment, during first year post-dx*	465 participants; 69% female; mixed types 26% breast, 24% lymphoma, 20% gynecological; mixed stage 60% at high risk for anxiety/ depression 2 groups (CBT, TAU)	Prevention of anxiety and depression in high-risk patients. CBT group half as likely to be diagnosed with anxiety or depression; Odds ratio = .54	3 weekly sessions (1, 90-min, face-to-face; 2, 45 min by phone) plus educational booklet CT manualized Low accessibility	1 nurse 1 social worker specialized training biweekly supervision	92% (465/506) of eligible agreed 67% (313/465) completed study High trainability

(Continued)

Table 6.1. Continued

	Study Characteristics		Ease of Dissemination[a]		
Citation/ Clinical Course	**N, Diagnosis, Stage/ No. of Groups**	**Results/Outcomes**	**Intervention Description, Theory, Accessibility[c]**	**Therapist Characteristics**	**Percent Acceptability/ Trainability[b]**
Strong et al. (2008) *Post-treatment survivor*	200 participants; 72% female; mixed types; 43% breast, 35% other; 16% gynecological, mixed stages; major depressive disorder; 2 groups (DCPC, TAU)	Reduction in depression symptoms at 3, 6, and 12 months Small effect (d = .34) at 3 months collaborative care intervention feasible, cost effective	2–10, 45-min sessions, over 3 months + 3 months telephone follow-up PST plus collaboration with PCP Manualized Low accessibility	3 oncology nurses + weekly supervision with psychiatrist	60% (200/334) of eligible agreed 84% (85/101) completed 12 months High trainability
Savard et al. (2006) *Metastatic disease*	45 participants; Stage IV breast cancer, 2 groups (CT, WL)	Clinically significant reduction large effects (d = 1.68) for depression posttreatment, maintained at 3, 6 months follow-up	8, 60–90 minute weekly sessions + 3 booster sessions CT Low Accessibility	2 licensed psych. (5 and 15 years experience)	74% (45/61) of eligible agreed 82% (37/45) completed study Low trainability
Mishel et al. (2005)	509 participants; breast cancer, stage unknown;	Better management of uncertainty, small to medium effects (d = .18 to .52), used audiotape and manual >2 times/month	4 weekly phone calls regarding cognitive-behavioral strategies, + 3 audiotapes, 125 pg.	Nurses	55% (575/1,053) of eligible agreed 88% (509/575) completed study

Long-term survivor	5–9 years posttreatment; 2 x 2 design (interv, WL) x (White, AA)		pt. manual; Uncertainty theory Manualized-RTIP High accessibility		High trainability
Chochinov et al. (2011) *End-of-life care*	441 participants; terminally ill, <6-month life expectancy; 3 groups (interv, client-centered care, TAU)	No significant difference in distress, depression, desire for death or suicidality self-reported improved experience of end of life; no effects on primary outcomes	1–3, 60 min sessions (pt. responds to 9 questions, response transcribed, bequeathed to family/ key persons Existentialism, Generativity Manualized Medium accessibility	1 psychiatrist, psychologist 1 palliative care nurse, 3 day training	50% (441/883) of eligible agreed 74% (326/441) completed study High trainability

NOTE. Best available research evidence is always evolving and changing. These selected exemplars were identified as "best available" between May 2011 and December 2013.

[a]Ease of dissemination is operationally defined as an intervention <12 sessions, provided by one qualified provider such as a social worker, psychologist, or nurse (adapted from Jacobsen & Jim, 2008).

[b]Trainability is an estimate of how easy an intervention is to train to others—operationally defined as High = manual available + nondoctoral provider, Moderate = manual available OR treatment provided by nondoctoral provider, Low = no manual and treatment provided by doctoral-level provider (taken from Chorpita et al., 2011).

[c]Accessibility of manual: High = online, Medium = published manual/book/workbook, Low = from researcher only, None = no manual available.

[d]Rated as highly trainable despite lack of a manual since intervention is an orientation tour.

AA, African American; Ca, cancer; CASPT, cognitive, social processing theory; CBT, cognitive-behavioral therapy; CT, cognitive therapy; DCPC, Depression Care for People With Cancer; GS, graduate students; L & F, Lazarus and Folkman's cognitive model of stress; PMR, progressive muscle relaxation; PST, problem-solving therapy; RCT, randomized controlled trial; rec/mets, recurrence or metastases; RTIP, Research Tested Intervention Programs; SC, supportive counseling; SMT, stress management training; TAU, treatment as usual; WL, waitlist.

mixed types of cancer, two are of women with breast cancer (Mishel et al., 2005; Savard et al., 2006), and one of gynecological cancers (Manne et al., 2007). Six of the nine are of patients with either mixed or unreported stages, while two are of patients with advanced disease (Manne et al., 2007; Savard et al., 2006) and one is end-of-life care (Chochinov et al., 2011). Sample sizes range from 45 to 509, with half of the studies having greater than 350 participants.

Results and Outcomes Measured

The primary outcomes measured in these nine studies are psychosocial distress, anxiety, and depression. These represent the majority of individual interventions in psycho-oncology (Jacobsen et al., 2006). Some secondary outcomes include quality of life, vitality, role limitations, fatigue, insomnia, knowledge, dignity, and patient–provider communication. Costs were reported in two studies (Jacobsen et al., 2002; Strong et al., 2008), both reporting reasonable cost benefit.

Overall, these studies report a range of effects from no differences (Chochinov et al., 2011) to very large effect sizes (d = 2.04 to 4.49; Nezu et al., 2003). Most report small to medium effects with two studies (McQuellon et al., 1998; Savard et al., 2006) showing large effects. Most positive outcomes are over the short term, although three studies (Manne et al., 2007; Savard et al., 2006; Strong et al., 2008) report maintenance of benefits over 3- to 12-month follow-ups.

An Introduction to Dissemination

Dissemination is a component of translational research that focuses on transportability of findings to real-life everyday clinical settings. Multiple disciplines in health care are recognizing the significant science-to-practice gap and the need for greater attention to the processes of translating newly discovered science to daily practice (McHugh & Barlow, 2012d). One component of this larger translational process is to consider issues of diffusion, dissemination, and implementation when accessing and appraising background and foreground knowledge. Thus, Table 6.1 includes information about ease of dissemination as evaluated by considering three different components of a studied intervention—components closely tied to the three pillars of evidence-based practice (EBP):

- the intervention itself (i.e., the evidence),
- the therapist/provider (i.e., clinical expertise), and
- the patient preferences and willingness to participate (i.e., patient characteristics).

Characteristics of the *intervention* of importance include

a. its frequency, duration, and overall length;
b. its use of known theoretical approaches and their accompanying techniques;

c. the existence and ease of accessibility of a detailed manual that specifies how to implement the intervention; and
d. the process of training professional staff to implement the intervention.

Characteristics of the *therapist/providers* used in the study are also important, specifically for comparison to those available within a typical psycho-oncology setting. These include characteristics such as the therapist/provider's

a. profession,
b. level of expertise/degree of experience, and
c. need for additional training and/or supervision in the provision of the intervention.

Finally, *patient characteristics* such as their

a. preferences,
b. willingness to participate, and
c. overall acceptance of the intervention

are also important. Calculating the percent of eligible patients who agree to participate in a study and the percent who complete the studied intervention can approximate patient acceptability.

Recommendations have also been offered (Jacobsen & Jim, 2008) about characteristics of studies most likely to increase ease of dissemination. These include the following characteristics of the intervention:

- Should be completed within 12 or fewer sessions
- Should be implemented by one staff person trained at the undergraduate or master's level
- Should be provided with use of an easily accessible manual
- Should include widely known theoretical approaches and techniques
- Should be learned with minimal training and/or supervision
- Should be preferred and acceptable to most patients

Table 6.1 provides ratings of these characteristics of dissemination. Accessibility to a manual, trainability, and patient acceptability are rated. *Accessibility of the treatment manual* is rated from high to none based upon the ease of accessing the manual:

- Online availability is rated as *high*.
- Availability from well-known professional book publishers is rated as *medium*.
- If access is only available by directly contacting the original author, access is rated as *low*.
- If there is no manual, access is rated as *none*.

Trainability of an intervention has been defined (Chorpita et al., 2011) as a combination of ease of access to the treatment manual, plus the level of training (undergraduate, masters, doctoral) of the providers in the original study.

- Trainability is rated as *high* when there is a manual available and the intervention is provided by non-doctoral-level providers.
- *Moderate* trainability is when there is either a manual available or a nondoctoral provider.
- *Low* trainability is when there is no manual and a doctoral-level provider provides treatment.

Finally, *patient acceptability* addresses the key EBP principle of patient characteristics, preferences, values, and context. Acceptability can be estimated by looking closely at the percentages of eligible patients who agree to participate in a study and by the percentage of patients who complete a study intervention. High participation and completion rates imply patient acceptability.

Ease of Dissemination of Individual Interventions

Intervention Descriptions

The interventions described in Table 6.1 range from one to ten sessions, with a mean of 4.6 sessions. Overall minutes per intervention range from as little as 20 minutes in only one session to 900 minutes spread over 10 sessions. The most common frequency is weekly. The majority of sessions took place in the oncology setting, although four of the nine studies also included planned telephone contacts, three of which were for follow-up or booster sessions (Manne et al., 2007; Pitceathly et al., 2009; Strong et al., 2008), while one study was provided exclusively via telephone (Mishel et al., 2005). One study was a single-session clinic tour and orientation (McQuellon et al., 1998), and another single-session study (Jacobsen et al., 2002) was offered in two formats: professional and self-administered.

Theoretical Approaches

The nine studies are heavily influenced by cognitive and cognitive-behavioral theory. Two studies (Pitceathly et al., 2009; Savard et al., 2006) cite cognitive therapy (CT) of Aaron Beck (Beck et al., 1979) as their theoretical foundation; one cites cognitive-behavioral therapy (CBT) (Jacobsen et al., 2002); another cites cognitive, affect, social processing theory (CASPT) (Manne et al., 2007); and one cites problem-solving theory (PST) (Nezu et al., 2003). Lazarus and Folkman's (1984) cognitive model of stress is cited as the theoretical basis for one study (McQuellon et al., 1998), while uncertainty theory, the guiding framework for another study (Mishel, 1990), has its roots in Lazarus and Folkman's model. Two exceptions to this dominance of CBT include (1) the dignity therapy study by Chochinov and colleagues (Chochinov et al., 2011), which is grounded in existentialism and the developmental concept of generativity, and (2) a supportive counseling intervention used as one of the treatment interventions in the Manne and colleagues (2007) study of women with gynecologic cancers. As further background knowledge, basic explanations of each theory and their hypothesized mechanisms of change (i.e., how they work) are described next.

Cognitive-Behavioral Therapy

Jacobsen and colleagues' (2002) study of two forms of stress management training—as preparation for chemotherapy—incorporates traditional behavioral techniques (abdominal breathing, progressive muscle relaxation, coping self-statements) for managing stress with the goal of preserving quality of life. With an improved set of specific coping strategies, it is hypothesized that patients will use these skills at various times throughout their experience with cancer treatment to maintain quality of life and remain actively involved in daily activities, and to experience less disruption to daily roles, less pain, and fewer other physical problems. The mechanism of change to decrease distress, anxiety, and depression is through the use of specific cognitive-behavioral coping skills.

Cognitive Therapy

Two studies (Pitceathly et al., 2009; Savard et al., 2006) cite CT as the theoretical framework for their interventions. One utilized CT techniques to prevent anxiety and/or depressive disorders, with patients identified as "at risk" for either mental disorder. In three individual sessions, patients were encouraged to tell the story of their cancer experience while the therapist, in collaboration with the patient, helped to identify illness-related concerns/problems and their underlying thoughts and beliefs. These patient-generated examples were then used to identify the effectiveness of existing coping strategies. The cognitive model of emotion was explained and related educational information was provided, targeted at identifying potential maladaptive thoughts and the development of more effective cognitive coping strategies. The other study (Savard et al., 2006) was a direct adaptation of Beck's CT for depression for use with women with Stage IV metastatic breast cancer, who had been screened for the presence of significant symptoms of depression. The adaptation involved identifying specific needs of women with metastatic cancer and establishing goals of maintaining daily activities, identifying negative thoughts, and using cognitive restructuring to modify dysfunctional or irrational thoughts. As in traditional CT, the mechanism of change is thought to be the experience of less negative and more positive emotions by first awareness of and, next, alteration in thought processes related to a range of emotions, particularly those thoughts identified as dysfunctional, irrational, unrealistic, or, in other forms problematic. This same mechanism is hypothesized to be applicable in these studies to both prevent the onset of clinical depression (Pitceathly et al., 2009) and to treat already existing clinical levels of depression (Savard et al., 2006).

Cognitive Model of Stress

Lazarus and Folkman's well-known and highly useful cognitive model of stress is directly cited in one of the studies (McQuellon et al., 1998) and serves as the foundation for the theory of uncertainty in illness (Mishel, 1990), as used in another study (Mishel et al., 2005). The model specifies a cognitive process in which people engage in reaction to life stressors. Two forms of appraisal—*primary* and *secondary*—are noted in which primary appraisal involves a focus on the nature of the stressor(s) and a determination if they are meaningful to the individual and if they are likely to cause harm, threat, or a challenge to the individual's overall well-being. Secondary appraisal involves the cognitive process of evaluating one's coping skills and abilities as they relate to the specifics of the stressful event. The balance between primary (perception of the nature of a stressful event) and secondary (perceived skills, abilities, and resources a person brings to the event) appraisal determines the level of distress. Thus, when a cancer patient encounters a stressful event, if her primary appraisal is high and her secondary appraisal is low, she will experience a high degree of distress; conversely, if secondary appraisal of skills and resources is high and the stressful event is appraised as low, her distress is low or absent. This model also focuses on coping strategies organized into two broad types: *problem-focused*, use of active, engaged, problem-oriented strategies that look for solutions; and *emotion-focused*, more passive internal strategies designed to manage emotional reactions. Both are very applicable to coping with the many problems and emotions associated with the experience of cancer.

Hypothesized mechanisms of change in this model include increased awareness of the appraisal processes; alterations of thoughts within the appraisal processes; and the recognition, development, and enhancement of coping resources and strategies. Thus, in the McQuellon and colleagues study (1998), the cancer diagnosis and initial clinic visit are the stressful events and successful participation in the clinic orientation results in more knowledge, comfort, and familiarity with the setting, thus altering cognitive appraisals and increasing coping resources and skills.

In the uncertainty management intervention (Mishel et al., 2005), the theory proposes that uncertainty is likely when components of an illness include characteristics such as inconsistency, randomness, unpredictability, and/or lack of information, all common characteristics of breast cancer, particularly for long-term survivors. Life events that trigger uncertainty do so as a result of primary and secondary appraisal processes in which the patients' abilities to cope are perceived to be insufficient relative to the perceived demands of the situation. This imbalance results in distress, anxiety, and/or depression. Thus, in the uncertainty management study, a variety of emotion-focused and problem-focused coping strategies were taught, with change hypothesized to occur via altered appraisal of both the demands of the situation and available resources, skills, and abilities.

Cognitive-Affective-Social Processing Theory

Cognitive-affective-social processing theory (CASPT) proposes that successful adaptation to difficult life events like cancer involves actively dealing with all three of the components of the experience—the cognitive, affective, and social.

Cognitive processing involves coping with life assumptions that are challenged by cancer, *affective processing* involves learning to express emotions and to tolerate negative emotional experiences that come with cancer, and *social processing* involves talking with others about one's experiences. Helpful processing of any of the three types is thought to be enhanced by good communication with others, receipt of social support, venting of emotions, learning to tolerate negative emotions, use of acceptance and positive reframing, and less use of avoidance and denial. In the CBT intervention with women with gynecologic cancers (Manne et al., 2007), six weekly sessions plus one telephone booster session focused on a variety of skills to better process cognitive, affective, and social experiences associated with cancer. The proposed mechanism of change is thought to occur via enhanced processing of cognitive, affective, and social experiences associated with gynecologic cancer, resulting in less distress and better quality of life.

Problem-Solving Therapy

Problem-solving therapy (PST) has been modified and adapted for use with cancer patients predominantly as an individual intervention in a project titled Project Genesis (Nezu et al., 2003). Project Genesis conceptualized the experience of cancer as both a significant source of stress and a series of sometimes ongoing problems and daily hassles. Taken together, these sources of stress increase the likelihood of a person experiencing significant distress, such as depression. However, if one is good at problem solving, this skill can serve as a moderator/buffer of the relationship between cancer stressors to distress. As noted earlier, PST found very large effect sizes (d = 2.04 to 4.49). The PST model conceptualizes improved problem solving as a mechanism of change as it moderates the degree of distress a person diagnosed with cancer may experience. In the Nezu and colleagues' (2003) study, they directly tested this mechanism by noting whether improved problem solving was associated with less distress, noting that this was the case. This is thus one of the few studies where a hypothesized mechanism of change was directly tested; decreased distress was associated with improved problem solving.

Existential Theory and Generativity

Theoretical concepts from existential philosophy (Yalom, 1980) and the developmental concept of generativity (Erikson, 1950) are key concepts in dignity therapy (Chochinov & McKeen, 2011), a novel psychotherapy for use with terminally ill patients. The existential concerns of isolation, meaning, loss of freedom, and particularly death are all highlighted when experiencing cancer, particularly at the end of life. Generativity, an important developmental task of later life, emphasizes the desire to contribute, to give back something meaningful to those persons loved and, by so doing, have a sense of a lasting legacy that may live beyond oneself. Dignity therapy is designed to address these major existential issues. It is a structured psychotherapeutic intervention with persons at the end of life, in which the therapist helps a dying patient reminisce, consider his or her most cherished values—that which has made life most meaningful—and to generate a legacy document that communicates these ideas, and prepares it to be bequeathed to significant others. In so doing, the hypothesized mechanism of change is to use time at the end of one's life to experience a greater sense of generativity that can serve to maintain a sense of dignity, marked by respect, honor, meaning, and quality of life.

Supportive Counseling

As discussed in Chapter 3, the paradox of supportive counseling/psychotherapy in cancer care is that it has been considered "the single most important tool of the psycho-oncologist" (Lederberg & Holland, 2011, p. 3), and yet it is also the least understood. There is no consensus on its components, very little agreement on how to define it or what its mechanisms of action are, and very little empirical support for its use (Lederberg & Holland, 2011). However, in Table 6.1, the Manne et al. (2007) study of women with gynecologic cancer used supportive counseling as one of the three experimental conditions, and it was found to be better than the CBT intervention and the usual care condition for a subgroup of the sample—for those women with more physician-rated physical symptoms and/or those women who were more likely to express positive emotions. In the Manne and colleagues' (2007) study, mechanisms of change in SC were thought to be encouraging emotional expression, validation, support of coping strategies, and improved self-esteem and autonomy. In a later analysis (Manne et al., 2008), SC was associated with cancer-related emotional expression, emotional processing, positive reappraisal, and seeking instrumental support, but only positive appraisal was found to be a mediator for fewer symptoms of depression.

Collaborative Care Model

Although collaborative care is not a theoretical approach in the typical sense, it is important to note that one study from Table 6.1 (Pitceathly et al., 2009) utilized a research approach that tested a collaborative care model. Despite the development of NCCN Guidelines for the management of distress in cancer care, few studies have been designed to test a comprehensive, complex *system of care* for cancer patients (Jacobsen, 2009), in which screening is followed by the use of an evidence-based protocol for treatment that includes close collaboration between specialty and primary care and careful follow-up to measure long-term effects. Pitceathly and colleagues (2009) have tested such a model, taking from a much longer tradition of research in collaborative care of depression in primary care (Gilbody et al., 2006). Their findings note that a collaborative care model offering a complex, nurse-delivered intervention is feasible, cost-effective, and decreases symptoms of depression in cancer patients at 3, 6, and 12 months. The mechanism of change may be at the systems level, where change within the health care delivery model results in improved identification and more effective psychosocial and pharmacologic interventions to reduce depressive symptoms.

Dissemination Conclusions

Taken as a whole, the nine studies in Table 6.1 show good to very good dissemination potential. Nearly all have manuals available (two online); most interventions are short term with high trainability, very good patient acceptability, and they represent interventions spread out across the clinical course of the disease. Two studies (Jacobsen et al., 2002; Mishel et al., 2005) stand out as relatively easy to disseminate because their treatment manuals and a variety of related materials are freely available online through the Research Tested Intervention Programs (RTIP) Web site.

- The Jacobsen and colleagues' (2002) study of a stress management intervention for patients preparing to start chemotherapy is easily disseminated because of (a) the ease of availability of resources via RTIP; (b) the familiarity by most health care professionals of the intervention components of paced abdominal breathing, progressive muscle relaxation, and use of coping self-statements; and (c) its cost-effectiveness when provided as a patient self-administered intervention.
- The Mishel and colleagues study (Mishel et al., 2005)—also available via RTIP—is easy to disseminate; the patient audiotapes, instruction booklet, and patient manuals are first given to patients and the intervention is then provided via four telephone calls by nurses.

One other study, the McQuellon and colleagues (1998) one-session cancer center orientation tour, is also easy to disseminate. Although no manual is provided, this should not slow dissemination because the nature of each clinic's setting, physical facility, clinical procedures, and support programs dictates the development of unique, center-specific booklets. Also, the one-session orientation provided by non-doctoral-level providers makes this orientation intervention easy to disseminate. The selection of which studies to try to disseminate may also be determined by where, on the clinical course, interventions are most needed. As indicated, the studies are implemented from the very first appointment, through active treatments, into posttreatment survivorship and at the end of life. Reference citations for manualized interventions and related resources are provided in Box 6.1.

Summary of the Evidence Base for Individual Interventions

The evidence base for individual interventions, as represented by nine selected exemplars in Table 6.1, indicates that there are a number of effective, potentially disseminable interventions that decrease the distress, anxiety, and depression experienced by cancer patients diagnosed with a variety of types and stages of disease. PST for mixed-type patients, prescreened for significant psychological distress (Nezu et al., 2003), was found to have very large effect sizes; CT for advanced breast cancer patients (Savard et al., 2006) and a brief orientation to the oncology clinic (McQuellon et al., 1998) report large effect sizes; while most other studies found small to medium effects. One study has no demonstrated efficacy (Chochinov et al., 2011) on primary outcomes but has demonstrated feasibility to provide a unique approach to end-of-life care. Various theoretical approaches

Box 6.1

Accessibility of Manuals: Reference Citations for Manualized Interventions and Related Resources From Exemplars of Best Available Individual Interventions

At First Appointment

McQuellon et al. (1998)—No manual.

At Start of Chemotherapy

Jacobsen et al. (2002)—Manualized—Program manual available online via Research Tested Intervention Programs (RTIPs). Retrieved December 20, 2014, from http://rtips.cancer.gov/rtips/programDetails.do?programId=289799

Related Resources for Professionally Administered Stress Management Training

Burish, T. G., Snyder, S. L., & Jenkins, R. A. (1991). Preparing patients for cancer chemotherapy: Effect of coping preparation and relaxation interventions. *Journal of Consulting and Clinical Psychology, 59*, 518–525.

Carey, M. P., & Burish, T. G. (1987). Providing relaxation training to cancer chemotherapy patients: A comparison of three delivery techniques. *Journal of Consulting and Clinical Psychology, 55*, 732–737.

Meichenbaum, D. (1985). *Stress inoculation training.* New York, NY: Pergamon Press.

Turk, D. C., Meichenbaum, D., & Genest, M. (1983). *Pain and behavioral medicine: A cognitive-behavioral perspective.* New York, NY: Guilford Press.

On Active Treatment

Manne et al. (2007)—Manuals available from the authors.

Nezu, A. M., Nezu, C. M., Felgoise, S. H., McClure, K. W., & Houts, P. S. (2003)—Manualized.

Nezu, A. M., Nezu, C. M., Friedman, S. H., Faddis, S., & Houts, P. S. (1998). *Helping cancer patients cope: A problem-solving approach.* Washington, DC: American Psychological Association.

Metastatic Disease

Savard et al. (2006)—Manual adapted from:

Beck, A. T., et al. (1979). *Cognitive therapy of depression.* New York, NY: The Guilford Press.

Long-Term Survivorship

Mishel et al. (2005)—Study indicates manualized, but no indication of manual availability.

End-of-Life Care

Chochinov et al. (2011)—Manualized.
Chochinov, H. M. (2012). *Dignity therapy: Final words for final days*. New York, NY: Oxford University Press.

---

are used, yet most are influenced by cognitive and cognitive-behavioral theory. Supportive counseling has been shown to be beneficial and an existential approach to end-of-life care is feasible. One novel study tested a collaborative care model, an important step forward in demonstrating efficacy of integrative care in oncology. Trainability of these interventions is good as manuals are available and the predominant approaches are generally well known among mental health providers. Finally, patient acceptability seems particularly high among these interventions, as dropout rates were quite low.

CASE EXAMPLES: HOW TO DO EVIDENCE-BASED PRACTICE OF INDIVIDUAL INTERVENTIONS

In addition to recommended interventions across the clinical course, this chapter offers, in significant detail, two case examples of how to do EBP. The case examples show how to do EBP in psycho-oncology by combining the six core competencies: AAA TIE (ask, access, appraise, translate, integrate, evaluate) across components of the disease continuum. As noted by Norcross and colleagues (2008), when making clinical decisions on how to integrate research evidence, clinical expertise, and patient characteristics, clinicians ultimately have three options regarding the evidence: adopt, adapt, or abandon. The two case examples in this chapter illustrate a straightforward adoption of best available evidence and a more complex adaptation using two concurrent interventions to augment the primary treatment. Both examples are written in second person, as has been done in other EBP training programs, to highlight the internal clinical decision-making process of an experienced psycho-oncologist.

Case Example 1—KM: Normal Adjustment to Initial Diagnosis of Gynecologic Cancer

Referral Information

In the midst of a busy day at the Cancer Center, you happen upon Dr. Smithson, a medical oncologist with whom you have worked for a number of years. He quickly launches into an explanation of a patient he has just seen earlier this morning. You wish you had more time and privacy to talk, but know that is not likely to happen given the rush of the day. He explains, "The patient, KM, is a 62-year-old, White, married female, referred to me after her PCP did some of the initial workup and suspected a malignancy. I need to finish the workup, but at this point, I suspect it's some type of gynecologic cancer, most likely ovarian or uterine. Although she was pretty well informed and seemed to understand what was going on, once I mentioned further scans, she just got really tearful and explained that she feels overwhelmed, has little support, and has been crying a lot. She seemed pretty depressed. She is married, but it sounds like her family and husband are not very helpful. So I explained about you and suggested she schedule with you. She is thinking about it, and I think she probably will. Thanks! Oh, if you think she needs an antidepressant just let me know."

Although you have a few more questions, Dr. S is gone before you can think to ask them, and you begin the process of preparing to see this new patient. You check your calendar and see that she did schedule in about a week. Before doing any formal preparation, you find yourself thinking back about other patients you have seen with ovarian, fallopian tube, cervical, or other gynecologic cancers, and you realize there is quite a variety in type, seriousness of the disease, and prognoses. You will need to gather some general background information first.

You Begin the Evidence-Based Practice Process

Step 1: Ask Specific Clinical Questions, Both Background and Foreground

You identify the following *biomedical* background questions:

- What are the various types of gynecologic cancers and how serious are they?
- What are the varying prognoses for various types?
- What is involved in the initial workup for most gynecologic cancers?
- What treatments might be recommended: surgery, chemotherapy, radiation?
- How rigorous are the treatments in terms of recovery time, side effects, and overall impact on quality of life?

These initial background questions focus on the biomedical or disease component of this patient's experience, and you consider looking for answers in various easily accessible, traditional sources. You might look for an electronic medical textbook, the NCI's PDQ statement specifically about gynecologic cancers, or even the American Cancer Society's (ACS) Web site with basic information on cancer types. You decide to begin with the ACS site (http://www.cancer.org/Research/CancerFactsFigures/), where you can find up-to-date facts and figures as well as easy-to-read basic information. You read about gynecologic cancers, and you see that uterine cancers are more prevalent (6% of all new cancers in women) than ovarian cancer (3%), but the prognosis for uterine is better (5-year survival rates of 84%) than ovarian (5-year survival rates of 46%). You also find information about cervical cancer, and note that its prevalence is less than uterine or ovarian and its prognosis is similar to uterine (5-year survival rates of

72%). In looking at survival rates, you realize you will first need to know the stage before arriving at very meaningful information, and you decide to move on, knowing you can eventually get staging information from Dr. Smithson later. You also note on the ACS site some helpful explanations of various diagnostic procedures via imaging (CT scan, MRI, chest X-ray, PET) and you quickly review them, anticipating your patient might have questions about these. You also quickly look over the general treatment information for ovarian, cervical, and uterine cancers. You notice again that without staging information, it is hard to know specifics. However, you note that for all three gynecologic cancers, surgeries, chemotherapy, and radiation therapies are possible.

You also identify the following *psychosocial background* questions:

- What is the best way to screen and assess for overall distress?
- What is the prevalence of depression in cancer patients?
- What is the best way to evaluate symptoms of distress such as anxiety and depression?
- What is the best way to distinguish different levels of severity of distress?
- What would be considered normal adjustment given the current biomedical realities?
- You find yourself again asking a classic psychotherapy question—What treatment (i.e., techniques) and by whom (therapist characteristics) is most effective for this particular patient (i.e., patient characteristics) (Paul, 1967), experiencing her specific concerns, at this point early in the diagnosis of some type of gynecologic cancer?
- What is the best available evidence for treatment of distress/anxiety/depression for patients with gynecologic cancers? Is any particular treatment better than others?
- What types of social support are available for cancer patients, and are any types more important than others?

You already know answers to some of these questions from you prior clinical experience. You are very familiar with the NCCN Distress Guidelines (National Comprehensive Cancer Network, 2014), and you are knowledgeable about the general psychotherapy literature—particularly the research on empirically supported relationships (ESRs) (Norcross, 2002, 2011), empirically supported treatments (ESTs) (Chambless & Hollon, 1998), and the skills of the psychotherapist (Crits-Christoph et al., 1991). You realize little consensus exists on the relative contribution of each of these components to effective psychotherapy (Norcross & Lambert, 2011), yet you know recent findings support their integration by attention to both the general elements of effective therapy relationships and patient characteristics on which to modify these general elements. You have been using a recommended format for the assessment of psychosocial adaptation (see Chapter 5) that is a semistructured, supportive clinical interview (Nicholas & Veach, 2000), and you routinely evaluate symptoms of anxiety and depression.

However, you do need to search for answers to some of the other psychosocial background questions, so you first look for filtered resources that might help (see Figs. 4.3 and 4.4). You wonder if there are national guidelines for treatment of depression in cancer patients. You realize there are a number of good sources of information such as the NCI's PDQ Depression statement (http://www.cancer.gov/cancertopics/coping/emotionaleffects#Depression) or the small Quick Reference for Oncology Clinicians (Holland, Greenberg, & Hughes, 2006), and so you check the National Guidelines Clearinghouse (http://www.guideline.gov/browse/by-topic.aspx) and find a guideline for depression in adults with chronic health problems (http://www.guideline.gov/content.aspx?id=15522&search=depression#Section396). In the "scope" section of this guideline, it mentions cancer as one example of a chronic health problem. It recommends a stepped-care approach to treatment of depression, emphasizing the severity of symptoms from subthreshold with mild to moderate symptoms through treatment-resistant and severe symptoms with appropriate steps indicated. The guideline reminds you of the importance of attending to co-occurring anxiety and to routinely assess for symptoms of suicide. You also know from past familiarity with NCI's PDQ statement on depression that about 15%–25% of cancer patients experience depression and from the PDQ statement on "normal adjustment" the distinction between normal and pathologic levels of anxiety and depression in recently diagnosed cancer patients.

You wonder about literature specifically on gynecologic cancers, and you check out the Cancer Control P.L.A.N.E.T. site, where you have previously learned that some of the Research Tested Intervention Programs (RTIP) (http://rtips.cancer.gov/rtips/searchResults.do) have been helpful. However, this time you do not find any literature specifically targeted to women with gynecologic cancers. You do find some meta-analytic review articles (Osborn et al., 2006; Rehse & Pukrop, 2003) indicating a number of effective psychosocial interventions for cancer patients in general. You believe you have enough basic background information, and you move on and formulate some *foreground questions.*

- If the patient is, in fact, experiencing depression, how severe are her symptoms? Is she also experiencing comorbid anxiety symptoms?
- Is this patient interested in participating in ongoing psychotherapy/counseling to alleviate symptoms of distress?
- If so, would she prefer any particular psychotherapeutic approach? Would she prefer individual or group?
- What does she think/feel about taking medication for depression or anxiety symptoms?
- Does she have any past experience with mental health services and, if so, what were they and how did they go? Do these experiences influence her current treatment preferences?
- Are there any demographic, cultural, disease, developmental, or treatment-related factors that might influence her treatment preferences?

The first clinical interview: Assessment of psychosocial adaptation, initial establishment of psychotherapy relationship with general elements of empathy, alliance, and collaboration on goals/tasks.

You meet KM and escort her back to your office. She is unaccompanied and looks both frightened and tired. You begin your psychosocial assessment interview with a brief description of

- *who you are;*
- *what the intent of this first appointment is (i.e., hear her story, validate her experience with cancer to date, assess the severity of any psychological symptoms, if feasible answer questions regarding further workup/treatment, set goals for future appointments if needed); and*
- *then you explain confidentiality and its limits, and you have her sign your consent-for-treatment forms.*

You then begin the interview by asking her to tell you the story of her recent medical care and diagnosis. She hesitates, becomes a bit choked up, and simply says, "It's been very scary, such a shock. I was fine, my health was good, and then all of a sudden this!" You learn that she had been having some vague, nonspecific abdominal pains for a few months and went to her family physician who treated her for gastroenteritis and irritable bowel. When her symptoms did not improve, her physician started additional tests. Then she says, "They found something on a scan that looked alarming, and they did a biopsy. It came back cancerous, and now Dr. S wants me to do more scans so they can know more details. I have been very upset, I can't sleep, I have been crying almost all day, every day, and my family—particularly my husband—doesn't seem to understand the seriousness of this! They just don't seem to get it!"

Throughout this early part of the interview, you adopt a supportive, patient-centered approach, as you want to be certain to allow the opportunity for her to feel comfortable to express her emotions. As the "telling of the story" section of the interview begins to end, you become more directive in asking specific questions, assessing particular symptoms (overall distress, depression, anxiety, any physical complaints), checking any past history of mental health services, asking about how family is doing, and evaluating her perception of emotional, instrumental, and informational support with the goal of determining overall psychosocial adaptation—defined as consisting of three parts (continued involvement in daily life, minimizing disruptions to life roles, and managing expected emotional distress).

From Karen, you learn that her symptoms of anxiety seem within the normal range (worried about upcoming scans, possible future treatments, long-term prognosis, and what this will all mean for her future and her family) as they are focused on the uncertainties and unknowns of the future. She acknowledges that her anxiety will probably get better when she gets more medical information. Her symptoms of depression are very closely interwoven with those of anxiety and include frequent sad mood, very frequent tearfulness, some sleep disturbance (early morning wakening), decreased appetite, and thoughts of death. You carefully evaluate for suicide and learn that she has not been having any suicidal ideation, nor plan or intent, but rather her thoughts of death are if her cancer was not treatable or of an advanced stage. She clearly does not want to die and indicates she has lots of reasons to live.

At the end of the interview, she completes the Hospital Anxiety Depression Scale (HADS) and the PHQ-9 and GAD-7 self-report screening questionnaires for additional data to both assist in diagnosis and ongoing measurement of outcome. Her HADS total score of 23 (anxiety = 13, depression = 10), PHQ-9 score of 10, and GAD-7 of 14 indicate symptoms of depression and anxiety within a moderate range.

Ultimately, you determine that her symptoms of distress (anxiety and depression) are subthreshold to any mental disorder, and although they are of concern, she does not meet full criteria for any anxiety or mood disorder. By the end of the interview, she seems a bit calmer and indicates she found it helpful to have a chance to talk to someone other than family/friends who listened, allowed her to express her feelings, and validated her experience. She agrees with you that it might be of help to continue to do so in the future, particularly if she gets more bad news or faces difficult treatments. You also learn she has never had any prior mental health services and that she has no particular preference regarding counseling/psychotherapy approaches. She would prefer to avoid any antidepressant medication for now, since she is concerned that she will probably be taking other new medicines for her treatments. You support that opinion by sharing with her your thoughts that antidepressants probably are not warranted right now anyway because she is only reporting mild to moderate symptoms of depression. You both agree to meet again in 2 weeks. By then she expects to know more and you anticipate knowing the disease stage and potential treatment plan from Dr. S.

Post–Psychosocial Assessment Interview: Summary of Key Patient Characteristics

- 62-year-old, White, married female, high school graduate, employed
- Recently diagnosed gynecologic malignancy
- Moderately severe symptoms of anxiety and depression, determined to be subthreshold for any mental disorder
- Poor emotional social support from husband and family
- No past history of mental health services or counseling/psychotherapy
- Not inclined to try antidepressant medications

Step 2: Accessing the Best Available Research Evidence

The filtered, secondary resources (guidelines clearinghouse, PDQ statements), although helpful for general background information, did not answer specific foreground questions. Thus, you design a search strategy of the unfiltered primary literature, using the sequential steps recommended by Gibbs (2003).

Step 1 is to formulate a PICO question. The two closely related PICO questions are formulated to guide your search. The first question has no C (comparison treatment or comparator) as it asks the absolute efficacy question.

> *For a 62-year-old female, recently diagnosed with gynecologic cancer, with mild to moderate symptoms of depression and anxiety and poor emotional support, what is the best available counseling/psychotherapy for alleviating symptoms of distress and maintaining psychosocial adaptation?*

The second PICO question asks a relative efficacy question by adding a comparison treatment component.

> *For a 62-year-old female, recently diagnosed with gynecologic cancer, with mild to moderate symptoms of depression and anxiety and poor emotional support, is supportive counseling better than cognitive-behavioral therapy for alleviating symptoms of distress and maintaining psychosocial adaptation?*

You chose to search for these two approaches since you are competent to provide either. *Step 2* involves listing keywords or terms that correspond with each of the four PICO components, and *step 3* involves listing possible synonyms or known terms from various controlled vocabulary databases (e.g., PsycINFO, CINAHL, and PubMed).

P—gynecologic(al), ovarian, uterine, cervical, distress, depression, anxiety, cancer, neoplasm, oncology
I—psychosocial, counseling, psychotherapy, psychological intervention, psychological treatment
C—supportive counseling, cognitive-behavior(al) therapy
O—adaptation, adjustment, quality of life

Step 4 is to begin the search, in this case of unfiltered, primary literature such as PsycINFO, CINAHL, and Medline. These can be accessed via many libraries by use of EBSCOhost. The search terms used were as follows:

> neoplasm OR cancer and SUBJECT (gynecolog* OR ovarian OR uterine) and SUBJECT (psychotherapy OR supportive counseling OR psychological intervention OR cognitive-behavioral therapy)

Twenty different articles were identified. Of the 20, 6 were studies of genetic testing/counseling, 5 were nonintervention studies, 2 were pilot or feasibility studies with small sample sizes (n = 24–33), 1 was a study with low-income Latinas, 1 was a guided imagery intervention, 1 was a qualitative study that did not report quantitative outcomes, and 1 had no abstract available. The remaining three were all part of a study testing two different psychotherapies against usual care (Manne et al., 2008, 2010; Manne, Ostroff, & Winkel, 2007). In this study, 353 women with gynecological cancers were randomly assigned to one of three groups: (a) supportive counseling, (b) a form of cognitive-behavioral therapy focused on coping and enhanced communication, or (c) usual care. Seven, 1-hour, weekly sessions of the two primary interventions were provided. The Manne and colleagues (2007) articles appear most relevant and may prove to be best available evidence. Further appraisal is needed.

Step 3: Appraising the Research Evidence

A series of recommended steps for appraising the research evidence (see Chapter 4) were applied to the Manne and colleagues study (2007). As an APA publication, the journal follows the JARS (American Psychological Association [APA] JARS Working Group, 2008) reporting standards and has good transparency and details of procedures used. Using a critical appraisal form from the Evidence-Based Mental Health Web site in the United Kingdom (http://cebmh.warne.ox.ac.uk/cebmh/education_critical_appraisal.htm), it was determined that participants were randomly assigned, stratified for level of depression at baseline, but not "blinded" to which group they were in (not unusual for this type of a study since it is not feasible to blind therapists and often not desirable to blind participants).

Participants were *not* selected to participate based upon elevated scores on any measures of depression or distress, suggesting this is not a study of patients diagnosed with a mental disorder, but rather a study of patients experiencing a range of severity of distress and depression. No significant differences were found in pretreatment demographic and medical characteristics across groups and treatment attendance (>60% attended at least five of seven sessions), and treatment integrity (a procedure to evaluate adherence to and quality of interventions) was good (90% across six sessions). The two experimental treatment groups were treated equally and were compared against "usual care," which was only minimally described and does not appear equal to the two treatment groups. The interventions are described in good detail and access to the treatment manuals is available. Outcome measures used are well described, frequently used in similar research, and are valid and reliable. Intent-to-treat analyses were done, indicating all participants who began the trial were accounted for.

Results showed that participants in both intervention groups reported fewer depressive symptoms than those in the usual care group at 6- and 9-month follow-ups. Also, women whose physical symptoms increased over time and/or were more expressive of positive emotions did better with the supportive counseling intervention. Given the location and participant characteristics, this study has pretty good generalizability to community cancer centers and to settings where many participants may not have college degrees. Finally, both interventions were rated as very acceptable and highly regarded by participants. Your appraisal of this study indicates that it is well done and is good empirical evidence for use of either supportive counseling or the cognitive-behavioral (CBT) form of psychotherapy.

Session 2—First Counseling Session: Focus on Treatment Planning and Patient Collaboration

Two weeks have passed and you have your second appointment with KM. During the past 2 weeks, she has completed the additional workup and now has a diagnosis. She explains, "Unfortunately, the doctors are telling me this is most likely ovarian cancer, and I am now scheduled for surgery next week. As I understand it, it won't be until after the surgery that they know for sure what the stage is, but given my earliest symptoms in my stomach, they think it's probably spread outside the ovaries and so would be a more advanced stage." She seems relatively composed when telling you this, but then, "I catch myself telling others this and it seems surreal, like I am talking about somebody else . . . it can't be me, I'm not even very sick!" She does acknowledge, however, that she thinks she is a little less distressed than 2 weeks ago, since "at least I know what it is and what we are dealing with." She explains, "Don't get me wrong, I hate this, but at least it's no longer a complete mystery."

After listening attentively and paraphrasing and reflecting Karen's thoughts and emotions, you then move on to discuss your ideas on how counseling might be of help. You explain to her that you found good research that suggests two different forms of counseling/psychotherapy have been found helpful for women just recently diagnosed with ovarian cancer and experiencing distress (i.e., symptoms of depression). She asks you about the two forms and how they differ. You explain that in many ways they are very similar, but one is more structured than the other. In the more structured form (CBT), "We would be talking about specific coping strategies. I would be teaching you certain skills and strategies that we would practice in here, and you would be asked to do some practice at home. You will learn about stress management, problem solving, specific ways of coping, the impact that ovarian cancer may have on you, and generally how to cope effectively. In the less structured form, I would be mostly listening to you and helping you understand, express, and deal with the emotional aspects of what you are going through. You will be encouraged to talk about what is most important to you about what you are experiencing, identify how you feel about what you are experiencing, and how to express those feelings. I will mostly help you identify your ways of coping and encourage effective coping strategies."

By the end of the session, Karen indicates she thinks she would be more interested in the less structured form where she could simply come in and talk about whatever she had been experiencing lately. She seems particularly interested in the potential for emotional support from counseling because she continues to indicate she has not gotten much from her husband and family. She is leery of having to learn and practice anything new because she feels like her life is going to be very busy soon with cancer treatments. Then she asks, "I have heard about others who have kept journals—written about what they are going through—during treatment. Do you think that would be any help?" In general, you indicate probably, yes, but that you would look into it. You plan to meet again after she has completed and is beginning to recover from the surgery (probably 3 weeks or so), at which time you explain you both will know more of the details of her treatment plan, you will know more about journaling, and the two of you can begin the supportive counseling that you explained today.

Post Session 2: Summary of Key Patient Characteristics

- 62-year-old, White, married female, recently diagnosed with ovarian cancer, stage unknown, but likely advanced (Stage III or IV)
- Moderate symptoms of anxiety (GAD-7 = 14) and depression (PHQ-9 = 10), determined to be subthreshold for any mental disorder
- Insightful, willing and able to express emotions
- Poor emotional social support from husband and family
- No past history of mental health services or counseling/psychotherapy
- Not inclined to try antidepressant medications
- Interested in supportive counseling over CBT
- Curious about benefits of "journaling"

Post Session 2—Additional Accessing Literature Regarding "Journaling"
Step 1 involved formulating another PICO question:

> *For a 62-year-old female, recently diagnosed with gynecologic cancer, moderate symptoms of depression and anxiety and poor emotional support, is "journaling" (writing about the emotional aspects of her experience) better than not "journaling" for alleviating symptoms of distress and maintaining psychosocial adaptation?*

As before, steps 2 and 3 are to list keywords/terms, their synonyms, or related known terms from various controlled vocabulary databases (e.g., PsycINFO, CINAHL, and PubMed) that correspond with each of the four PICO components such as:

P—gynecologic(al), ovarian, uterine, cervical, distress, depression, anxiety, cancer, neoplasm, oncology
I—journaling, writing, emotion*
C—no comparator in this question
O—adaptation, adjustment, quality of life

Step 4 is to begin the search, in this case of unfiltered, primary literature such as PsycINFO, CINAHL, and Medline. Once again this was done via EBSCOhost. The search terms used were as follows:

neoplasm OR cancer and SUBJECT (journal* OR writing) and
SUBJECT (emotion* OR express*) AND randomized AND controlled AND trial AND gynecologic*

With this search strategy, no results were found. The search term gynecologic* was removed and five results were found. Of the five studies, two were on women with breast cancer, one was with children, one with grief and bereavement, and one with persons with fibromyalgia. Thus, it appears there are no retrievable studies on "journaling" in women with gynecologic cancers. Although not an ideal fit with KM, the two studies (Low, Stanton, Bower, & Gyllenhammer, 2010; Stanton et al., 2002) with women with breast cancer were appraised. In both of these studies, the intervention group wrote about the "deepest emotional" aspects of their cancer experience, compared to a control group who wrote about the factual aspects of their cancer experience. Both groups wrote at home for 20 minutes on four occasions over a 3-week period. Their research designs were appropriate for the questions asked, their abstracts indicated they closely followed required journal reporting standards, and both are in highly respected, peer-reviewed journals. A quick review of their abstracts noted that the most recent of the two studies (Low et al., 2010), with its main outcome measure of depression and its test of different levels of perceived social support, was more relevant to KM, so it was appraised further. Results of this study noted that although there were no significant differences between the two groups, there were differences in outcome for those women reporting low levels of emotional support. Those reporting lower levels of social support had lower levels of intrusive thoughts about their cancer. Thus, although it is a study of women with metastatic breast cancer and therefore a different population than KM, it may have some relevance for her, and there does not appear to be any evidence of harm in "journaling."

Step 4: Translating the Research to a Particular Patient

As discussed in Chapter 4, the process of translating research findings to the needs of a particular patient is challenging—particularly in mental health care (Norcross et al., 2008). Research focuses on group findings that need to be translated to individual patient contexts. A clear understanding of the various meanings of "local context" is essential to effective translation (see Chapter 4). Use of journal reporting standards (see Table 4.6) and considering questions of local context (Chapter 4) help translate research to a particular patient.

In the current case example, the question is *How well do the findings of the Manne and colleagues study (2007) translate (generalize) to KM?* Comparing the list of key patient characteristics from earlier with the description of the study in the methods section of the study reviewed should answer this question.

KM is a few years older (62) than the mean ages of the study participants (56), but marital status, race, and educational status are all comparable to the majority of those in the study. KM's cancer type (ovarian) is the same as 81% of study participants, and her anticipated stage (III) is consistent with 45% of the participants. Her presenting problem of depression and her preference for supportive counseling over CBT is acceptable since both groups were effective in alleviating symptoms of depression. Your clinical judgment that she is insightful and willing to discuss and express her emotions matches well with the process of supportive counseling. Regarding clinical expertise, as an experienced psychotherapist you are familiar with and are competent to provide supportive counseling. If needed, you can also access the treatment manual from the authors of the study, and you have frequently reviewed the chapter by Lederberg and Holland (2011) as a helpful resource. You have chosen to use the PHQ-9 and the GAD-7 as outcome measures. These are different than the outcome measures in the study (BDI and IES), but they are all commonly used measures of distress (i.e., depression and anxiety—see Mitchell, 2010b). Finally, regarding patient characteristics, the lack of husband and family emotional support and her employment status with consideration for retirement are two life context variables of importance to attend to. In summary, it appears that the Manne and colleagues study translates pretty well to KM.

Step 5: Integration—Pulling It All Together and Developing a Treatment Plan

Integration involves pulling together all three components of EBP: (1) accessed and appraised best available evidence, (2) clinical expertise, and (3) patient characteristics, culture, and preferences. As discussed in Chapter 4, there is often "dynamic tension" (Norcross et al., 2008) among these components, most commonly between the degree to which the available evidence best matches with the patient characteristics and preferences. Norcross and colleagues (2008) refer to this as tension between *fidelity* and *fit*. Fidelity strives to provide a treatment intervention in a manner most like that provided in the original research, while fit strives to "make it work" with each client by adapting or modifying it in effective ways. Clinical expertise, contained within specific competencies (see Table 4.7) involves the skillful and flexible integration of best available evidence with patient characteristics in ways to maximize both fidelity and fit—and to do so repeatedly in an iterative manner, attending closely to feedback about patient self-reported outcomes. Ultimately, integration results in one of three possible clinical decisions: adopt, adapt, or abandon (Norcross et al., 2008).

In the present case example, the available evidence regarding the primary intervention of supportive psychotherapy seems to fit well, and thus you consider (after collaborating with KM at her next appointment) *adopting it* with very little need to modify it. There seems little tension between fidelity and fit since both the CBT-based and the supportive counseling interventions were effective, allowing you to choose either to match patient preferences. The available evidence matches well with patient characteristics (demographic and medical variables) and preferences (supportive counseling over more structured CBT), and you have the training and expertise to provide the intervention. Thus, the treatment plan is to provide a seven-session supportive counseling intervention timed around KM's cancer treatments. Potential goals are to alleviate symptoms of overall distress (i.e., anxiety and depression) and to maintain psychosocial adaptation as defined by active involvement in daily life, minimizing disruptions to roles and regulating expected emotional distress.

Regarding the question about journaling, the degree of fit of the Low et al. study (2010) is fair to good. Internal validity of the study was very good, yet its generalizability to KM is not perfect. However, to match her interest and preference to try journaling, the details of the intervention will be explained to KM along with the differences in populations studied. She will be told how to focus her journaling on her "deepest emotional experiences" and that the typical instructions suggest 20-minute periods of time. It will be offered as an option for her, to do on her own at home, and attention to change in frequency of "worry" (items 2, 3, and 7 on GAD-7) will be monitored on the periodic GAD scores.

Session 3. Discuss Treatment Plan, Collaborate on Goals and Treatment Tasks, and Begin Supportive Counseling

Karen returns in 3 weeks. She has now completed her surgery and, although still in some pain, can see that she is feeling a little better and is "on the mend" from the surgery. You heard from Dr. S that the staging has been complete and it is Stage IIIb. Karen explains, "Yes, they told me Stage III, which I know is not good, but also that it could be worse."

Before beginning the supportive counseling, you explain that you looked into the idea of journaling, and in one well-done study in patients with breast cancer, it wasn't helpful for everyone but "It was helpful in reducing symptoms of depression in patients who felt that they didn't have much social support—like you have mentioned—I think it's worth considering." You explain how it is done. "What they did in this study was instruct patients to write about their deepest emotions in regard to their illness experience. In the study, the participants wrote for 20 minutes each time, so that might be a reasonable thing to try. What do you think?" KM agrees and indicates she is kind of intrigued by the idea and eager to try it.

Next you collaborate on goals. You explain that her scores on the questionnaires she filled out at the first appointment indicated that her feelings of anxiety and depression are considered to be in the moderate range of severity, and you suggest that, between the two of you, each time you meet, one of your goals will be to see how she is doing with any feelings of anxiety and depression. Have they changed, stayed the same, or gotten worse? You explain that the best way to monitor this is to periodically fill out the same questionnaires again.

She agrees that these are reasonable goals, but she has questions about how she will accomplish them since she feels like she still has much to face now, with recovering from surgery, then getting through chemotherapy—which she says "scares me to death!" and who knows what else later. How "she gets there" are the tasks, and so you explain how supportive counseling works. You explain that during the counseling sessions, her task will be to talk about what she is going through, to consider how she feels about what she is going through, to consider how she is/or might cope with it, while as the counselor, your job is to listen attentively, to be empathic and try to understand her feelings, to reassure, to identify already existing coping skills, to validate, to be encouraging, and to help her explore what she is going through.

In general ways, she seems to understand. You reassure her that if at any time she feels like the supportive counseling is not helpful, to be certain to let you know and you can discuss it. You have transitioned into supportive counseling by simply continuing to talk about her recent experiences, how she has been feeling, her coping efforts, concerns for her family, and so on. The remainder of this first session is devoted to providing supportive counseling. You agree to meet again in 1 week.

Step 6: Evaluation of Evidence-Based Practice

Monitoring Patient Outcome: Repeat Administrations of PHQ-9 and GAD-7

In the final EBP step, the evidence-based practitioner evaluates the effectiveness of the entire EBP process. Although evaluation can occur at various levels (institution, profession, etc.), the emphasis here is on patient outcome and an evaluation of varying degrees of emphasis on the three EBP components. Patient outcome will be monitored by the PHQ-9 and GAD-7, which will be administered at Sessions 3 and 6 of the seven-session supportive counseling. Given baseline measurement of moderate severity—subthreshold for any mental disorder—their repeated administration is being used to assess change in symptom severity due to the counseling intervention and to monitor closely any worsening of symptoms. Worsening of symptoms could push KM over the threshold into the severity range of either major depressive disorder (MDD) or generalized anxiety disorder (GAD), which would then require reevaluation and reconsideration of the treatment plan (e.g., consideration of antidepressant medication). Lastly, using clinical judgment, you will be monitoring KM's overall psychosocial adaptation (i.e., continued involvement in daily life, minimization of disruption to life roles, managing expected emotional distress).

Evaluation of Evidence-Based Practice Components

Ongoing use of EBP also requires case-by-case consideration of the varying degrees to which each of the three components converge. The current case serves as a prototypic example of ideal convergence where all three components are equally involved in the clinical decision-making process. Very good fit and fidelity was achieved as the best available evidence fit the patient characteristics and preferences, while the psycho-oncologist had the necessary clinical expertise to provide the supportive counseling intervention with journaling.

A final evaluation of the EBP steps includes the intentional archiving of the literature searches from the earlier case as critically appraised topics (C.A.T.s) as described in Chapter 4. A completed CAT includes a well-organized summary of the entire EBP process, including the clinical bottom-line results, the citation, clinical question, search terms, study description, and evidence summary as appraised. Develop and save a CAT for this case in your Dropbox folder.

Case 1—KM: Evidence-Based Practice Across the Clinical Course

The development and collaboration with the patient regarding the initial treatment plan is just the start of the ongoing, recursive process of EBP. Considering possible "twists and turns" in the KM case example, the clinical expertise of the practitioner is essential in making clinical decisions regarding when, how, or whether to adapt, adopt, or abandon best available evidence, as the clinical course evolves and changes. As Norcross and colleagues (2008) (pp. 210–211) aptly explain,

> we will need to make dozens of minidecisions, and there will never be empirical research to guide all of them. There remain many problem constellations and clinical situations for which empirical data are sparse. We cannot possibly expect that every practitioner's action will flow from research data (Chambless & Crits-Christoph, 2005). In such instances, clinicians use their clinical expertise and the best available research evidence to develop coherent, realistic treatment strategies (American Psychological Association, 2006).

As the ongoing iterative EBP continues, interventions as listed in Table 6.1 may prove to be best available evidence if KM's disease process were to proceed in certain directions, resulting in different combinations of interventions across the clinical course of the disease. For example, she may ask how to prepare for the emotional aspects of chemotherapy and find that self-administered stress management training (Jacobsen et al., 2002) helps her lower overall distress. Here would be the intersection between an individual intervention (self-administered or brief professional intervention) at the start of chemotherapy for normal adaptation. If KM's disease were to progress and she experiences depressive symptoms sufficient for a diagnosis of major depressive disorder, then cognitive therapy for depression (Savard et al., 2006) may be warranted. Depending on how KM's disease progresses, the other exemplars in Table 6.1 may also be utilized that illustrate a wide variety of intersection between specific interventions across the clinical course of the disease.

Case Example 2—WD: Metastatic Prostate Cancer and Complicated Grief

Referral Information

You receive a call from a former patient, WD, whom you saw about 10 years ago following an original diagnosis of Stage II prostate cancer, asking if he can schedule to see you once again. At the time of his original diagnosis you saw him for eight sessions of supportive counseling for moderate to severe distress (i.e., subthreshold for any mental disorder) during his course of external beam radiation treatment (EBRT). As his EBRT treatment progressed, his overall distress and fears of the disease decreased, and he was coping well, continuing to work, and experiencing good support from family, particularly his wife.

He is now a 66-year-old, married, White male with a rising prostate-specific antigen (PSA) level. After consulting with his radiation oncologist, who agreed with the treatment plan of his urologist, he is now trying to decide what to do next. On the phone he tells you that "the doctors tell me I need to take some hormone shot." He does indicate he has heard from friends about some "weird" side effects. You agree to see him and schedule an appointment for next week.

Later that week you run into his radiation oncologist and you mention the call from this patient. The oncologist responds, "Oh good, I'm glad he is going to see you since he seemed very upset when I saw him last, mostly about his wife having died." You learn this happened about 13 months ago, and you are surprised that WD hadn't mentioned that to you during the phone conversation.

You Begin the Evidence-Based Practice Process

Step 1: Ask Specific, Clinical Questions: Both Background and Foreground

You identify the following *biomedical* background questions:

- Is it very typical for Stage II disease to recur after 10 years?
- What is the patient's long-term prognosis?
- What is hormone therapy and, specifically, what are common and not-so-common side effects of the medications?

For quick answers to these questions, you access the ACS Web site again and search for information on prostate cancer (http://www.cancer.org/cancer/prostatecancer/index). After about 15 minutes you have some interesting information. Included is information regarding treatment options (e.g., salvage radical prostatectomy, hormonal therapy, immunotherapy, cryosurgery, chemotherapy) and side effects for each. You learn that androgen deprivation therapy (ADT) blocks production of androgen to prevent it from interacting with cancer cells. Side effects include bone flare (a temporary increase in bone pain resulting from the drugs blocking production of testosterone), swelling and tenderness of the breast, impotence, nausea, fatigue, osteoporosis, diarrhea, hot flashes, loss of sexual desire, and weight gain. Regarding general information about prognosis, you quickly search the ACS site for survival rates for prostate cancer (http://www.cancer.org/Cancer/ProstateCancer/OverviewGuide/prostate-cancer-overview-survival-rates) and learn that the 5-year survival rate for "distant metastases" (i.e., outside the prostate or prostate bed/pelvis) is 31%. You cannot easily find information about how common recurrence is after 10 years, so you wait and plan to ask his oncologist later. Your primary concern is the potential complications his illness experience might have on any common grief reaction he may be experiencing.

You identify the following *psychosocial* background questions:

- What is normal grief/bereavement?
- What are the symptoms of complicated or prolonged grief?
- What is known about individual treatment options for complicated or prolonged grief?

Your general knowledge includes awareness that the *DSM-5* changed the criteria for "bereavement" and removed it as an exclusion criterion in major depression. You need to look more closely in the *DSM-5* at these changes. You learn that within the diagnostic criteria for major depression, there is discussion about how grief is different from major depression—normal grief has predominant symptoms of loss and emptiness; the sadness is likely to decrease in intensity over days to weeks and it occurs "in waves," rather than persistently. However, it is also noted that both major depression and normal grief can both occur together, and if a patient meets criteria for major depression, even though it is after a significant loss, the major depressive disorder should be diagnosed.

Another important addition to *DSM-5* is a diagnosis provided for further study, titled, "persistent complex bereavement disorder." It is listed in the back of the manual for consideration for future use, but it can be helpful at present. You notice that it defines a time frame for grief-related symptoms of greater than 12 months for grieving adults and 6 months for children. Grief-related symptoms are to have persisted more days than not for at least 12 months before being considered a persistent, complex bereavement disorder.

You plan to include close attention to these differential diagnostic questions during your clinical interview.

You have stayed current on literature related to complicated or delayed grief reactions, so you check for bereavement via the National Guidelines Clearinghouse to see if there are any consensus-based standards of care. You search for "grief" (http://www.guideline.gov/content.aspx?id=14423&search=grief) and find only a brief mention in a clinical guideline for quality palliative care and conclude there does not appear to be any consensus on specific interventions for grief in cancer patients. Next, you check the text *Psycho-Oncology* (Holland et al., 2010), where you find a chapter on bereavement (Lichtenthal, Prigerson, & Kissane, 2010) that includes literature on supportive counseling, psychodynamic/interpersonal psychotherapies, and cognitive-behavioral therapy for grief, as well as a very helpful discussion of complicated grief. You review risk factors for complicated grief and note that cumulative losses is a risk factor.

With these background questions answered, you formulate foreground questions, anticipating the clinical interview.

- What is/are his primary concern(s) at this time?
  - coping with his metastatic disease
  - fears of the uncertain future and/or death
  - grief over the death of his wife
  - frustration with treatment side effects
  - overall quality of life, existential concerns, and so on
- What level (normal, mild-moderate, moderate-severe) of severity of distress (i.e., anxiety, depression, trauma-related symptoms) is he experiencing?
- Does he meet diagnostic criteria for any *DSM* diagnoses, such as major depressive disorder, posttraumatic stress disorder, generalized anxiety disorder, or the proposed persistent complex bereavement disorder?
- Are there any demographic, cultural, disease, developmental, or treatment-related factors that might influence his treatment preferences?

Session 1—*The first clinical interview: Assessment of psychosocial adaptation, and reestablishment of psychotherapy relationship with elements of empathy, alliance, and collaboration on goals/tasks.*

You meet WD in the waiting room, and you greet each other warmly, recalling the last time you saw each other. He appears thinner and is clearly moving much slower than you recall from 10 years ago. You escort him to your office, and he sits down and immediately begins to tell you the story of his prostate cancer. He was doing fine, with no symptoms and all of his follow-up appointments with his doctor showed no evidence of any cancer. Things were getting back to normal, and he returned to work. About 6 years ago (age 60) he retired, and he and his wife were looking forward to plans to do some traveling, spending time with their three adult children and grandchildren.

He then skips up to about 4 weeks ago when he explains that his children were worried that he missed several appointments with his family doctor (his family doctor was checking his PSA periodically). They insisted that he go and so he did. That's when he learned his PSA had been rising. He then was referred back to his urologist, who consulted with WD's former radiation oncologist. Both doctors agreed that WD ought to try "these hormone shots." You listen closely, paraphrasing, reflecting, and summarizing his thoughts and feelings. There is a fairly long pause . . . before you ask, wondering about the side effects, "How have the hormone shots been for you?" He seems uncomfortable and eventually explains, "I am not taking them." You are surprised and ask for clarification. WD explains, "I just don't want to go through all of this again, I just don't really care anymore!" You realize it has been about 20–25 minutes in to the session and he hasn't mentioned his wife—and so you ask. "I understand that your wife died."

With tears beginning to flow, he explains how his wife of 41 years died. It is obviously difficult for him to talk about it. He hesitates frequently—even seems to want to avoid the topic—but with your encouragement and empathy, he offers the following. "About 5 years ago, when she was around 62, she was diagnosed with leukemia. She was tired a lot, would wake up at night all hot and sweaty with a fever. She went to our family doctor who did some blood work and referred her to a medical oncologist. She had some chemo. I think she was in remission for a while, but it never seemed to last very long. . . . She would have a few good months, and then her blood counts would drop and she would again go through more treatments. Eventually there just weren't any more treatments that were working. We had hospice come in." You try to probe a bit about the details of the last few days of her life, but he "just doesn't want to go there!"

You eventually learn that throughout all of his wife's illness, he didn't pay much attention to his own health. When his children learned that he had missed some appointments, they insisted that he go. Even now he says, "I haven't decided yet whether I am going to do these hormone shots, I really don't care if I live or die."

You recall from your past sessions with WD that you felt he was not only very close to his wife, but maybe even overly dependent on her. She was the one who convinced him to see a doctor when he was having symptoms and to undergo his radiation therapy. She was with him at nearly every treatment; she usually drove him to and from treatments and, although that could of course simply represent strong support, the more you learned the more you recall that she made lots of pretty basic decisions for him. This information becomes more salient and important now, in the face of her death.

You switch your focus to his decision-making process and ask further about where he is in trying to decide about the hormone therapy. You learn that he hasn't done much of anything in the way of trying to decide, but rather indicates, "I just don't care anymore." It has been 3 weeks since his doctors recommended the hormone therapy, and his children are concerned that he hasn't made any decision.

You focus your interview on current symptoms and evaluate for major depression, generalized anxiety, and posttraumatic stress symptoms, being attentive to the differences between prolonged grief disorder and these related disorders. He also completes the PHQ-9 (total = 20, Severe) and GAD-7 (total = 7, Mild). You conclude that he meets criteria for major depression (significant anhedonia, lots of sadness and crying most every day, periodic guilt, difficulty concentrating and decreased energy, sleep disturbance, and some weight loss), but not for generalized anxiety. You would like to know more about the details of the last few days of his wife's life, as they may be relevant to any posttraumatic stress symptoms, but you conclude you will need to wait for a later appointment when he may be more willing to talk about that time period.

You wonder about the benefit of an antidepressant and you ask. He explains that his family doctor prescribed one for him, somewhat at the insistence of his children, and that he has been taking it for about 7 months now. He offers, "I can't really tell much difference, but I have been taking it every night."

For now, moving on to goals, you suggest that the first thing you ought to collaborate on is decision making about hormone therapy. He somewhat reluctantly agrees, and only after you discuss it more and you remind him that he called you to make this appointment on his own, indicating to you that he must want to make some decision or he would not have shown up for the appointment. You recognize some urgency in this decision, and you schedule another appointment in 2 days. He agrees.

Post First Interview: Summary of Key Patient Characteristics

- 66-year-old White male
- Wife died 13 months ago
- Prior EBRT for prostate cancer
- Rising PSA
- MD is recommending hormone therapy
- Grieving, possibly complicated grief (i.e., persistent complex bereavement)
- Meets criteria for major depressive disorder, severe
- Mild anxiety
- Avoiding decision making about hormone therapy

Prior to your next appointment you have two foreground questions:

- An Intervention Question—Are decision aids for advanced prostate cancer available (e.g., online), and if so, are they beneficial in helping patients decide?
- An Intervention Question (PICO format)—For a 66-year-old male with advanced prostate cancer, is the use of a decision aid better than no decision aid, in making a decision about which treatment to pursue?
- A Diagnostic Question—What is the best way to assess complicated grief (i.e., persistent complex bereavement)?

Step 2: Accessing the Best Available Research Evidence

For these specific questions, you do a quick search of filtered literature. For your first intervention question, you try the Cochrane Library, using the search terms "decision aid" AND "prostate cancer." You do not find any reviews that appear relevant, and you try a broader search by use of the terms "decision aid" only, and you find one relevant review of RCTs (O'Connor et al., 2009) titled *Decision aids for people facing health treatments or screening decisions* (http://onlinelibrary.wiley.com/o/cochrane/clsysrev/articles/CD001431/frame.html). A quick review of the abstract indicates that such aids do better than usual care in terms of (a) increased knowledge, (b) lower decisional conflict about feeling uninformed and about personal values, and most important, (c) an increased number of people make a decision. For the diagnostic question you recall your review of *DSM-5*, and you go back to the chapter in the *Psycho-Oncology* text (Lichtenthal et al., 2010) where they discuss an earlier proposal of "prolonged grief disorder" which you review, while also noting a reference for a self-report questionnaire to assess complicated grief (Prigerson et al., 1995), the Inventory of Complicated Grief (ICG). You learn that it is not available electronically, so you order it via interlibrary loan.

Since you have another appointment in two days, you postpone Step 3: Appraising the evidence, for later, after you have a more complete psychosocial assessment, particularly regarding possible complicated grief.

Session 2: Completion of Psychosocial Assessment

WD returns for his second appointment, during which your primary focus is (1) on his grief reaction—differentiating it from major depression, generalized anxiety, and any posttraumatic symptoms—and (2) decision making regarding the recommended hormone therapy. You realize that he was very tentative and somewhat avoidant of talking about his wife's death at the last appointment, but your hope is that with more time together and stronger rapport and alliance, he will be more willing to talk about her death. You therefore make a clinical decision to wait until later in this session to ask about her death and begin the session with a focus on his decision regarding hormone therapy. You ask, "So, have you had time to think further about a decision?" He indicates he is still not very motivated to do anything, finds it hard to concentrate, and continues to be very sad and tearful almost every day.

You see this admission of sadness and tears as a potential opening to ask further about his wife, and so you alter your plans and decide to ask about her death now. You gently ask, "Tell me, what were the last few days of her life like?" Once again, he is very hesitant and looks down to the floor, tears welling up, before he quietly murmurs, "It was awful!" You reflect, "awful?" "Yea," he responds. "Even though we had Hospice involved, I really didn't have much of any idea that she was close to dying. I knew she was very tired, sleeping a lot more, was hardly ever very alert, but I don't know, I guess maybe I just didn't want to think about her not being here with me, and I figured I would have time to talk to her still, be with her more. Then, one morning the Hospice nurse came and indicated she thought that my wife might not last too many more days. My children seemed to understand, but I just couldn't accept that and pretended, I guess, that the nurse was wrong and that I would have time to visit and spend more time with my wife. Then, on May 18, about 3 o'clock in the afternoon, I was outside in the garage when my daughter came out and told me, 'You better come in and see mom,' her breathing was shallow and light. The Hospice nurse was coming, and I was pretty scared and decided to wait until the nurse got there, but by the time the nurse arrived, my wife had already died. The nurse went in and checked on her, came out and told me that she died, and I guess 'I lost it.' I don't really remember much of it, but I've been told I went in the bedroom, tried to wake my wife up, started shaking her, pulled out the IVs, was mad, hollering at everyone and nearly tore up some of the furniture. I didn't know what I was doing!

My kids and the nurse were scared; they didn't know what to do so they called the police, who came and had to almost physically restrain me. I eventually calmed down, but I was terrified and felt helpless. It was a terrible scene. Fortunately the police didn't charge me with anything, and I felt terrible later and very embarrassed. The funeral was just about as bad. I couldn't stop crying. I just couldn't face being there, and for most of the wake, I stayed in the side room and went home as soon as I could. I almost thought I would be better off dead if I couldn't be with her. My kids did get me to go to the cemetery for that part of the funeral, but I wanted to get out of there as quick as I could. For days and weeks after, I just kept thinking, this can't be real, it just can't!"

He continues to tell you the story of the next few days, the funeral and how the past 13 months have gone. Prominent throughout the story are signs of complicated grief:

- *His tears and sadness are almost exclusively related to missing his wife.*
- *He has lots of intrusive thoughts and images about the last times he saw her at home and in the casket. When he pulled out her IVs, the blood spilled out; some of it got on him, and this was very traumatic for him.*
- *He cannot stop thinking about those last few days and is mad at himself and feels guilty for not talking to her about some things. ("If I could only have one more chance to talk to her.")*
- *He still seems emotionally numb, bitter, and angry about her leaving him.*
- *He has yet to go back to the cemetery, even though his children have been encouraging him to.*

- *He rarely leaves the house and feels as if his life is meaningless, worthless, and not really worth living.*
- *About his only pleasure is daydreaming about times with his wife, acting as if he is back then with her when she was alive.*

He eventually stops telling the story and seems exhausted to have reexperienced some of it by telling you about it. This long and detailed story takes up most of this session, and you only have a brief time to explain to him what you learned about decision aids and ask if he would be willing to do one, with your help. Although he seems minimally interested, he does agree to at least look at it with you, during the next appointment in 1 week. He completes the Inventory of Complicated Grief (ICG) and scores a 30.

Post Second Interview: Summary of Key Patient Characteristics

- Further assessment determines complicated grief (prolonged grief disorder) rather than major depressive disorder
- Possibly some symptoms of posttraumatic stress
- Avoidance of going out of the house, reminders of his wife
- Possibly a generalized (not just since wife died) avoidant coping style
- Willing to try a decision aid, but not likely to do on his own

Step 2: Accessing the Best Available Research Evidence (cont.)

You make a clinical decision that the better treatment plan would be to focus primarily on the complicated grief, and you begin a search for best available evidence. You also want to continue your search regarding access to decision aids, preferably online so that you can complete one with WD during a session if necessary.

You design a search strategy of the unfiltered, primary literature, using the sequential steps recommended by Gibbs (2003).

Step 1 is to formulate a PICO question:

> *For a 66-year-old widowed male—13 months post death of his wife of 41 years—recently diagnosed with advanced prostate cancer, experiencing complicated grief, what is the best treatment for relieving symptoms of complicated grief?*

Steps 2 and 3 are to list keywords/terms, their synonyms or related known terms from various controlled vocabulary databases (e.g., PsycINFO, CINAHL, and PubMed) that correspond with each of the four PICO components, such as:

P—complicated grief, mourning, bereavement, loss, prolonged grief

I—psychosocial, counseling, psychotherapy, psychological intervention, psychological treatment, cognitive-behavioral therapy

C—none
O—depression, anxiety, trauma, distress, complicated grief

Step 4 is to begin the search, in this case of unfiltered, primary literature such as PsycINFO, CINAHL, and Medline, via EBSCOhost. The search terms used were as follows:

(grief OR mourning OR bereavement) and (complicated OR prolonged) and (counseling OR psychotherapy OR psychological treatment OR cognitive behavioral therapy) and randomized trial

All three databases were restricted to search for review articles only, from 2000 to 2011. The search identified 17 articles, 7 of which involved treatment modalities other than individual counseling/psychotherapy, such as group (n = 4), Internet-based (n = 2), or family (n = 1), and 3 were focused on special populations (2 on persons with intellectual disabilities, and 1 on alexithymia). Interestingly, the remaining seven articles were all from the same research group. They include an original randomized trial (Shear, Frank, Houck, & Reynolds, 2005), one book chapter, and five other articles that were secondary analyses of data from the original study. You return to the chapter on bereavement in the *Psycho-Oncology* text (Lichtenthal et al., 2010) to check its reference list and find one other treatment specifically for complicated grief (Boelen, de Keijser, van den Hout, & van den Bout, 2007). These two treatments (Boelen et al., 2007; Shear et al., 2005), developed specifically for complicated grief reactions, are most relevant and require further appraisal.

Step 3: Appraising the Research Evidence

You decide to use two different forms for appraising this research evidence because each seems to contribute a slightly different perspective. First, you use the 25-item checklist from the CONSORT extension to RCTs of nonpharmacologic intervention (Boutron, Moher, Altman, Schulz, & Ravaud, 2008a). Both articles are very transparent and contain nearly all of the 25 items from the checklist. You find that the Shear et al. (2005) article does not have many details about the therapists (how many, academic degrees, disciplines, how allocated to treatment groups) and no quantifiable method for evaluating treatment fidelity (therapist adherence), but rather it is indicated that group supervision, with use of selected audiotaped sessions, was provided. The two treatment interventions are adequately described. Likewise, the Boelen et al. (2007) article has good transparency with nearly all 25 items included. One concern is the randomization procedure used (minimization method) to allow for a more balanced group assignment for some prognostic factors (i.e., violent/nonviolent death, death of a child/other relative). Some systematic bias could have been involved in group assignment because it was not done blindly and was done by the first author. However, this randomization method is explained to be a limitation to the study results and does have some support for use in studies with small sample sizes (Scott, McPherson, Ramsay, & Campbell, 2002). The allocation was done after a brief screening was completed and was based only on the two identified prognostic factors (i.e., violent death and death of a child).

The results of both studies support the notion that complicated grief is a unique phenomenon, separate from major depression or other mental disorders, and that interventions designed specifically for it can be developed. Shear et al. (2005) tested a proven empirically supported therapy (EST) for depression (interpersonal therapy [IPT]) against a novel treatment for complicated grief (CGT). CGT consisted of three phases (similar to IPT) and was based on the dual-process model of adaptive coping to loss (Stroebe & Schut, 1999). Its unique components include a "revisiting" procedure, modeled after in vivo and imaginal exposure in PTSD, in which patients are asked, with eyes closed, to tell the story of the death, in detail. Therapists audio record the telling of the story, and patients listen to the audiotape at home. In addition, intervening for the distress symptoms (yearning, reveries) was done via attempts to enhance a sense of connection with the deceased through in-session imaginary conversations with the deceased, use of memory questionnaires inviting reminiscence, and so on. CGT was compared to the typical three-phase approach of IPT and its focus on loss, role transitions, and interpersonal relationships (Weissman, Markowitz, & Klerman, 2000).

The Boelen et al. study (2007) compared two forms of cognitive-behavioral therapy with a nonspecific supportive counseling (SC) intervention. The CBT components of cognitive restructuring (CR) and exposure therapy (ET) were provided in two different orders. Thus, the study had three groups: supportive counseling, CBT with exposure first, and CBT with cognitive restructuring first.

Second, you use the Quality of Study Rating Form (QSRF) (Gibbs, 1989; see Appendix B) to rate the overall strength of results in both studies. The QSRF and its accompanying instructions show how to initially rate various study components, similar to the CONSORT, and how to measure effect sizes, absolute risk reduction, and number needed to treat (NNT). In the Shear et al. study, 51% of all participants responded to the CGT treatment, while 28% responded to the IPT. Pretreatment to posttreatment changes in symptoms of complicated grief had effect sizes of 1.64 for those who received all sessions and 1.35 for all patients in the intent-to-treat analysis. However, attrition for each treatment was fairly high with 27% of the CGT group (n = 13) and 26% (n = 12) of the IPT group. Some of the attrition was due to refusal to participate in the CGT imaginal exposure exercise. The number needed to treat (NNT)—an estimate of how many patients would need to receive the treatment to show a difference in outcome from the control group—for this study was 2.9 for those who competed all sessions and 4.3 for all participants in the intent-to-treat analysis. In the Boelen et al. study (2007), the intent-to-treat analysis found that 45% responded to the CBT intervention where the exposure therapy was presented first (cognitive restructuring second), 22% to the

CBT with the reverse order (cognitive restructuring first, exposure second), and 0% to the supportive counseling. For those who completed all sessions, the percentages were larger (50%, 31%, and 0%) and in the same order. Effect sizes for pretreatment to posttreatment changes were 1.80 for those receiving all sessions and 1.29 for those in the intent-to-treat analysis. NNT were 2.2 for completers and 4.5 for all participants.

The overall appraisal suggests that CGT, CBT (both forms), and IPT are all effective treatment interventions for complicated grief. In CBT, exposure first and cognitive restructuring second is better. Effect sizes of >1.00 are considered large and clearly beneficial. CGT and CBT with exposure therapy presented first are the two most effective therapies. Supportive counseling was not effective. Regarding a literature search on decision aids, you return to the TRIP database and search for "shared decision making" and "cancer." The search identifies 14 systematic reviews in Medline, and one seems most applicable given its title, *Decision making in oncology: A review of patient decision aids to support patient participation* (http://www.ncbi.nlm.nih.gov/pubmed/18755939). You review its abstract and learn that, in general, decision aids such as the one on the ACS Web site are effective in increasing patient involvement in decisions and that there is no current evidence suggesting any one aid is better than any others. You decide to proceed with suggesting use of the ACS Web site decision aid.

Session 3—Focus on Goals, Treatment Planning, and Patient Collaboration

Your third session with WD begins by checking in on how his week has been and if he has thought any more about making a decision regarding his treatment. He indicates, "About the same. . . . I still don't feel like doing much of anything, crying some, but mostly just feel numb and don't care about much of anything."

You proceed with a discussion about counseling goals and the importance of the two of you collaborating on these goals. WD seems to understand but continues to be "underwhelmed" by the whole discussion. He is difficult to engage in any collaborative decision making, and you find yourself hypothesizing that his difficulty in collaborating could be either the result of the complicated grief symptoms, or the result of an avoidant coping style, or he just needs more time to consider his options and is simply not ready yet to make a decision. You know that the interventions for complicated grief were between 12 and 16 sessions over 12–19 weeks and that it is clearly not in his best interest to wait until his grief symptoms remit before making a decision about further treatment. You decide to suggest a first goal of helping him decide about the prostate cancer treatment by use of an online decision aid. He has a few questions, but ultimately agrees to proceed with that during today's session.

Before proceeding, you explain to him the options for the treatment of his complicated grief. First, you begin by explaining to him what complicated grief is and some of the factors that seem to have made his grief more difficult to cope with (e.g., the long-term, very close relationship between WD and his wife; her relatively quick death; his reaction at the time of her death; and his difficulties in adapting since her death). He doesn't really seem much interested, but he accepts your explanation. You then explain, "There are some specific forms of counseling designed to help with more complicated forms of grief, like yours." You explain, in understandable language, that these therapies involve trying to better understand the connection between thoughts and emotions, and that they involve examining his thoughts about his wife's death, both at the time she died and over the past 13 months. You explain the two-part emphasis in this therapy is on both adjusting to the loss, while simultaneously working on reengaging with life—looking ahead to the future. You offer that "I realize that may seem difficult to do right now, but maybe not in the future." You also explain that these therapies involve a procedure where the two of you will talk about and "revisit" the story of her death, and that you will want to hear about all of the details again. He looks worried when you mention this, but you explain that you realized—last session when he was telling you the story—that those last few days of her life were very traumatic for him and that you think getting over some of the trauma of her death is maybe the most important part of the therapy. Again, he seems skeptical but somewhat grudgingly agrees that "Maybe you're right." For now, you suggest he just think about these therapies, and next time you can talk about his preferences.

For now, you want to show him an example of an online decision aid to help him decide what to do about treatment for his cancer. He agrees, and you show it to him on the computer in your office. He seems to understand the idea and agrees to look it over at home.

Step 4: Translating the Research to a Particular Patient

After accessing and appraising the literature, you have identified four potential evidence-based treatments for complicated grief: CGT, CBT (two forms that vary by which component provided first), and IPT. You have also assessed, via clinical interview and self-report questionnaire (ICG), the presence of complicated grief in the context of the need to make a decision about further treatment (i.e., hormone therapy) for his prostate cancer. Thus, the match between the interventions and the diagnosis of complicated grief is pretty good.

However, there are lots of differences between WD and the samples of the two studies reviewed. How well do either of these studies generalize to the specific needs of your client? First, neither is a study of cancer patients and the mean participant age in both studies (mid-40s) is nearly 20 years younger than WD, and the mean time since loss for both studies combined (2.75 years) is much longer than for WD (13 months). A number of patients in the CGT treatment refused to do the exposure component, and you question whether WD is motivated enough to actively participate in exposure, with its homework component and potential for reexperiencing some of the trauma. One similarity between your patient WD and the studies is that a large percent of both studies were persons whose grief was from loss of a spouse.

You conclude that you must be aware of these differences between the studies from which the evidence comes and your client, but that these four forms of treatment for complicated grief have strong evidence with effect sizes (1.80 to 1.29) that are quite impressive.

The clinical interviews to date suggest that WD is showing avoidance behaviors in multiple contexts that may be part of his complicated grief, readiness to change, and/or coping style (Norcross, 2011). In future sessions, attention to these competing hypotheses is important.

You need to continue to collaborate with him to identify his attitude and opinions toward treatment options and continue to consider if there are any other demographic, cultural, disease, developmental, or treatment-related factors that might influence his treatment preferences.

Step 5: Integration—Pulling It All Together and Developing a Treatment Plan
Integration involves pulling together all three components of EBP: (1) accessed and appraised best available evidence; (2) clinical expertise; and (3) patient characteristics, culture, and preferences. In this case the tension between fit and fidelity is notable. There is strong evidence of fidelity, but questionable fit, as based upon sample characteristics relative to patient demographics. The strength of the evidence is strong (effect size), suggesting that the treatment should be provided with close attention to fidelity (i.e., close adherence to treatment components), but treatment may require adaptation or modification to fit this patient to make it work. Some of the characteristics upon which to consider adaptation include WD's status as a cancer patient facing recurrence, co-occurring distress over decision making regarding hormone therapy, willingness to comply with treatment components such as the exposure therapy, overall avoidance tendencies and/or readiness to change, trauma-like symptoms at time of wife's death, recency of loss (13 months), and older age than study participants.

The integration of clinical expertise is also relevant. As an experienced psychotherapist with specific experience in CBT, exposure-based interventions, and grief counseling, you feel competent to provide the CBT components and, given the description of how exposure (i.e., "revisiting") was provided in the CGT study, you feel competent to provide either the CGT or the CBT with exposure therapy. You also realize you do not have any formal training in IPT. Therefore CGT and CBT are the two therapies you will explain to WD in his next session, to elicit any preferences he may have. Additional flexibility and clinical expertise/skill is likely to become necessary as treatment proceeds and may need to be adapted via modifying the intervention to specific patient characteristics.

Brief Session 4. Decision Aid, Further Collaboration About Treatment Plan

This session is held in conjunction with an appointment that WD has with his radiation oncologist who wanted to see him about his decision regarding the recommended hormone therapy. You see WD prior to this appointment. He indicates that he is feeling about the same and that he continues to be unable to decide what to do about the hormone therapy. He did look over the decision aid (https://www.cancer.nexcura.com/Secure/ToolBox.asp?CB=265) but found it a bit long and hadn't finished it. You ask if he read the information about side effects of hormone therapy, and he says he had and that they were "about what he had heard from other guys." The idea of swelling and tenderness of the breasts and hot flashes "seems weird," and the side effects related to sexuality "don't really matter much to me anymore." The others weren't very worrisome. He agrees to finish the decision aid this week, see what his oncologist has to say later today, and then bring all of this new information with him next week.

You then explain the treatment options for complicated grief, and he listens closely. You emphasize that this is a form of counseling that usually takes a while (4–6 months) and that you would recommend meeting weekly. You and he will talk both about the details of his wife's death and about the future. You will ask him to do some things at home, in between appointments, like making lists of thoughts, his future plans, and recalling memories of his wife. You explain, "As you know, it might not be easy to remember back and experience some of the pain of losing her, but most all counseling for grief recommends doing that." You note that he is listening intently and thinking about whether he wants to do this. (This focus seems qualitatively different from other recent sessions during which he seemed distant and disengaged.)

WD pauses a bit, thinking, and eventually says, "Well, OK, I guess so, it's certainly no good the way things are now, and you were helpful to me when I first went through treatment years back. I know I can trust you." This has taken most of the 30 minutes you had scheduled prior to his appointment with his oncologist, and so you finish and schedule for 1 week.

Step 5: Integration—Pulling It All Together and Developing a Treatment Plan (cont.)

Now that you have his agreement to proceed with the complicated grief treatment (Patient Preference), you decide to proceed with the CBT and ET/CR (Boelen et al., 2007) format (Best Available Evidence). You choose this over the Shear et al. (2005) study because it is less intense than the exposure treatment (Clinical Decision), and you have concern that if exposure were to result in temporary increases in distress, he might not comply (as did a number of participants in the Shear et al. study). You also recognize that your prior experience is with CBT and not IPT, which was the conceptual framework (i.e., three-phase treatment, focus on life transitions, loss, etc.) for CGT in the Shear et al. study (2005) and, thus, you were not competent (lack of Clinical Expertise) to proceed with the IPT components of the CGT treatment. Other considerations for the treatment plan include concern about the urgency to make a decision about hormone therapy, and you reconsider your three competing hypotheses about why he is taking a long time to decide—symptoms of complicated grief (life is meaningless without his wife, guilt related to the loss, stunned/shocked/numb), coping style of avoidance, and readiness to change (Norcross, Krebs, & Prochaska, 2011). You note that you will need to continue to monitor his decision-making process and integrate this with the complicated grief treatment.

WD Initial, Tentative Treatment Plan and Ongoing Case Formulation

The treatment plan for WD involves a process of adapting best available evidence by a form of modification in which the primary treatment of complicated grief (Boelen et al.'s CBT with exposure therapy presented first, prior to cognitive restructuring) is augmented with the use of a decision aid to enhance knowledge of prostate cancer treatment options and side effects. Given the urgency to make a decision about hormone therapy, you plan to incorporate these two interventions concurrently, mixing in components of each during the first few sessions, or until he has made his decision.

Although there is some tension between fit (patient differences from study participants) and fidelity (augmenting the CBT plus ET/CR with a prostate cancer decision aid), the strength of the evidence, as indicated in the effect sizes for both treatments reviewed, indicates that these are effective interventions that should be helpful for WD, despite his status as a cancer patient, older age, and shorter time since loss. A complicating factor is the current need to decide about hormone therapy and the likely ongoing distress reactive to his recurrent prostate cancer (neither of which was part of the studies reviewed). Thus, the initial treatment plan is to adapt the best available evidence by concurrently providing the grief treatment, augmented with time to use the decision aid to assist in decision making. In all likelihood as a result of this adaptation, the normal weekly 12 sessions of CBT with ET/CR will be extended and take longer to implement successfully. The treatment protocol calls for three sessions of ET, followed by three sessions of CR. Given the additional complexity of a decision to be made regarding hormone therapy and the recurrence of his prostate cancer, the pace and total number of sessions will be modified as needed. You will monitor outcome by periodic completion of the ICG.

Session 5. Completion of Decision Aid, Start of Complicated Grief Treatment

WD returns to the next session, having met with his oncologist and having finished the decision aid in the past week. He brought the report from the ACS that is generated at the completion of the decision aid. You ask what his oncologist had to say, and WD indicates that the doctor is still recommending hormone therapy and he "wants me to decide as soon as possible." Despite these recommendations, WD offers, "I just still don't know if it's worth it! Now that I know more about the side effects, I keep thinking, why bother?" You reflect these feelings: "Sounds as if you feel somewhat hopeless, as if it's not important to make a decision, now that your wife is gone." He responds, "Yea, that's pretty much it. I just can't get past why all of this happened now, and even more than a year later, there are times when it still doesn't even feel real . . . like it didn't even happen. Sometimes I get very mad at myself." You ask, "Mad? Why mad at yourself?" He goes on to explain that during much of the last few months of his wife's life, he just wasn't paying close attention to her. He thinks she had been much sicker than he ever noticed, but he was just not very attentive to her. In fact, he gets particularly teary-eyed when he explains about a couple of incidents in which she, although probably feeling very poorly herself, asked how he was feeling . . . if he was okay . . . if he was in any pain or discomfort from some of the prostate symptoms he continued to experience. He explains, "That really gets to me. Here she was—close to dying—and she was watching out for me, and I wasn't even hardly thinking about her."

You recognize that this particular component of WD's grief—anger at self, guilt, and remorse—is particularly important to attend to in future sessions. For the remainder of this session, he tells more of the story of her death—what symptoms she first noticed, how/when she sought medical care, hearing from her oncologist that her treatments were no longer effective, the decision to seek hospice care, the eventual increasing decline, and once again, the last few days and hours of her life.

With more of the story now told, you recognize that during the time of her illness and death, he was very avoidant. He acted as if much of this wasn't happening. His children made many of the decisions about her care. He was physically present, but rarely emotionally available to support his wife or children. He only rarely went in to his wife's bedroom where the hospital bed and other medical paraphernalia were. ("It was just too hard!") He only minimally attended the funeral proceedings. Now, since her death, he has had multiple regrets, feels remorseful, and is angry with himself. He is avoiding lots of situations that might remind him of her—has yet to do anything with any of her possessions, rarely goes into the room where the hospital bed was, sleeps in another room/bed, tried to go back to church once but didn't return. He also shares that he has little structure to his day, feels very lonely, indicates he can't figure out what he should be doing with his life, and hasn't thought much at all about anything regarding his future. All of this confirms your diagnosis of complicated grief and you begin the CBT with the exposure therapy component presented first.

In this first actual treatment session you explain the rationale for exposure. You suggest to him that maybe he is continuing to have a difficult time with her death because it has been difficult to do things that remind him of her (going through her possessions such as clothes, books, etc.) and that it is important to gradually do these things again (i.e., stop avoiding and confront these reminders). You reassure him that you are confident he can do these, but it will take some time and planning. You ask that this week he write down some of the things he has noticed that he has avoided doing, both internal things like thinking of her, as well as external things like going places, seeing certain people, and doing certain things. You explain, "For now, just make a list of both types and we will look at it next time." He agrees.

In the final 10 minutes of the session, you return to the decision about hormone therapy. You look over the decision aid report with him, explaining that it seems to clearly recommend hormone therapy over the other treatment options (surgery, immunotherapy, chemotherapy). He simply says, "I'll think about it." You recall your competing hypotheses about the delay in decision making and for now speculate that maybe it is mostly the result of many grief-related symptoms interfering with a decision.

Sessions 6–8 (2–4 of grief therapy)

Throughout the next three weekly 1-hour sessions, you integrate components of both CBT with ET/CR grief therapy with efforts to "move him along" in making a decision about hormone therapy. In Sessions 6 and 7, you more formally begin the exposure. You take the written list of internal and external stimuli that he notes he has been avoiding and collaboratively create the hierarchy from least to most difficult to approach. In sessions, you ask him to sit with eyes closed and to imagine (see himself doing) the external situations listed, first with those at the bottom of the hierarchy, working up to those higher on the hierarchy. You also do the imaginal exposure to the internal (thoughts, images, memories) stimuli. As you process how these individual exposure sessions are going, you incorporate homework assignments asking him to increase the frequency of actually doing some of these same activities at home, between sessions.

At Session 6 you note change on the complicated grief with a decrease of three points (not clinically significant) on the ICG as it drops to 27. He is moderately compliant to the homework assignments and is beginning to talk a bit more about his future. However, there is no change on the decision regarding hormone therapy. You need to modify the treatment plan.

WD Continued Case Formulation and Treatment Planning (cont.)

After Session 6, utilizing past knowledge and experience with issues of ambivalence and resistance to change, you make a clinical decision to begin conceptualizing his delay in decision making as a readiness-to-change issue, utilizing the transtheoretical model and its stages of change: Most voluntary behavior proceeds through a series of stages from precontemplation (it is not a problem), to contemplation (maybe it is a problem), to preparation (I am getting ready to make changes), to action (I am changing), and to maintenance (I have changed and am now trying to maintain it) (Prochaska & DiClemente, 2005)—with motivational interviewing (MI) (Miller & Rollnick, 2002) as a potential intervention. You have a background question:

- Is there any empirical literature testing motivational interviewing with cancer patients?

In your personal library you have Miller and Rollnick's (2002) *Motivational Interviewing*. You briefly review its table of contents and quickly skim two relevant chapters on use of MI in medical settings and a review chapter on its efficacy. From these you conclude that there is little, if any, empirical literature on use of MI with cancer patients. However, you are uncertain about more recent literature, since 2000. You have one foreground PICO formatted intervention question:

> *For a 66-year-old widowed male—13 months post death of his wife of 41 years—advised to begin hormone therapy for metastatic prostate cancer, but delaying making a decision, is motivational interviewing an effective intervention, compared to no intervention, for making a decision?*

You search unfiltered, primary literature (PsycINFO, CINAHL, and Medline) from 2000 to 2011 with search terms:

> *motivational AND interviewing AND neoplasm AND randomized trial*

Seven articles were identified, six were studies of health behavior change (smoking cessation, diet, physical activity) and one was on colorectal cancer screening.

As anticipated, none was on cancer patient treatment decision making. Despite the lack of empirical evidence with prostate cancer patients and decision making, MI has significant empirical evidence with a variety of other populations (Burke, Arkowitz, & Menchola, 2003), and its focus is on *ambivalence*. Miller and Rollnick (2002) define MI as *a client-centered, directive method for enhancing intrinsic motivation to change by exploring and resolving ambivalence* (p. 25). Its four major principles are to express empathy, develop discrepancy, roll with resistance, and support self-efficacy. When looking for markers of success in its use, you recall that it is important to listen for *change talk*—expressions by the client indicating some consideration of making a change in behavior—even if there is no strong commitment toward changing. You are very familiar with its foundation in Rogerian (Rogers, 1961) client-centered therapy and it is consistent with empathy and alliance—general elements of effective psychotherapy relationships that have been a part of all prior sessions—so you decide to utilize it for part of Session 7.

Session 7. Combined Intervention on Complicated Grief and Ambivalence Regarding Hormone Therapy

At the start of this session, you check in on the past week and WD indicates he has done pretty well with the grief-related homework. He has made some changes around the house (put back up some pictures of him and his wife he had earlier removed) and began a few tasks related to going through his wife's things. He notes that he felt good about giving some of it away to friends and family who knew her. He still doesn't want to give her clothes to just anyone. You encourage him to continue with these types of "reengagement in life" activities and note the improvement over the last couple of weeks.

You ask about his cancer treatment decision and, as anticipated, find no change. You decide to begin MI, and you briefly explain to him that for today, you would like to talk more about where he is regarding a decision. WD seems surprised, but when you ask if that is okay he agrees. You begin, "Tell me about your concerns with waiting to decide." He offers, "Well, I'm not really concerned about it; most of the time I don't really think about it, but every once in a while, particularly when I come here to the Cancer Center, I am reminded that I haven't made any decision. Plus, my kids are always on me about it." You reflect, "Much of the time you don't think about it until someone or someplace reminds you of it?" "Yea." You ask, "Tell me about your children's concerns." WD explains, "They're worried that the cancer will spread and I'll die." "And what about you?" "Well, sure that worries me, but not as much as them." "So what about that worries you?" "I don't want to die, although I know that I have been saying I don't really care, ever since my wife died. But deep down, I know I don't, but mostly I wouldn't want to be sick, laid up, feeling lousy and, of course, nobody wants to be in pain . . . yea, I guess I worry about being in pain if the cancer spread." You summarize, "So somewhat like your children, you do worry about what might happen if you don't start the hormone therapy, particularly if your health will decline, if you'll get sick, and mostly you don't want to be in pain." "Yea, I guess I have been just trying to avoid thinking about it all." You summarize, "What I hear you saying then, is that on one hand, there is a part of you that wishes you could just avoid all of this, sort of bury your head in the sand and hope it will go away, but on the other hand, another side of you realizes it isn't gonna go away, huh?" "Well when you put it that way, it just sounds pretty stupid of me!," he responds.

You note that maybe you overdid it with the "head in the sand" analogy, so you try to back up a bit, particularly since he already feels guilt and remorse in regard to his way of coping with his wife's death. You respond with more empathy, "Well, no, not stupid, but it makes sense to me that you would have lots of mixed feelings about whether to bother to go on or not. On one hand, life hasn't seemed hardly worth continuing lately, and then, on the other hand, it sounds like you realize the cancer isn't likely to just go away, even though you wish it would, and that if you ignore it, it's likely to get worse and may result in some pretty significant health changes." He reacts, "Yea, I guess I have been pretty mixed up about what to do, wishing I didn't even have to think about it and some of the time, just avoiding thinking about it since I haven't felt like doing much, but the last thing I want is to worry my kids anymore, they've been through a lot already." You seize the opportunity and reflect, "Yea, sounds like you wouldn't want your kids to have to face another loss anytime soon. So what do you think your options are?" From here he suggests some reasonable options like talking again to his children, but this time more genuinely sharing his mixed emotions. He indicates he feels like he has enough information after completing the online decision aid, but maybe it would be helpful to go back over that, even combining the two ideas and showing it to his children as part of the discussion. You reassure, encourage, and work to maintain this discussion about reasonable options (i.e., change talk) in hopes that he will move from contemplation to action. By the end of the session, you incorporate this new information about decision making with his other grief-related homework and suggest that in addition to his grief-related work, you think it sounds like he is ready to talk to his children about the hormone therapy. He seems to agree.

Sessions 8–12

In Session 8, he comes back and tells the story of having met with his children to talk about a decision. Overall, he says it went well. They understood his ambivalence, but still wanted him to go ahead with the hormone therapy. He also talked to a close male friend who had previously taken hormones, who indicated that at first it was unpleasant, but his body eventually adjusted and, considering the options of further disease progression, he was glad that there were still some treatments available. This feedback seemed to be very influential in WD deciding to call his oncologist and urologist and inform them that he has decided to go ahead with these treatments. You tell him you are pleased to hear this and glad he has made a decision. You also realize that in MI (Miller & Rollnick, 2002), one of the important principles to recall is that ambivalence never completely goes away, so you remind yourself to continue to check in periodically on how these treatments are going.

For the remainder of Session 8, as well as Sessions 9–12, you continue the CBT complicated grief therapy with the addition of cognitive restructuring during sessions 10–12. As is the protocol, you follow Beck's approach (Beck et al., 1979) of first introducing the basic ideas of identifying, challenging, and altering negative cognitions. You use homework sheets to facilitate the analysis of specific examples that the patient identifies.

Case 2—WD: Case Summary and Evidence-Based Practice Across the Clinical Course

This more detailed case demonstrates the iterative process of EBP and a form of adaptation of the evidence. The presenting problem of distress reactive to recurrent disease (and the need to make a decision about hormone therapy) was complicated by the death of his wife. The presenting symptoms of distress, initially conceptualized to be major depressive disorder, were later identified to be symptoms of persistent complex bereavement (i.e., complicated grief). Thus, the literature on treatment for complicated grief was accessed and appraised, and, although not a perfect match (notable fit-fidelity tension), the available evidence was appropriate to address his complicated grief. However, the need to make a decision about hormone therapy was urgent and could not be delayed. It was not clear whether his delay in decision making was influenced by his complicated grief or readiness to change. Thus, the primary intervention for complicated grief (CBT with ET/CR) was *augmented* with two other interventions: first, an online decision aid for patients with prostate cancer and, second, motivational interviewing (MI). Even after beginning the decision aid, WD continued to delay in making a decision and intervention components from MI (i.e., rolling with resistance, developing discrepancies, evoking change talk) were "woven" into the treatment. By Session 8 he had made a decision. Although it remains important to attend to any ambivalence that might resurface, in the remaining sessions the focus is on complicated grief.

This case demonstrates one way of adapting best available evidence and the recursive process of EBP (i.e., AAA TIE). As this patient's disease evolves, it could move along the disease continuum. If it does, other interventions, as represented in Table 6.1, may prove to be best available evidence.

Step 6: Evaluation of Evidence-Based Practice

Monitoring Patient Outcome: Repeat Administrations of Inventory of Complicated Grief

Evaluation of the EBP process at the level of the individual patient involves repeat administrations of the self-report questionnaire evaluating symptoms of complicated grief—the ICG. Patient outcome will be monitored by the ICG, which will be administered at Sessions 3, 6, and 9 of the anticipated minimum of 12 sessions. If more than 12 sessions are needed, readminister the ICG approximately every three sessions. In addition, using your clinical judgment, monitor the overall psychosocial adaptation (increased active reengagement in life).

Evaluation of Evidence-Based Practice Components: Relative Contributions

In Case 2, patient characteristics and preferences (avoidance of grief work and making a decision regarding needed prostate cancer treatment) resulted in the need for treatment adaptation and concurrent augmentation with the addition of MI and use of decision aids. Adaptation by concurrent augmentation was feasible given the clinical expertise of the psycho-oncologist. Patient characteristics and clinical expertise converge and contribute more than best available evidence.

Professional Evaluation of Evidence-Based Practices
Another way to evaluate the EBP process is to focus on the ongoing professional development that comes from EBP. Honestly appraise how frequently the EBP steps are followed by periodically estimating in what percent of patients a formal EBP process is followed, and by periodically inspecting the archived literature searches. As more clinical questions are asked, more literature is accessed and appraised and the number of archived searches grows. These searches are then available for future use in similar clinical situations, facilitating a more frequent use of EBP. The literature search on treatments for complicated grief, for example the case study of WD, is archived for future use via use of the Centre for Evidence Based Medicine (CEBM) Web site.

CHAPTER SUMMARY

This chapter focused on individual psychosocial health service interventions for adult cancer patients experiencing distress, anxiety, and/or depression. Given the need for the evidence-based practitioner to first have a general knowledge of relevant background knowledge from which to formulate relevant clinical questions, a review of best available evidence was provided, organized around a table of nine exemplar studies. Study characteristics (cancer type, stage, disease continuum) and ease of dissemination (theoretical approach, availability of treatment manual, intervention trainability, patient acceptability) is provided in Table 6.1. There are a number of effective individual interventions for adult cancer patients available to be offered across the clinical course of the disease that decrease distress, anxiety, and depression. The strength of these interventions varies from small to medium effects with a few showing large effects. Most show short-term improvement. Various theoretical approaches are offered, although many of them are strongly influenced by cognitive and cognitive-behavioral theory. Supportive counseling is one exception. Dissemination potential for individual adult interventions is good to very good. Nearly all reviewed studies have manuals available, and most interventions are short term, trainable, and possess good patient acceptability. Two detailed case examples were provided to show the process of using the sequential competencies (i.e., steps) of EBP. The first case illustrated a straightforward adoption of best available evidence plus some supplementation for a woman who experienced the initial diagnosis of gynecologic cancer. The second case illustrated a more complex process of adapting two interventions concurrently while also augmenting the primary treatment.

7

Group Psychosocial Health Service Interventions

This chapter provides background knowledge about group psychosocial health service interventions for cancer patients and offers a detailed example of how to do evidence-based practice (EBP) where the best available evidence suggests a group intervention. Like the previous chapter, the evidence-based practitioner will often begin an encounter with a new patient with a need for general background knowledge about group interventions. Background questions may include the following:

- Are group interventions for cancer patients effective?
- Are group interventions better than individual interventions for cancer patients?
- What theoretical approaches are used for group interventions for cancer patients?
- Which types of cancer patients (disease site, stage) have been studied in group interventions?
- What types of outcomes have been measured?
- Do interventions extend length of life?
- How long do most group interventions last?
- Are treatment manuals accessible?
- Do most patients seem to find group interventions acceptable?

The following summary of general background knowledge is designed to answer some of these background questions.

BACKGROUND KNOWLEDGE

Some of the earliest, most widely cited, and best-known psychosocial health service interventions in psycho-oncology have been group interventions (Spira & Casden, 2010). Bringing cancer patients together in a group where they are with others who share similar experiences can decrease isolation, heighten emotional support, buffer ongoing stressors, and provide opportunities to gain new knowledge. Group interventions can result in the acquisition of new coping skills as group members learn from expert presenters while also learning from one another. Group interventions also have the advantage of being both cost and time efficient and, thus, in combination with other known benefits, could be argued to be the treatment of choice.

Spira and Casden (2010) provide excellent background knowledge about facilitating groups with cancer patients. They note three *basic structures or goals* for groups: information-education, coping skills training, and social/emotional support, and three different *styles of facilitating group processes*: deductive or primarily therapist driven, inductive or primarily patient driven, and interactive—more evenly balanced. In combining these characteristics, Spira and Casden (2010) suggest three logical combinations:

- Information/education goals with deductive processes
- Social/emotional support with inductive processes
- Coping skills training with interactive processes

They suggest that the information-education goal is best facilitated by a deductive style in which cancer experts are providing information to patients via lecture or predominantly didactic presentations with the goal of new knowledge being acquired by patients. Little peer discussion or interaction occurs. This is often for patients with newly diagnosed disease and beginning treatment wanting to know more about side effects, treatment options, preventive measures, and/or future rehabilitation.

They recommend that the goal of providing social and emotional support is best facilitated by an inductive style in which any topics identified by patients as relevant and of importance to them are facilitated in such a way as to enhance the group's ability to provide social and emotional support. This style includes facilitating group processes that enable authentic, genuine expression of emotion between patients and therapists, within a supportive and cohesive group context.

Finally, they suggest that the coping skills training goal is best facilitated by an interactive style in which information about various coping strategies may be presented in a didactic style first, followed by practice at implementing the new skills, often by interacting with group members and/or by in-home practice between group sessions. This is for patients learning relaxation and imagery skills, communication skills with others (health care providers, family), effective cognitive coping strategies to reduce distress, and any other newly developing skills aimed at improved quality of life. Although these combinations are recommended, experienced facilitators will note that most groups include combinations that form various hybrids of these styles that may be predominantly comprised of one style over others. Thus, it is important to consider these characteristics as combinations that define group *processes*, facilitated within the entirety of various groups, rather than as rigid descriptions of how any particular group must be run. As more is known about group characteristics, it becomes important to distinguish and ask whether some groups are better suited for some patients over other patients (Helgeson, Cohen, Schulz, & Yasko, 2000). Future background questions will ask whether there are evidence-based recommendations that indicate a match between certain group approaches with certain types of patients that result in improved outcomes.

Group Versus Individual: Outcomes and Cost

Research has identified overall benefits for group interventions and some have been compared to individual interventions. Data have been collected on overall psychosocial outcomes, time efficiency, and cost. In general, results about whether group or individual interventions are better have been mixed, with many important questions still unanswered. However, group approaches have been found to be at least as effective as individual approaches for treatment of anxiety and depression (Sheard & Maguire, 1999). In a study of melanoma patients comparing similar interventions offered both individually and in a group (Fawzy, Fawzy, & Wheeler, 1996), the group intervention showed a greater magnitude of improvement and was clearly more time-efficient. Other studies have shown no differences on various psychosocial outcomes between individual and group interventions (Edgar, Rosberger, & Collet, 2001) or better outcomes for individual versus group interventions (Osborn et al., 2006). More comprehensive analyses of the costs of psychosocial interventions in psycho-oncology that include measures of variables such as medical cost offset have been encouraged (Carlson & Bultz, 2004), but few have yet been reported. Those that have been reported are encouraging (Lemieux, Topp, Chappell, Ennis, & Goodwin, 2006; Simpson, Carlson, & Trew, 2001), suggesting the possibility of reduced costs, particularly when studies preselect participants based on elevated levels of distress.

Participation in Group Interventions and the Growth of Online Resources

Despite positive benefits of group interventions, *the majority of cancer patients do not participate* in any structured, professionally led psychosocial group intervention. Very little research has been done on how many, who, or why cancer patients choose to participate in group interventions, but the majority of community cancer centers seem to universally report difficulties in maintaining viable and successful long-term, face-to-face support group programs. Studies conducted throughout the 1990s through the mid-2000s found that group participants were more likely to be female, of higher socioeconomic status, and younger, compared to nonparticipants (Grande, Myers, & Sutton, 2006). Although it might be assumed that participants would report having poor, or less than desired social support, results on this variable are mixed, with some studies reporting that group participants report having poorer social support than others, and other studies reporting that participants have better support (Hogan, Linden, & Najarian, 2002).

One way to reach more cancer patients with group interventions is via online community support programs (Gustafson et al., 2001). In recent years, a number of online support networks such as Cancer Care (http://www.cancercare.org/) CaringBridge, (http://www.caringbridge.org/) and the Cancer Support Community (http://www.cancersupportcommunity.org/) have developed quick, readily available sources of information and online support. Support provided is often from other cancer patients, as well as cancer care professionals, and some have begun research on the dissemination of online, professionally led synchronous (i.e., group facilitator and participants online at the same time) support groups, focusing on issues such as the transfer of training of psycho-oncologists (Stephen et al., 2011), strengths and weaknesses of online groups (Owen, Bantum, & Golant, 2009), and a randomized trial investigating different forms of online support (Lepore, Buzaglo, Lieberman, Golant, & Davey, 2011). Many ethical issues remain for cancer care professionals (e.g., most US licenses restrict practice across state lines) regarding provision of services online, but online access to group support, although different than face-to-face group support, is likely to increase as patient cohorts become increasingly familiar and comfortable with accessing online resources.

Research Evidence: Group Interventions

Although summaries of reviews of group interventions in cancer have been published (Andersen, 2002; Jacobsen & Jim, 2008; Faller et al., 2013) and guidelines for group treatment are available (Spiegel & Classen, 2000; Spira & Casden, 2010), reviews have seldom summarized empirical evidence by treatment modality. One meta-analytic review of group psychotherapies did summarize 42 randomized, controlled trials (RCTs) involving 5,428 patients (Faller et al., 2013) and reported small (d = .20) to medium (d = .50) effect sizes at posttreatment for emotional distress, anxiety, depression, and quality of life. These positive effects remained, yet were smaller at follow-up. Small effect sizes indicate that the patients receiving the treatments score between the 54th to 62nd percentile on treatment outcomes compared to those not receiving the treatment. The treated patients are 4 to 12 percentage points above the average patient not receiving the treatment. Small effect sizes also are interpreted to mean a 52%–57% success rate for those receiving the treatment. Medium effect sizes are comparable to a 66th–73rd percentile range or approximately 60%–64% success rate. More detailed knowledge of group interventions is available in the unfiltered primary literature.

The current chapter focuses on a few exemplars of best available evidence for group interventions with adult cancer patients reviewed and selected from 2010 to 2014 with publications from 1996 to 2010. This table is not intended to be a comprehensive review of group interventions but rather an exemplar of representative group interventions.

Unfiltered Primary Literature

Table 7.1 includes 13 studies. All are RCTs with sample sizes ranging from 71 to 353, with 7 of the 13 studies having more than 200 participants.

Study Characteristics

Cancer Type, Stage, and Disease Continuum

Nine of the 13 studies included in Table 7.1 are of women with breast cancer. Three (Lepore, Helgeson, Eton, & Schulz, 2003; Penedo et al., 2006, 2007) are of men with prostate cancer and one (Breitbart et al., 2010) is of mixed types of cancer. Of the studies of women with breast cancer, six (Andersen et al., 2004; Antoni et al., 2001, 2006; Helgeson, Cohen, Schulz, & Yasko, 2001; Kissane, Bloch, et al., 2003; Scheier et al., 2005) are of women with early-stage breast cancer, while three (Goodwin et al., 2001; Kissane et al., 2007; Spiegel et al., 2007) are of women with late-stage, metastatic breast cancer. The one mixed-cancer study is of patients with advanced prostate, lung, breast, or colorectal cancers (Breitbart et al., 2010). In these 13 studies, the locations along the disease continuum vary from prior to the start of treatment to advanced metastatic disease. Studies of women with early-stage disease typically received the intervention within weeks after their surgery, often while receiving other cancer treatments. Some studies start later but almost always within a year of diagnosis. Men with prostate cancer typically received their treatment within a few months to a year and a half after either surgery or radiation therapy. Interventions for metastatic breast cancer usually occur between 9 and 24 months after the onset of recurrence.

Results and Outcomes Measured

The 13 studies in Table 7.1 include varied outcomes. Psychological, psychosocial, and biobehavioral outcomes, as well as time to recurrence and survival time, have been measured. For psychological outcomes such as anxiety, depression, benefit finding, intrusive thoughts, and mood states, outcomes show small to medium estimated effect sizes (d = .11 to .55). Small to medium effect sizes (d = .25 to .42) are also reported for psychosocial outcomes such as social support, family functioning, and quality of life.

Existential outcomes such as meaning, spiritual well-being, and sense of peace show large effect sizes (d = .72 to .74) in the MCGP study (Breitbart et al., 2010), and large effects appear to be possible when measuring acquisition of new knowledge (Lepore et al., 2003) or self-reported physical well-being/functioning (Penedo et al.,2007; Scheier et al., 2005).

As a whole, these interventions show overall efficacy of group interventions. Novel results include the improved health behaviors and immune changes in the biobehavioral intervention (SIBCP) (Andersen et al., 2004, 2007), the improvements in optimism and benefit finding in the cognitive-behavioral stress management (CBSM) study (Antoni et al., 2001), and the improved spiritual well-being and sense of meaning in the meaning-centered group psychotherapy (MCGP) study (Breitbart et al., 2010).

Table 7.1. Exemplars of Best Available Evidence for Group Interventions for Varied Cancer Types and Stages: Study Characteristics and Ease of Dissemination

Study Characteristics			Ease of Dissemination[a]		
Citation/ Location	N, Diagnosis, Stage/ No. of Groups	Results/Outcomes	Intervention Description, Theory, Accessibility	Therapist Characteristics	Patient Acceptability/ Trainability[b]
RCTs of group, cognitive-behavioral, stress management approaches <u>for women with early-stage breast cancer</u> with psychological, health behaviors, immune system, and benefit-finding outcomes					
Andersen et al., 2004, 2007 *Midwest US*	227 women breast (90% Stage II, 10% Stage III) postsurgery, 2 groups (SIBCP, TAU)	Reduced anxiety ($d = .29$), improved support ($d = .34$) and dietary habits, decreased smoking; emotional and health behavior changes paralleled immunity; distress reduction primary mechanism	18, 1.5 hr group ($n = 13$) sessions weekly for 4 months + 1 monthly for 8 months. CBT, problem solving + diet, exercise, assertive communication, adherence to cancer treatments. Medium accessibility	2 clinical psychologists, all cotherapy	57% (227/401) of eligible randomized 93% (106/114) completed 12 months High trainability[d]
Antoni et al., 2006 *Florida, US*	199 women breast (52% Stage 0–I, 48% Stage II–III) postsurgery, 2 groups (CBSM, 1-day seminar)	Reduced cancer-specific thought intrusion—($d = .43$ and .55) for 6 and 12 months; decreased overall distress ($d = .33$ and .43); decreased interviewer-rated anxiety ($d = .74$)`	10, 2-hour weekly group sessions. CBT, relaxation/imagery audiotapes, group support, assertion training, emotional expression. Medium accessibility	female, post-doctoral fellows and advanced trainees in clinical psych, cotherapy	57% (227/401) of eligible agreed 85% (78/92) completed intervention High trainability

(*Continued*)

Table 7.1. CONTINUED

Study Characteristics			Ease of Dissemination[a]		
Citation/ Location	**N, Diagnosis, Stage/ No. of Groups**	**Results/Outcomes**	**Intervention Description, Theory, Accessibility**	**Therapist Characteristics**	**Patient Acceptability/ Trainability[b]**
Antoni et al., 2001 *Florida, US*	136 women, breast (10% Stage 0, 48% Stage I, 41% Stage II) postsurgery, 2 groups (CBSM, 1-day seminar)	Reduced prevalence of moderate levels of depression; increased benefit finding ($d = .43$) and optimism ($d = .02$)	10, 2-hour weekly group sessions. CBT, relaxation/imagery audiotapes, group support, assertion training, emotional expression. Manualized Medium accessibility	female, post-doctoral fellows & advanced trainees in clinical psych, cotherapy	92% (125/136) completed intervention, 85% (116/136) 3 months follow-ups, 73% (100/136) 9 months follow-ups High trainability
RCTs of group, cognitive-behavioral, stress management approaches <u>for men with early-stage prostate cancer</u> with psychological, quality of life, sexual functioning, perception of stress management skill, and benefit-finding outcomes					
Penedo et al., 2006 *Florida, US*	191 men, prostate (Stage I or II); 41% Hispanic, 18% Black mean age 65.1 years post-RP or RT, 2 groups (CBSM, 1-day seminar)	Increased benefit finding and quality of life (small effects, $d = .17, .33$) Stress management skills a possible mechanism	10, 2-hour weekly group sessions. CBT, various relaxation procedures, prostate-specific stress management skills Manualized Medium accessibility	master's or doctoral trained in clinical psychology, cotherapy	88% (235/267) eligible randomized 80% (107/133) completed intervention High trainability

Penedo et al., 2007 *Florida, US*	71 men, prostate (Stage I or II) Spanish speaking, mean age 65.5 years, post-RP or RT, 2 groups (CBSM-Spanish, 1-day seminar)	Improvements in physical (*d* = .90), emotional (*d* = .53), and overall (*d* = .42) well-being, and sexual functioning (*d* = .27)	10, 2-hour weekly group sessions. Spanish-translated CBT, various relaxation procedures, prostate-specific stress management skills, culturally adapted Manual-modified Low accessibility	PhD clinical psychologist and graduate student in health psychology, cotherapy Fluent in Spanish	34% (93/271) of screened randomized 77% (41/53) completed intervention Moderate trainability
RCTs of group existential (focus on life purpose, meaning-making, spirituality) approaches <u>for women with metastatic breast cancer</u>, with psychological, emotional, social well-being, mental disorders, sense of meaning/purpose, and survival time as outcomes					
Spiegel et al., 2007; Classen et al., 2001 *West Coast, US* 1991–1996	125 women, metastatic/recurrent breast, 25 months from time of recurrence, 2 groups (SEGT, Educ)	decline in traumatic stress (*d* = .25), no differences in mood disturbance; no survival difference	90-minute sessions, weekly, 1–8 years, Existential psychotherapy, social support, education, expression of emotions, self-hypnosis for pain/stress management Manualized Medium accessibility	specially trained psychologist, psychiatrists, social workers, all cotherapy	81% (125/155) eligible were randomized 98% (122/125) at least 1 year of the intervention High trainability
Goodwin et al., 2001 *Canada, Multi-Sites* 1993–1998	235 women, metastatic breast, 20 months from time of recurrence, 2 groups (SEGT, Educ)	Decrease in negative moods (small effects, *d* = .11 to .19); women most distressed at baseline benefitted most; no survival differences	90-minute sessions, weekly, at least 1 year Existential psychotherapy, social support, education,expression of emotions Manualized Medium accessibility	Specially trained psychiatrists, psychologists, social workers, nurse clinicians, all cotherapy	76% (120/158) of randomized completed 1 year 67% mean group attendance High trainability

(*Continued*)

Table 7.1. Continued

Study Characteristics			Ease of Dissemination[a]		
Citation/ Location	**N, Diagnosis, Stage/ No. of Groups**	**Results/Outcomes**	**Intervention Description, Theory, Accessibility**	**Therapist Characteristics**	**Patient Acceptability/ Trainability[b]**
Kissane et al., 2007 *Melbourne, Australia* 1996–2002	227 women, metastatic breast (Stage IV), 9.4 months from recurrence, 2 groups (SEGT, relaxation)	Improved and *prevented* depressive disorder (small effect, $d = .20$ to .24); reduced helplessness, hopelessness, and trauma symptoms; improved social functioning; no survival differences	90-minute sessions, weekly, at least 1 year Existential psychotherapy, social support, education, expression of emotions PMR/imagery. Manualized Medium accessibility	Specially trained psychiatrists, psychologists, social workers, all cotherapy	47% (227/485) of eligible randomized 76% (112/147) at least 1 year 72% mean group attendance High trainability
RCTs of group existential (focus on life purpose, meaning-making, spirituality) approaches <u>for women with early-stage breast cancer</u>, with psychological, emotional, family functioning, therapist differences, and survival time as outcomes					
Kissane et al., 2003, 2004 *Melbourne, Australia*	303 women, breast, early stage (12% Stage I, 88% Stage II) 1/3 with depression, receiving chemo., 2 groups (CEGT, relaxation)	Trend toward decreased anxiety, sustained family relationships, small effects ($d = .21, .25$); no survival differences, psychologists best therapists ($d = .51$)	90-minute sessions, weekly, 20 sessions. CEGT + relaxation, 6 identified goals Manualized Low accessibility	15 therapists—psychiatry, psychology, social work, oncology nursing, occupational therapy	62% (303/491) eligible randomized, 88% (136/154) completed >6 sessions High trainability

RCTs of group existential (focus on life purpose, meaning-making, spirituality) approaches for patients with mixed-type, solid tumor cancers with psychological, spiritual, sense of meaning, desire for death outcomes				
Breitbart et al., 2010 *NYC, US*	90 patients, advanced (63% Stage IV) solid tumor cancers, 61% prostate, breast, lung, or colorectal; 51% females, 2 groups (MCGP, SGP)	Improved spiritual well-being (*d* = .72) and sense of meaning/peace (*d* = .74); decreased anxiety and desire for death	90-minute sessions weekly, 8 sessions Frankl's logotherapy Manualized Medium accessibility	Specially trained psychiatrists, psychologists, psychology doctoral students, all cotherapy	56% (90/160) of eligible were randomized 71% (35/49) Completed MCGP 8-week intervention High trainability
RCTs of group psychoeducational interventions (less theoretically guided, more lecture/didactic presentation of information, +/- peer discussion), for women with early-stage breast and men with prostate cancer, with psychological, adjustment, knowledge, health behavior, sexual health, employment outcomes				
Helgeson et al., 1999, 2001 *Pittsburgh, US*	312 women, breast early stage (25% Stage I, 69% Stage II, 6% Stage III) prior to or early chemo, 4 groups (Educ, PD, Combined, TAU)	Enhanced adjustment in education groups: mental health (*d* = .21) physical health (*d* = .27) no benefits to discussion groups results maintained at 3-year follow-up	8 weekly sessions, 45 minutes (Educ) 60 minutes (PD) No manual No accessibility	1 masters-prepared oncology nurse and 1 oncology social worker, cotherapists for all groups	70% (312/445) of eligible randomized 62.5% (5/8) mean group attendance Low trainability
Lepore et al., 2003 *Pittsburgh, US*	250 men, prostate nonmetastatic, treatment within 1 month (56% prostatectomy) 3 groups (Educ, Educ + PD, TAU)	Both treatment groups increase knowledge (*d* = .82) Educ + PD group improved health behaviors (*d* = .29) Patients with no college benefitted most	6 weekly sessions, 60 minutes (Educ only) 105 minutes (Education for 60 + 45 for PD) SCPM No manual No accessibility	Male clinical psychologist, content experts (e.g., oncologist, urologist, dietitian)	77% (279/362) of eligible randomized 90% (250/279) completed study Low trainability

(*Continued*)

Table 7.1. Continued

Study Characteristics			Ease of Dissemination[a]		
Citation/ Location	**N, Diagnosis, Stage/ No. of Groups**	**Results/Outcomes**	**Intervention Description, Theory, Accessibility**	**Therapist Characteristics**	**Patient Acceptability/ Trainability[b]**
Scheier et al., 2005 *Pennsylvania, US*	252 women, breast, younger age (<50), early stage (I–III) recently completed adjuvant therapy, 3 groups (Educ, Nutrition, TAU)	Fewer depressive symptoms (d = .41) and better physical functioning (d = .91)	Four monthly, 2-hour sessions Education—info about psychosocial aspects of breast cancer; Nutrition—info about low-fat, high fruit/vegetable diet No manual No accessibility	Content experts (endocrinologist, psychologist, minister, oncology nurse, social workers, dietitian)	78% (252/325) of eligible randomized, 89% (224/252) completed study (79% nutrition, 72% Educ, 90% TAU) Low trainability

[a]Ease of dissemination is operationally defined as an intervention <12 sessions, provided by one qualified provider such as a social worker, psychologist, or nurse (adapted from Jacobsen & Jim, 2008).

[b]Trainability is an estimate of how easy an intervention is to train to others—operationally defined as High = manual available + nondoctoral provider, Moderate = manual available OR treatment provided by nondoctoral provider, Low = no manual and treatment provided by doctoral-level provider (taken from Chorpita et al., 2011).

[c]Accessibility of Manual—High = online, Medium = published manual/book/workbook, Low = from researcher only, None = no manual available.

[d]An NCI-funded dissemination study is ongoing.

CBSM, cognitive-behavioral stress management; CCOP, community clinical oncology program; CEGT, cognitive-existential group therapy; d = *Cohen's d* = standardized mean difference scores as reported or calculated using Wilson, D.B. online effect size calculator; Educ, educational group, 45 minutes, 8 topics, expert provided lecture-format, discussion discouraged; MCGP, meaning-centered group psychotherapy; PD, peer discussion, 60 minutes, professionals facilitated discussion, encouraged self-disclosure, emotional expression, mutual support; PMR, progressive muscle relaxation; RP, radical prostatectomy; RT, radiation therapy; SCPM, social cognitive processing model; SEGT, supportive-expressive group therapy; SGP, supportive group psychotherapy; SIBCP, stress and immunity breast cancer project.

Do Group Psychosocial Interventions Extend Length of Life?

This intriguing question has been studied since the original and unanticipated findings of Spiegel and colleagues (1989), reporting on a Yalom-style group therapy (Yalom, 1980) done with women with metastatic breast cancer in the 1970s (Spiegel et al., 1989). They reported an average 16-month survival advantage for participants in their supportive expressive group therapy (SEGT). This finding was eventually questioned (Fox, 1998), and it was suggested to be the result of an inadvertent sampling error, in which the average survival time of the participants from the *control group* of the SEGT study was much shorter (2.8% vs. 32% survival at 5 years) than typical. However, despite this possibility of sampling error, the original 1989 study spawned replication efforts in the United States (Spiegel et al., 2007), Canada (Goodwin et al., 2001), and Australia (Kissane, Love, et al., 2004). These replications efforts, of women with metastatic breast cancer receiving a manualized (Spiegel & Classen, 2000) intervention, failed to find any survival time advantage. Despite these failed replication efforts, interest in the possibility of a psychosocial intervention affecting disease endpoints, such as time to recurrence and/or overall survival time (Andersen et al., 2008; Kissane, 2011; Spiegel, 2012), continues. Kissane (2011) summarized 15 randomized clinical trials reporting survival outcomes, noting some methodological flaws and other relevant issues, and concluding that the preponderance of the evidence suggests that psychosocial interventions do not extend survival.

More recent interest appears to have shifted away from survival to understanding potential mechanism(s) of change that might explain the connection between interventions and disease endpoints. Potential mechanisms have included the following:

- *Immune system changes*—consistent with hypotheses suggesting stress reduction could affect key immune system changes (e.g., increased natural killer cell activity), which ultimately could affect cancer cell growth.
- *Behavioral changes*—consistent with hypotheses suggesting improved health outcomes such as decreased time to recurrence and/or increased survival time could be the result of improved health behaviors such as increased physical activity or improved diet, but most important, enhanced adherence to cancer treatments.

At present, ongoing randomized trials investigating the question of survival time have decreased, and interest has shifted to other potential mechanisms such as the roles of untreated depression, social support, health beliefs, health behaviors, and social disparities and their possible connection to survival via the behavioral mechanism of adherence to cancer treatments (Kissane, 2011).

Ease of Dissemination of Group Interventions

Taking results from well-designed RCTs and transporting them to a community cancer center is part of translational research and includes dissemination and implementation. As previously discussed in Chapter 6, ease of dissemination is important background knowledge. Thus, Table 7.1 includes information about ease of dissemination by providing a brief description of each intervention, its theoretical foundation, availability/accessibility of a treatment manual, therapist characteristics, patient acceptability, and how easy or difficult it is to train competent professionals to provide the intervention.

However, even when best available evidence includes effective group interventions, and the interventions are effectively disseminated, implementation of such interventions in real-world oncology settings continues to be difficult. Very few implementation research projects have been completed. In most community settings, resources for such implementation are limited. Thus, when evaluating the EBP of *group* psychosocial interventions, EBP models that also emphasize *other resources*—local administrative support, therapist time, availability of group therapy rooms, or routine patient referral for group interventions—are highly relevant. Without such resources (even when clinical expertise is good), best available evidence can be effectively disseminated, but still not effectively implemented.

Intervention Descriptions

The studied interventions in Table 7.1 have varied by number of sessions, session length, and frequency. The fewest number of sessions is 4 and the most is approximately 50 (weekly for at least 1 year). The most common session length is 90 minutes, with 120 minutes being next most common. Only 3 of the 13 studies in Table 7.1 were less than 90 minutes. All but one study met for weekly sessions. The total number of intervention hours varied significantly from as few as 8 hours to as long as over 4,500 hours. Other than session length being relatively standard at 90–120 minutes, the number of sessions varied tremendously, mostly due to the theoretical approach and subsequent group processes used. Psychoeducational group interventions, mostly utilizing the education-information process, were the shortest at four to eight, 60- to 90-minute sessions. The existential SEGT studies, mostly utilizing the social/emotional support process, were the longest at weekly 90-minute sessions for at least 1 year. The cognitive-behavioral therapy (CBT) approaches, using an interactive, coping skills training approach, were typically weekly, 90- to 120-minute sessions for 10 to 26 sessions.

Theoretical Approaches

The group interventions highlighted in Table 7.1 include different theoretical approaches, often consisting of similar intervention techniques and yet varied hypothesized mechanisms of action. Five different approaches are represented.

Cognitive-Behavioral Stress Management

The group approaches of Andersen and colleagues (2004, 2007) and Antoni and colleagues (2001, 2006) are most representative of cognitive-behavioral stress management techniques. Andersen's biobehavioral model—also referred to as the stress and immunity breast cancer project (SIBCP)—proposes that a psychological intervention can affect disease outcomes (time to recurrence/metastasis, survival) via varied mechanisms such as psychological (decreased distress, anxiety, depression), behavioral (improved compliance to cancer treatment, increased physical activity/exercise, healthy diet), and biologic (immune system parameters) changes (Andersen et al., 1994). The studies by Antoni and colleagues (2001, 2006) and Penedo and colleagues (2006, 2007) (see Table 7.1) propose that their intervention affects overall quality of life and physical health via improved cognitive appraisal of stressors, enhanced self-efficacy, improved awareness, and expression of emotions, increased perception of social support, and the resulting declines in stress-related hormones (Antoni, 2003). The group goals and processes in these CBT approaches most closely fit with coping skills training goals, facilitated by an interactive style.

Social-Cognitive Processing

In his work with men with prostate cancer, Lepore (2001) proposes a social cognitive processing (SCP) model, a model focused on the consequences of traumatic life events such as a diagnosis of cancer. SCP notes that the emotional distress that accompanies trauma is due to the individual's change in perception of himself or his world, and the meaning inherent in the trauma. The hypothesized mechanism of change occurs within the process of confronting, contemplating, and reevaluating the aversive events. This process of talking about the events and one's emotions and reactions, within a supportive group context, is proposed to facilitate adaptation and integration of these traumatic events into existing and newly evolving models of self or the world. The group processes in these CBT approaches include a combination of interactive skills training as well as occasional use of inductive social/emotional support.

Existential Group Therapy

Spiegel and colleagues (Classen et al., 2001; Spiegel et al., 2007), and subsequent replication studies, are the primary representatives of the adaptation of existential therapy to cancer, as represented in their supportive-expressive group therapy (SEGT) (Spiegel & Spira, 1991) with women with *late-stage metastatic* breast cancer. As attempts at replication of the original model, this approach is also represented in the work of Goodwin et al. (2001) and Kissane et al. (2007). As explained by Spiegel, "cancer activates the 'ultimate concerns of existence' which Yalom (1980) describes as isolation, meaning, freedom and death" (Classen & Spiegel, 2011, p. 107). Living with cancer can be an isolating experience and can be perceived as a reminder of the potential aloneness of death, while generating questions of meaning (e.g., "Why me?") and also experiencing a sense of loss of freedom and control. Participating in a group is proposed to counteract these existential concerns. The proposed mechanisms of change in SEGT are to confront these existential issues by enhancing social support; encouraging emotional expression and openness; helping to integrate a sense of a changed self, body image, and world; improving communication with health care providers; reordering life priorities; and "detoxifying" the fears of death by direct, open, supportive discussion. Active group participation, facilitated by a skilled group therapist, helps to achieve these goals. In Kissane and colleagues' explanation of the SEGT group process (Kissane, Grabsch, et al., 2004), they note that SEGT "transforms existential ambivalence into creative living, evidenced by humour, celebration, assertiveness, altruism, new creative pursuits and eventually courageous acceptance of dying" (p. 755). The primary group process in these groups is social/emotional support process.

Cognitive-Existential Group Therapy

This approach combines cognitive-behavioral and existential approaches as explained by Kissane and colleagues (1997) in their work with women with *early-stage* breast cancer. In this approach they highlight the group development through three phases—beginning, middle, and end—explaining how the two theoretical approaches are integrated throughout the group phases. The beginning phase involves the development of group cohesion to combat the sense of isolation and aloneness and thus emphasizes existential therapy, while middle and later phases involve confronting common themes (e.g., fear of recurrence, communication with health care providers, coping with side effects), during which cognitive coping strategies are emphasized. During the final phase, when the group is ending, issues of loss and reordering of priorities arise and are thus approached with existential therapy. This combined existential-cognitive model is thought to be more appropriate for women with early-stage cancer, while SEGT is more appropriate for those with advanced disease. As a combined theoretical approach, varied group processes are used in CEGT with a primary mix of social/emotional support and coping skills training.

Meaning-Centered Group Psychotherapy

This existential intervention is based upon the work of Viktor Frankl and his concept of logotherapy ("logo" is the Greek word for meaning). According to Frankl, the primary motivation in life is to find a sense of meaning, even in the face of life's most difficult situations (he was a concentration camp survivor). Inspired also by the work of Irving Yalom (1980), Breitbart and Applebaum (2011) developed an 8-week intervention designed to help advanced cancer patients. Participants report a loss of meaning, despair, hopelessness, and a desire for a hastened death. Meaning-centered group psychotherapy (MCGP) helps participants recognize and acknowledge the importance of spiritual well-being and meaning-making, particularly at the end of life. Key concepts related to Frankl's ideas include the following:

- *The meaning of life*—life has meaning that has, and always will, continue to exist, and those experiencing a loss of meaning have become disconnected to it, not that it no longer exists.
- *A will to meaning*—all human beings have an innate desire to find and create meaning.
- *Freedom of will*—we have the right and responsibility to find meaning and to choose how we will make sense out of suffering (i.e., "choose our attitudes toward suffering").

- *Sources of meaning*—four primary sources of meaning come from creativity, experience, attitude, and legacy.

Within the context of the 8-week group psychotherapy experience where particular themes as described here are highlighted each week, a number of didactic presentations, discussions, and experiential exercises have been developed. These group experiences, drawing from the major principles of logotherapy, are hypothesized to result in an enhanced sense of meaning by recognizing, acknowledging and capitalizing on a variety of sources of meaning, which in turn improves quality of life, while reducing psychological distress and despair.

Dissemination Conclusions

The studies provided in Table 7.1 vary in ease of dissemination with most having high trainability and moderate accessibility to a treatment manual. Most providers were doctoral-level psychologists or psychiatrists and so the level of training may make those studies more difficult to disseminate. Treatment length varied considerably. However, in considering theoretical approach and treatment length together, it is clear that the longer interventions were three SEGT approaches with a typical length of weekly sessions for at least 1 year (>52 sessions). Considering the other 10 studies, treatment length varies from 4 to 20 sessions with a mean of 10. Thus, on the average, considering all of the studies in Table 7.1, ease of dissemination is good. Many of the studies show a treatment length of 2–3 months of weekly sessions, theoretical approaches (e.g., CBT, SEGT) that are generally familiar to most mental health professionals, manuals that are accessible from traditional book outlets, and high trainability. Patient acceptability of the interventions also seems good. Once a patient agrees to participate in an intervention (about 6 in 10 agreed), it appears that the vast majority (83%) received a large percentage of the intervention. The doctoral training level (psychologists, psychiatrists) of many of the providers makes dissemination somewhat more difficult, but given the cotherapy used in all of these studies, that might be less of an impediment to dissemination. Lastly, it is important to recognize that even with reasonable dissemination, as discussed earlier, when local resources in support of group interventions are lacking, implementation remains difficult. Reference citations for manualized interventions and related resources are provided in Box 7.1

Summary of the Evidence Base for Group Interventions

The majority of group interventions for cancer patients have been for women with either early- or late-stage breast cancer and for men with prostate cancer. A variety of psychological, psychosocial, and biobehavioral outcomes have been studied with improvements noted in overall quality of life such as decreased

Box 7.1

Accessibility of Manuals: Reference Citations for Manualized Interventions and Related Resources From Exemplars of Best Available Evidence, for Group Interventions

For Women with Early-Stage Breast Cancer (Cognitive-Behavioral, Stress Management Approaches)

Andersen et al. (2004, 2007)—Manualized.

Treatment manual and patient guidebook available as part of NCI-funded dissemination and implementation study for trainees attending 2-day training, *Cancer to Health C2H.*

Related Resources

Andersen, B. L. (1992). Psychological interventions for cancer patients to enhance the quality of life. *Journal of Consulting and Clinical Psychology, 60*, 552–568.

Andersen, B. L. (2002). Biobehavioral outcomes following psychological inerventions for cancer patients. *Journal of Consulting and Clinical Psychology, 70*, 590–610.

Antoni et al. (2001, 2006)—Manualized.

Antoni, M. H. (2003). *Stress management intervention for women with breast cancer.* Washington, DC: American Psychological Association.

For Men With Early-Stage Prostate Cancer (Cognitive-Behavioral, Stress Management Approaches)

Penedo et al. (2006)—Unpublished manual.

Penedo, F. J., Dahn, J. R., & Antoni, M. H. (2001). *Cognitive-behavioral stress management (CBSM) intervention for prostate cancer.* Unpublished manual, University of Miami, Department of Psychology.

Penedo et al. (2007)—Manual adapted from:

Penedo, F. J., Antoni, M. H., Dahn, J., Molton, I., Gonzalez, J. S., . . . Kinsinger, D. (2000). *Cognitive-behavioral stress management in men treated for prostate cancer.* Unpublished intervention manual.

Related Resources

Antoni, M. H. (2003). Stress management effects on psychological, endocrinological, and immune functioning in men with HIV infection: Empirical support for a psychoneuroimmunological model. *Stress, 6*, 173–188.

Antoni, M. H., Baggett, L., Ironson, G., August, S., LaPerriere, A., Klimas, N., Fletcher, M. A. (1991). Cognitive-behavioral stress management intervention buffers distress responses and immunologic changes following notification of HIV-1 seropositivity. *Journal of Consulting and Clinical Psychology, 59*, 906–915.

For Women With Metastatic Breast Cancer (Existential)

Spiegel et al. (2007), Classen et al. (2001)—No manual.

Related Resources

Goodwin et al. (2001)—Manualized.
Kissane et al. (2007)—Manualized.
Spiegel, D., & Classen, C. (2000). *Group therapy for cancer patients: A research-based handbook for psychosocial care.* New York, NY: Basic Books.
Spiegel, D., & Spira, J. (1991). *Supportive/expressive group therapy: A treatment manual of psychosocial intervention for women with recurrent breast cancer.* Stanford, CA: Stanford University School of Medicine.

For Women With Early-Stage Breast Cancer (Existential)

Kissane et al. (2003, 2004)—Manualized.
Kissane, D. W., Bloch, S., Miach, P., Smith, G. C., Seddon, A., & Keks, N. (1997). Cognitive-existential group therapy for patients with primary breast cancer techniques and themes. *Psycho-Oncology, 6*, 25–33.

Patients With Mixed Type (Existential)

Breitbart et al. (2010)—Manualized (meaning-centered group psychotherapy).
Breitbart, W. S. (2014a). *Meaning-centered group psychotherapy for patients with advanced cancer: A treatment manual.* New York: Oxford University Press.

Related Resource: Manual Adapted for Individual Modality

Breitbart, W. S. (2014b). *Individual meaning-centered psychotherapy for patients with advanced cancer: A treatment manual.* New York: Oxford University Press.

For Women With Early-Stage Breast Cancer and Men With Early-Stage Prostate Cancer (Psychoeducation)

Helgeson et al. (1999, 2001)—No manual.
Lepore et al. (2003)—No manual.
Scheier et al. (2005)—No manual.

---

distress/anxiety/depression and improved well-being. A few novel positive outcomes include improved health behaviors and immune system changes, optimism/benefit finding, and spirituality/sense of meaning. Two theoretical orientations—cognitive behavioral and existential—have dominated this literature, while a few psychoeducational interventions have de-emphasized theory in favor of didactic presentations and acquisition of new knowledge. Overall ease of dissemination is good, with published manuals, treatment lengths that average 2–3 months of weekly sessions, theoretical approaches well known by many mental health professionals, and good patient acceptability.

CASE EXAMPLE: HOW TO DO EVIDENCE-BASED PRACTICE OF A GROUP INTERVENTION

The following case example provides a detailed illustration of how to do EBP where a group intervention is warranted. This case emphasizes:

1. The need for repeat development of PICO questions, literature searches, and appraisal of the literature as the case evolves and clinical questions change.
2. The importance of monitoring patient progress with the use of self-report questionnaires and their use as feedback to therapists to avoid treatment failures.
3. The use of patient feedback to prompt discussion and consultation with the patient that results in the modification of a treatment plan.
4. The use of a mix-and-match strategy in developing a modified treatment plan.

Case Example 3—KG: Individual Supportive Psychotherapy for a 48-Year-Old Male With Stage IIIA Colorectal Cancer

Referral Information

One of the RNs in the chemotherapy infusion area contacts you to make a referral of a patient she saw yesterday. The RN gave the patient a distress thermometer screening and the patient indicated a score of 6 on the 10-point scale, adding that "I guess I could use someone to talk to about all of this." The patient is a 48-year-old, White married male who was recently diagnosed with Stage III colorectal cancer. In reviewing his medical oncology chart, you note that he had surgery, the cancerous tumor was removed, and he is now receiving chemotherapy labeled FOLFOX4. The nurse indicated that it seems he is experiencing distress mostly over the seriousness of his disease, but she also wonders if he has much social support because he has only had someone drop him off and pick him up for most of his chemotherapy treatments; no one has stayed with him. She also explains that he has had some difficulties with managing the ambulatory pump that is a part of his chemotherapy; he has to wear this for about 24 hours after he finishes his onsite chemotherapy.

You Begin the Evidence-Based Practice Process

Step 1: Ask Specific, Clinical Questions: Both Background and Foreground

Relevant *biomedical* background questions include the following:

- How serious is Stage III colon cancer?
- What is the likely long-term prognosis?
- What is FOLFOX4 chemotherapy?
- What side effects might be associated with it?

- Is there any family history, and is colon cancer a hereditary form of cancer?

An excellent and quickly accessible online source of information of background knowledge is the NCI's PDQ Web site. From this site, which you access by Googling "cancer.gov" and then searching the PDQ statement on "colon cancer treatment," helpful information is obtained, written for both health care professionals and patients. For ease of understanding, you switch back and forth between the two PDQ versions, and using the NCI Dictionary link, it is feasible to get most of the aforementioned questions answered.

Stage III is serious, but further information would be helpful since it is divided into substages A, B, or C based upon whether and how far the tumor invaded the internal lining of the intestines, and if any lymph nodes were found to be positive. FOLFOX4 chemotherapy involves three different drugs (oxaliplatin, leucovorin, and fluorouracil [5-FU]) given on two consecutive days, weekly. One unique aspect of the treatment is the administration of some of the 5-FU via an ambulatory pump that the patient wears for 22 hours, every other week. Some of the more common side effects are neutropenia (lowered white blood cells)—and thus concern about infections—and peripheral neuropathy (pain, numbness, tingling, weakness in parts of the body, often in the hands or feet), which is generally reversible once chemotherapy is over but sometimes lingers long term. In regard to prognosis, the PDQ site indicates 6-year survival rates for patients receiving the FOLFOX4 treatment are about 73%. It is also indicated that colon cancer is sometimes hereditary and that groups who have a higher than normal risk are those with a first-degree relative with colon cancer and those with some specific hereditary conditions.

Relevant *psychosocial* background questions include the following:

- Are there any psychosocial concerns unique to treatments for colon cancer?
- What types of social support are most important for colorectal cancer patients?
- Are there any postsurgical complications that might result in psychosocial distress for colon cancer patients (e.g., colostomy)?
- Are there particular forms of psychosocial distress, such as fears of death, that may be more prevalent with more advanced Stage III cancers?
- Is there empirical evidence for any specific psychosocial health service intervention recommended for colorectal cancer patients?

You have general knowledge applicable to some of these questions, but it is important to review some relevant resources. You look through sources of background knowledge that include the textbook *Psycho-Oncology* (Holland et al., 2010), the *Quick Reference for Oncology Clinicians* (Holland et al., 2006), and the *Handbook of Psychotherapy in Cancer Care* (Watson & Kissane, 2011). The *Quick Reference* has a list of psychological concerns in colorectal cancer that includes

(a) guilt over delay in doing a screening colonoscopy, (b) adjustment difficulties to stoma/ostomy, (c) burden of possible familial increased risk, (d) anxiety/embarrassment about chronic bowel difficulties, (e) depression, and (f) delirium during end-of-life care. Of particular help is a chapter in the *Psycho-Oncology* textbook titled *Gastrointestinal Cancer* (Krouse, 2010), which provided a quick overview. From this source you note that colorectal cancer is the most common of the gastrointestinal cancers (i.e., esophagus, stomach, colon, rectum, pancreas) with nearly equal prevalence in men and women. Stage is a major factor in overall quality of life, and the patient's health-related quality of life is a major consideration. Areas of potential problems include (a) nutritional status, eating, bowel functioning; (b) the stigma associated with bowel problems; (c) isolation, withdrawal, depression; (d) loss of social support and the impact on family relationships (particularly related to food, eating, dinner times, etc.); (e) need or not for an ostomy, either temporarily or permanently; and (f) and impact on sexuality. These quality-of-life problems are usually more common and more serious for patients with rectal cancers than colon cancers and are often due to the consequences of surgery. It will be important for you to collaborate with other health care providers such as the oncologist, surgeon, chemotherapy nurses, and possible pain specialist. As you anticipated, this book chapter confirmed that with more advanced disease, there are likely to be more concerns about death and dying. From the *Handbook of Psychotherapy in Cancer Care* (Watson & Kissane, 2011), you note that no specific counseling or psychotherapy intervention has been uniquely developed for patients with colon cancer. Two meta-analytic reviews (Meyer & Mark, 1995; Rehse & Pukrop, 2003) readily available online via the Cancer Control P.L.A.N.E.T. portal note improved quality of life for most cancer patients who participate in psychosocial interventions. Colorectal cancer patients participated in some of these studies, but none had intervention components specifically developed for concerns unique to colon cancer.

You then searched the National Guidelines Clearinghouse (NGC) for background information about distress in cancer care by use of the search term *distress AND cancer* and the most relevant guidelines were those from the Oncology Nursing Society (ONS) titled *Putting Evidence Into Practice.* The ONS has a series of clinical guidelines on a variety of oncology-specific concerns including anxiety, depression, fatigue, anorexia, nausea, lymphedema, dyspnea, peripheral neuropathy, and so on. You quickly reviewed the guidelines for depression (Fulcher, Badger, Gunter, Marrs, & Reese, 2008) and anxiety (Sheldon, Swanson, Dolce, Marsh, & Summers, 2008) and note that both recommend psychoeducation and psychosocial interventions, CBT, individual or group counseling/psychotherapy, and support groups.

Relevant *foreground* questions prior to the first session include the following:

- Is there a family history of colorectal cancers and, if so, has he undergone genetic testing?
- Did the patient need to have a colostomy, following surgery? If so, was it temporary?

- What is the nature of his relationships with others, particularly family and spouse?
- Has he become isolated, withdrawn from usual social contact? If so, why?
- Has his interest in sexual activity changed?
- How does he feel about frequency of bowel movements, or other GI-related symptoms?
- Does he perceive there to be less social support than he desires?
- How has he managed the time period, self-care, and related hassles when he has the ambulatory pump attached?
- How serious is his distress? Does it meet criteria for any specific mental disorder such as major depression, any anxiety disorders, or posttraumatic stress disorder?
- Is he interested in ongoing counseling/psychotherapy, and if so, does he have preferences about modality (individual, group, couples, family)?

Session 1

> *The first clinical interview: Assessment of psychosocial adaptation, establishment of psychotherapy relationship with elements of empathy, alliance, and collaboration on goals/tasks.*

The procedure for the semistructured psychosocial assessment of a newly diagnosed cancer patient (Nicholas & Veach, 2000), as described in Chapter 5, should be used for this patient.

You meet KG in the waiting room and escort him to the counseling office. You explain the purpose of this initial visit—to hear about his particular situation and to evaluate how well he is adapting to the various stressful situations he has faced. During this assessment, you will be listening to evaluate overall psychosocial adaptation as consisting of three components: maintaining active involvement in things of importance, minimizing disruptions to daily roles, and effectively managing expected emotional distress.

To start the interview, you ask to hear about his story. He explains that he was having a lot of stomach and bowel problems for a few months, initially thinking it was just irregularity, not enough fiber, or occasional "weird-flu" symptoms, until one day he noticed some pretty dark blood in his stool and lots of cramping. This scared him enough to set up an appointment with his family doctor, for the very next day. KG was not very familiar to his family doctor, as he tended to avoid going to the doctor unless he really felt lousy. He learned from his doctor that it was going to be necessary to have a colonoscopy—something he knew about, but didn't think he was old enough yet to worry about. He had the colonoscopy, and they discovered a colon mass that was biopsied and confirmed that this was cancer, an adenocarcinoma. Additional tests were run, including a CT scan of the abdomen and pelvis. It was decided that surgery was the first step and it generally went well. After some time to recover from the surgery, he met with his oncologist and learned that because some of his lymph nodes were involved, he would need to have chemotherapy. He was frightened and very disappointed that he had to do chemotherapy. He even thought about not doing it, but he was persuaded by his oncologist that it was very necessary. He is now doing chemotherapy, having completed two cycles. When asked, he didn't know the stage, although you now realize it is Stage IIIA because there was some evidence of cancer cells in his lymph nodes.

In proceeding with the psychosocial assessment interview, you learn that KG, although still legally married, has been separated from his wife for the last couple of years. They have two adult children (mid-20s), one living with his wife at her home and the other living on his own. He describes his relationship with his wife as "okay" but doesn't elaborate. In fact, he avoided the issue of whether they were separated, divorced, or living together at first, and eventually reported, "I guess I might as well be honest with you." He then explained that they have been separated for 2 years and were close to getting a divorce when he got sick. Although they now see each other more frequently, he thinks his wife only comes around because she feels guilty and sorry for him. They haven't talked about going ahead with the divorce since he got sick. Although she had been around more at the time of his initial diagnosis and surgery, he doesn't see her daily anymore. She does check in on him when it's time for his next chemotherapy. When directly asked about his assessment of social support, he responds, "Well, I guess it's okay, but I'm not sure what I should be expecting. I have been pretty much on my own these last couple of years. I live alone and go to and from work by myself, when I was working, so I've gotten used to being alone a lot, and don't really mind it too much." His two sons also check in on him, usually by telephone, about once per week. He also indicates there is no family history of colorectal cancer that he is aware of and no genetic testing.

Before getting sick, KG worked regularly as an insurance salesman in an office with about five other full-time employees. He admits that he misses those routine workdays and the chance to visit and talk to his coworkers. He has done well financially, as an insurance agent, but generally doesn't find it very challenging, meaningful, or stimulating anymore. He is on medical leave while finishing the current round of chemotherapy.

Other assessment procedures determined that he has a very good understanding of his disease, the treatment plan, and his prognosis by providing accurate, relevant details during the interview. His understanding is that the surgery "was successful" in getting the tumor and now he has to do chemotherapy "for a while." His medical oncologist told him the current survival rate for his type and stage are about 75% of those who complete surgery and the current chemotherapy. He offers that he was lucky that his surgery went well and he didn't have to have a colostomy. He is now on week three of his chemotherapy and hasn't had any major side effects, although he had to get some extra fluids one time, and he has been told to stay away from crowds on certain days after his treatment. He has just recently begun to notice some tingling and numbness in his toes, but it hasn't stopped him from doing his usual routine. He doesn't like the hassle of the ambulatory pump and bag part of his chemotherapy, but he has managed it pretty well by himself. The first time, he was really worried about all he needed to do, so he got his wife to come over and help him with some of it, but since then he has done it on his own. His current nutritional status, ability to eat regular meals, and bowel movements are somewhat problematic, but he says they are all getting easier to manage in recent weeks. He has lots of diarrhea, but manages it okay by himself. He does get embarrassed sometimes if he is out eating with others and has to worry about all of this, so he just hasn't gone out to socialize much at all lately, even turning down a couple of invitations. Because he has been separated from his wife, sexuality is not of concern to him, although he does indicate he hasn't had much interest at all since he got sick.

He completes the Hospital Anxiety and Depression Scale (HADS; Holland, Greenberg, & Hughes, 2006; Zigmond & Snaith, 1983), used frequently as a screening device to measure the presence of significant symptoms of anxiety or depression. His scores were 3 for anxiety and 4 for depression, indicating mild levels of both anxiety and depression, both subthreshold to any mental disorder. He has no prior mental health history or any prior experience with counseling or psychotherapy, but he is interested in trying it out with the initial goal of "having someone to talk to about all that has changed lately." You conclude that his overall psychosocial adaptation is fair to good. The disease and its treatment have interfered and altered his daily routine, and interrupted his typical roles (e.g., employee), as has his separated status (e.g., husband) and his children's age (e.g., no regular role as a father), but his ability to manage expected distress is good since he is currently reporting mild levels.

In a brief discussion about possible psychosocial interventions for him, you explain that both individual and group counseling might be of help for him and check to see if he has a preference. He indicates no particular preference, but he does wonder, "What will we talk about each time?" His next appointment is scheduled for 1 week.

Post Psychosocial Assessment Interview: Summary of Key Patient Characteristics

- 48-year-old, separated, White male
- Stage IIIA colon cancer, postsurgery
- Currently doing chemotherapy, weekly, two consecutive days
- Managing the ambulatory pump component of chemotherapy okay now
- Minimal to no regular social support; has declined some offers to socialize due to worry about eating, bowel habits, and so on
- Mild to moderate distress—does not meet criteria for any mental disorders
- Mild chemotherapy side effects
- No past experience with counseling or any preference for individual or group.

Step 2: Accessing the Best Available Research Evidence

You begin the process of accessing best available research by following the sequential steps recommended by Gibbs (2003). *Step 1* is to formulate a foreground PICO question, in this instance, with no C (Comparison).

For a 48-year-old male, currently undergoing chemotherapy for Stage IIIA colon cancer, what is the best intervention for decreasing distress and increasing social support?

Step 2 involves listing keywords or specific search terms that correspond with each of the four PICO components and *step 3* involves listing possible synonyms or known terms from various controlled vocabulary databases (e.g., PsycINFO, CINAHL, PubMed).

P—male, colon, colorectal, bowel, advanced cancer, neoplasm
I—psychosocial intervention, psychotherapy, counseling, psychological treatment
C—compared to no treatment
O—support, social support, anxiety, depression, distress

Step 4 is to search for filtered literature. You did this prior to the first appointment and identified evidence-based guidelines for distress from the Oncology Nurse Society, via the NGC, specifically for the treatment of anxiety and depression in mixed types of cancer patients. Although KG does not meet criteria for any specific anxiety or mood disorder, the guidelines remain relevant for mild to moderate distress. You did not find any clinical guidelines for psychosocial interventions specifically tailored to colon cancer patients. Thus, *step 5* involves searching unfiltered sources specifically for RCTs of psychosocial interventions and with the use of search terms that would identify any interventions targeted specifically for colon or colorectal cancer patients.

You complete an unfiltered literature search, accessed via EBSCOhost, using the search terms *colon cancer AND psychosocial OR psychological OR counseling AND intervention*, with use of the search limiters of *treatment outcome/clinical* for PsycINFO, *randomized controlled trial* for CINAHL and Medline, and the timeframe 1996–2014. This search identified 18 publications, 10 of which were studies of early detection/screening of colon cancer, 2 were of exercise interventions, 2 were virtual reality as distraction during chemotherapy interventions, 1 was on adherence to medications in patients at risk for colon cancer, and 1 was with a noncancer population. Only 2 of the 18 studies were psychosocial interventions, both were with newly diagnosed cancer patients, with mixed types (breast, colon, and lung cancers), and neither was specific to colorectal cancer patients. One of them (Edgar et al., 2001) found positive outcomes only for breast cancer patients receiving an individual intervention, and the other study (Rawl et al., 2002) used a study-specific, computer-based nursing intervention, which is not widely available.

Summary of Conclusions

- There do not appear to be any RCTs of psychosocial interventions uniquely tailored to colon cancer patients.
- There are clinical guidelines for psychosocial interventions for depression (Fulcher et al., 2008) and anxiety (Sheldon et al., 2008) for cancer patients in general, both of which recommend psychoeducation and psychosocial

interventions, and cognitive-behavioral therapy, offered via either individual or group modalities.

Given this patient's mild to moderate distress and minimal to no social support, you consider recommending a group intervention, but for now choose to proceed with individual supportive psychotherapy (Lederberg & Holland, 2011) and further assessment of coping strategies and treatment goals.

Session 2—First Counseling Session, Supportive Psychotherapy, Assessment of Coping Strategies and Treatment Goals via Patient Collaboration

You see KG for an individual counseling session, 2 days prior to his next chemotherapy. He is generally feeling well physically because he has had some time to recover from his most recent chemotherapy, and he notes how it seems easier to cope emotionally when he is feeling better physically. You affirm this observation and spend much of the initial part of the session listening attentively to KG, and you conclude that his level of distress is still about the same; he continues to spend most of his time alone, hearing from his sons every few days and his wife as the time for his chemotherapy gets closer. He estimates that he spends about 3–4 days per week pretty much by himself; he doesn't like this, but sees few options at the present time since he is starting to notice more fatigue following each chemotherapy and worries that he may be more susceptible to infections. He has turned down a couple of offers to go to dinner with friends, and he is still off from work. Throughout most of this session, your goal is to provide supportive listening, encouraging his recognition and expression of feelings, while continuing to assess current coping strategies and levels of distress. You conclude he has limited social support, which has altered his usual coping, and his levels of distress remain mild to moderate and subthreshold to any mental disorder.

Toward the end of the session, you shift the focus to more direct discussion of goals, treatment options, and KG's preferences. KG again identifies that he is a bit uncertain about what he wants to "get out of the counseling," although he does find it helpful to have a neutral source to talk to about how he is feeling and some of the ways he is coping. He is also concerned that he "not waste his time" if the sessions are not being helpful. KG directly asks, "How will you or I know if this is helpful for me?" Since you are familiar with outcome monitoring as a method of evaluating the effectiveness of psychotherapy in the more general psychotherapy literature, you suggest that maybe it will help to keep track each week of how much distress (anxiety or depression) he is experiencing on that particular week. He agrees, and you explain that you will look into the best way to monitor how counseling is going. Other agreed-upon goals include maintaining his current helpful coping strategies, and learning more about some possible new strategies, particularly if he experiences any worsening of physical symptoms or overall distress as his chemotherapy progresses. You schedule the next appointment for 1 week.

Post Session 2: Summary of Key Patient Characteristics

- 48-year-old, separated, White male with Stage IIIA colon cancer
- Currently doing chemotherapy and only minimal side effects

- Mild to moderate distress
- Minimal to no social support
- Agrees to routine monitoring of distress to evaluate progress
- Given his continued lack of contact with others, you begin to think that a group intervention might be best.

Post Session 2—Accessing the Evidence Base for Best Available Outcome Instrument to Monitor Progress in Psychotherapy

Background questions about routine monitoring of patient progress need to be addressed:

- Is there empirical support for routine outcome assessment to monitor progress in psychotherapy?
- Are there any clinical guidelines for the use of routine outcome assessment in either the broader oncology or psychotherapy literatures?
- Are there any specific self-report questionnaires recommended for use with cancer patients to monitor progress in counseling/psychotherapy?

You again review the filtered literature to access background knowledge—an example of the iterative process in EBP. The *Quick Reference for Oncology Clinicians* (Holland et al., 2006) has a chapter on screening instruments that explains the use of the Distress Thermometer, HADS, Zung Depression Rating Scale, Mini-Mental Status Examination, the Memorial Delirium Assessment Scale, the CAGE for screening of substance abuse, and the FICA for asking about spirituality. Most of these instruments are used for assessment of specific symptoms and are not commonly used as measures of progress in psychotherapy. They are offered in the *Quick Reference* as instruments to use for screening of general psychosocial distress and related symptoms, although some (e.g., HADS) are also described as capable of measuring change over time. The *Handbook of Psychotherapy in Cancer Care* has separate chapters explaining 21 different, well-developed interventions for use with cancer patients, and within each there is discussion about their efficacy but no direct discussion about routine monitoring of outcome. A chapter in *Psycho-Oncology* (Pirl, 2010) on various instruments in psycho-oncology discusses the selection of instruments, pointing out that it is important to consider the purpose for using the measure, the population, whether it has had psychometric testing to determine reliability and validity, its sensitivity to change, the burden for the patient to complete it, and its ease of scoring. The clinical practice guideline in psycho-oncology titled *A Pan-Canadian Practice Guideline* (Howell et al., 2010) provides much detail about when and how to screen and assess for anxiety and depression, along with suggestions for both pharmacologic and nonpharmacologic (i.e., psychosocial) treatments, but it does not directly talk about outcome assessment to evaluate benefits of psychotherapy. A special issue of the *Journal of Clinical Oncology* (Lyman & Levine, 2012) on comparative effectiveness research (CER)—obtained via online first by e-mail notification—includes an article on patient-reported outcomes in adult oncology, indicating that the importance of assessing patients' subjective experiences is essential to all of evidence-based cancer care.

In summary, this brief review for background knowledge concludes the following:

- The psycho-oncology specific literature on psychotherapy does not directly address routine measurement of patient outcome as a means of monitoring progress.
- There are clinical guidelines for when and how to screen to identify the presence or absence of anxiety and depression, but they do not directly discuss measurement of patient outcome as a means of monitoring progress.
- There are a variety of specific self-report questionnaires used with cancer patients for screening for distress, some that are capable of measuring change over time, but none have been routinely used for monitoring progress.
- In selecting instruments, it is important to consider their reliability, validity, sensitivity to change, and burden on patients.
- Assessment of patients' subjective experiences via use of patient-reported outcomes is an important issue in other areas (e.g., CER) of evidence-based cancer care.

You again begin the sequential steps for accessing best available evidence. *Step 1* of the search strategy is the development of a well-formulated PICO question regarding overall efficacy of outcome monitoring.

For a 48-year-old male, currently undergoing chemotherapy for Stage IIIA colon cancer, and receiving outpatient psychotherapy, is routine monitoring of progress more helpful than no monitoring for the relief of mild to moderate distress?

Steps 2 and 3 involve identifying the key words and potential synonyms from the PICO statement:

P—male, colon, colorectal, bowel, advanced cancer, neoplasm
I—outcome monitoring, psychotherapy, psychosocial intervention, counseling, psychological treatment
C—no monitoring
O—support, social support, anxiety, depression, distress

Steps 4 and *5* are to search for either filtered or unfiltered literature. You previously searched the filtered literature, when answering your background questions. This time you search the unfiltered, broader psychotherapy literature via EBSCOhost using the search terms *psychotherapeutic outcome AND anxiety OR depression OR distress*. You include CINAHL, Medline, and PsycINFO databases. The search was limited to 2008 to 2014 and 112 publications were identified, many of which were book chapters. To look for general overviews of outcome assessment in psychotherapy, you scan the titles and abstracts and find that one was most relevant (Lambert, Vermeersch, Brown, & Lent, 2008) as an introduction to measuring outcome. From this review, you realize that other search terms are relevant, and so you develop a second search strategy in which the search terms *treatment outcomes AND feedback OR progress monitoring OR progress tracking AND Lambert* were used. Nineteen references are identified and reviewed. Two important references from this search are a meta-analytic review of a psychotherapy quality assurance system (Shimokawa, Lambert, & Smart, 2010) and a brief guide to what measures have been developed for use in progress monitoring in psychotherapy (Overington & Ionita, 2012).

Search Summary

- The meta-analysis (Shimokawa et al., 2010) warrants further review and appraisal regarding the PICO question, as applied to the general psychotherapy literature.
- The brief guide (Overington & Ionita, 2012) is a helpful summary of what instruments are available for routine use in psychotherapy and indicates that despite the availability of a variety of psychotherapy progress monitoring systems, none has been developed for use with cancer patients.

To identify any possible additional references relevant to progress monitoring in cancer care, you develop another search strategy. This search is of Medline only for 2008 to 2014 with search terms of *colon cancer AND screening AND anxiety OR depression OR distress*. This search finds 22 abstracts. Review of these abstracts identifies a study evaluating sensitivity and specificity and cutoff score for the Distress Thermometer (DT) and the HADS, as compared to a structured diagnostic interview, in 99 patients with colorectal cancer (Patel, Sharpe, Thewes, Bell, & Clarke, 2011). Now that relevant literature has been identified, they need to be appraised.

Step 3: Appraising the Research Evidence

From the two formulated PICO questions and the three literature searches, three related questions can be answered form the accessed literature. First, what is the best available evidence for the effectiveness of a psychosocial health service intervention for patients with colon cancer? Second, what is the evidence for the use of psychotherapy outcome measures for monitoring of patient progress, and third, is there a preferred self-report outcome measure to use with cancer patients?

Given the lack of any psychosocial health service interventions tailored specifically for colon cancer patients, the best available evidence appears to be the broader research on psychosocial interventions for cancer patients experiencing distress, anxiety, and/or depression. In addition to a number of clinical practice guidelines (see Table 1.2 in Chapter 1) and the 2008 Institute for Medicine report (Institute of Medicine, 2008) recommending the need for such interventions, there have also been a number of systematic and meta-analytic reviews of psychosocial interventions with cancer patients (Faller et al., 2013; Lepore & Coyne, 2006; Meyer & Mark, 1995; Sheard & Maguire, 1999) that despite criticisms of methodological shortcomings (Coyne et al., 2006; Newell et al., 2002) conclude with the finding that the preponderance of the evidence suggests that there are a variety of psychosocial interventions that have been proven to be beneficial for a wide variety of cancer patients (Andrykowski & Manne, 2006; Manne & Andrykowski, 2006). These include various types of psychoeducation, CBT, and supportive psychotherapy offered in either an individual or group modality. Colon cancer patients have been participants in some of the psychosocial intervention trials. Thus, general guidelines suggest it is beneficial to provide such services to patients with colon cancer. However, these general guidelines do not provide specific details of the type of intervention.

In regard to the second question, use of patient monitoring of progress, the meta-analysis of Shimokawa and colleagues (2010) is relevant. It is a meta-analytic review of a specific psychotherapy quality assurance system that uses the Outcome Questionnaire (OQ-45; Lambert, Morton, et al., 2004). This review reports on six studies testing the efficacy of a system in which young adults, predominantly college-age students (mean age = 24; total $n = 6151$) receiving outpatient psychotherapy, were given the OQ-45 at each session, and after scoring and comparison to expected recovery curves, feedback was given to the psychotherapists who could alter their intervention, when needed, in an effort to avoid negative outcomes. In all six studies, the experimental group received the feedback and was compared to a treatment as usual (TAU) group that did not receive any feedback. This meta-analysis was appraised by both the PRISMA 27-item checklist (Liberati et al., 2009) and the Meta-Analysis Reporting Standards (MARS) of the APA (American Psychological Association JARS Working Group, 2008), indicating that it is a well-executed meta-analysis with results considered to be valid and reliable. Both intent-to-treat (ITT) and efficacy analyses were completed. The primary results indicate that the groups receiving feedback did better than those not receiving feedback. Feedback was effective in enhancing therapy outcome, as measured by the OQ-45, and two forms of feedback were successful in decreasing treatment failures. The aggregate effect size from the efficacy analysis for the groups where feedback to the therapist was given was .53 (95% CI [0.28–0.78]), generally considered a large treatment effect. This effect size is comparable to an improvement of 12 points on the OQ and is considered to be a clinically significant change. The aggregate effect size from the ITT analysis was .28 (95% CI [.47–.10]) considered to be a small to medium effect size. This is equivalent to an improvement of 6.4 points on the OQ. Thus, this evidence supports the routine use of outcome measures as a means of monitoring patient progress in psychotherapy, at least within the context of this particular OQ-45 quality assurance system. However, there is no evidence available regarding the use of the OQ-45 with cancer patients.

The evidence of most relevance to the third question—Is there a preferred outcome measure to use with cancer patients?—is the Patel and colleagues study (Patel et al., 2011). In this study, researchers evaluated 99 colorectal cancer patients for the presence of any anxiety or depressive mental disorder via the "gold standard" of a structured clinical interview—the Composite International Diagnostic Interview (CIDI). These same patients also completed the DT and the HADS. Researchers then compared the test results from the DT and the HADS with the clinical interview, to identify sensitivity (true positives), specificity (true negatives), and an optimal cutoff score. The results showed that the optimal cutoff score for the HADS was 10, resulting in sensitivity of 73% (percentage correctly identified as having anxiety/depression) and specificity of 72% (the percent correctly identified as not having anxiety/depression) for any anxiety or depressive disorder. Results for the DT was an optimal cutoff score of 4 with a sensitivity of 60% and a specificity of 67%. There were no overall statistically significant differences between the two instruments. However, in comparing the two, both were found to have acceptable sensitivity and specificity for depression, but the DT was not considered acceptable for anxiety (sensitivity dropped to only 50%). Researchers found them acceptable as screening instruments to be followed by more thorough clinical interviews for the assessment of mental disorders. Since this study was evaluating screening instruments for their accuracy in diagnosing depression or anxiety disorders, it was appraised by use of the 25-item checklist from the Standards for the Reporting of Diagnostic Accuracy Studies (STARD) (Bossuyt et al., 2003b). A majority (17 of 25) of the checklist items were reported in this study, suggesting that the reliability and validity of the results appear acceptable.

Thus, although either the DT or HADS is acceptable as a screening instrument for depression, only the HADS is recommended for anxiety. Neither is developed or used regularly for routine monitoring of progress in psychotherapy as in the OQ-45 quality assurance system, but they have been widely used in research studies measuring outcomes in randomized trials, thus indicating they are sensitive to measuring change. The OQ-45 has been tested with populations of primarily college-age students, while both the DT and HADS have been widely and routinely used in research with cancer patients. Lastly, the Patel study was of a sample of patients with colorectal cancer, as in the current case example.

Appraisal Conclusions

- The psycho-oncology outcome literature indicates that psychosocial health service interventions provide a variety of benefits (e.g., decreased distress) for patients with a variety of cancer types and stages, including colon cancer.
- Best available evidence indicates positive outcomes for a variety of interventions, including supportive psychotherapy, offered in either an individual or group modality.

- There is evidence that routine monitoring of patient progress in psychotherapy is helpful; this comes primarily from one quality assurance system (Shimokawa et al., 2010), but the broader oncology literature is also encouraging routine use of patients' subjective reports of progress (Lyman & Levine, 2012).
- Those instruments validated as strong measures of outcome in psychotherapy (e.g., OQ-45) have not been evaluated for use with cancer patients.
- Two other instruments (DT and HADS) have been tested as valid and reliable screening instruments with cancer patients, but they have not been tested as measures of monitoring progress in psychotherapy, and yet they have been used in many psychosocial research studies with cancer patients.
- Of the two instruments, the HADS (with use of a cutoff score of 10) is more reliable in identifying the presence of *both* anxiety and depression than the DT.

With these conclusions in mind, the next step is to translate the accessed and appraised literature to the specific needs of KG.

Step 4: Translating the Research to a Particular Patient

From the appraisal of the accessed literature, you conclude that (a) there are no psychosocial interventions targeted specifically to the needs of colon cancer patients, and (b) supportive psychotherapy is one of a variety of interventions shown to result in positive outcomes for many cancer patients. You are experienced in providing supportive psychotherapy and have been guided by authoritative literature (Lederberg & Holland, 2011).

Regarding the question of measuring outcome as a means of monitoring progress, there is mixed evidence. The well-tested OQ-45 quality assurance system has strong valid and reliable evidence for its use in improving patient outcomes when feedback is given to psychotherapists. However, it has never been tested with cancer patients. There are no data on any progress monitoring system for use with cancer patients. Instead, there are a number of instruments that have been widely used, for many years, as self-report questionnaires shown to be effective in screening for distress, anxiety, and depression, and to be valid and reliable instruments when used as outcome measures in psychosocial intervention research. Two were recently reviewed in a study of colorectal cancer patients (Patel et al., 2011), and the HADS was found to be the best for screening of depression and anxiety, with a recommended cutoff score of 10.

Step 5: Integration—Pulling It All Together and Developing a Treatment Plan

In the current case example of KG, the available evidence suggests supportive psychotherapy is an appropriate intervention. Regarding clinical expertise, you are experienced and well trained to provide supportive psychotherapy and will be following a general, authoritative guide (Lederberg & Holland, 2011), while also monitoring progress by collecting data from the HADS at each session.

Finally, the patient (KG) previously indicated he would be willing to defer any specific decision about best treatment to you. Thus, there do not appear to be any significant patient preferences relevant to choice of treatment intervention, but there are important patient preferences related to monitoring of progress. KG indicated that he does not want to "waste time" if the intervention is not proving to be of help. Given the earlier appraisal of the benefits of progress monitoring, you decide it is important to use it with KG. Thus, the routine session-by-session use of the HADS as a measure of patient progress will be implemented, and the feedback regarding the scores on the HADS will be used as a check against "wasting time" and/or symptom changes. This form of adaptation, where routine progress monitoring is added to the primary intervention, can be considered a *supplemental augmentation* (Ruscio & Holohan, 2006) of the original intervention, by adding a systematic method to monitor patient progress. The relative contribution of the three EBP components in the development of this initial treatment plan for KG is important to consider. In this case, clinical expertise is highlighted over patient preferences (deferred treatment selection to psycho-oncologist) and best available evidence (general outcome efficacy literature), although the evidence in support of progress monitoring is also influential in the current treatment plan.

Session 3

Prior to the start of Session 3, KG completes the HADS, after you provide a brief explanation of how to fill it out and how it will be used as a method of monitoring his progress. It takes him about 5 minutes to complete. His scores on the HADS are 4 for anxiety and 4 for depression. You explain to him that it will be important that he complete the HADS prior to each session. He agrees and recognizes it is a way to address his concerns about not wasting time.

Overall, KG reports he is doing about the same. "I survived my most recent chemo," and "It seemed a little bit easier than the earlier ones." He indicates he is still spending a lot of time by himself but is generally "doing okay." His mood is assessed as similar to prior sessions, where he acknowledges mild to moderate degrees of sadness and worry, but not at the level of any mental disorder, and generally within what would be expected as the normal range, given his overall life circumstance. You continue with supportive therapy, attending closely to his emotional reactions and existing coping strategies, affirming his overall experience and noting to him the coping strategies that seem to be helping. He is generally cooperative in sessions, but occasionally seems "stuck" and you note that the sessions seem to go slow and he seems to be only minimally responsive to your efforts to encourage expression of emotions. You both agree to meet weekly for a few weeks.

Sessions 4–6

Prior to each session, KG completes the HADS, and each week, the new scores are compared to the previous week's scores using the recommended cutoff of 10 as optimal for determining the presence of either an anxiety or depression-related mental disorder. His scores to date for anxiety, across these three latest sessions, are 5, 5, and 7 and for depression are 5, 6, and 7. Because they are all increasing and are now above the cutoff of 10, it becomes important to discuss these changes.

Session 6 Discussion

During this discussion, you ask KG for feedback on how he feels the sessions are going. He indicates that although he has come to like you for some reason, "the sessions just don't seem as helpful as when we first started." By asking about the change in HADS scores and soliciting feedback, you open up more direct discussion of in-session topics, techniques, and processes, trying to affirm, acknowledge, and reassure KG that his feelings and opinions about the sessions are "what matters most" when monitoring his progress. As a result of the open conversation and feedback, you both come to agree that the sessions, as planned, are no longer helping and something needs to change. KG is not sure what, but he does report "nothing much lately seems to matter or be of importance to me. I guess I have just never been able to make any sense out of why I am going through all of this, and it's really, really hard; much harder than I ever anticipated. Lots of the time lately, I find myself thinking why, why am I the one going through this?" You respond empathically, once again affirming that these feelings are understandable and make sense, and you note that much of what KG is saying sounds, "like it's been hard to find any meaning in what seems like a bunch of very meaningless events" KG responds with a slight bit more energy and awareness saying, "Yeah!, meaningless is a good word to describe it all. All of the time alone, conflict with my wife, distance between me and my kids, even the side effects of chemo . . . none of it seems to make any sense . . . . I am just going through the motions, and even lately think maybe it's not worth going through all of this!"

You again empathize and affirm these feelings, while also proceeding with a brief assessment of self-harm, and KG denies that he has ever gone so far as to think about hurting himself. He directly denies any suicidal ideation and indicates, "I couldn't ever do that to my kids"—a common statement indicating the presence of this protective factor. Lastly, you suggest that you will again look at what other treatment options are available, particularly now that maybe his key concerns have more to do with a sense of meaninglessness than earlier. You talk directly to KG, indicating that you wonder if maybe he would now be more helped by talking to other patients who may have experienced similar feelings; patients who also worry about the uncertainty of their future. KG agrees that maybe that would be helpful now, and so you both agree to discuss other treatment options soon. You explain that you will do some more investigation of the research and available local resources for group interventions, and you will be in touch via telephone.

Post Session 6

- Symptoms of anxiety, and particularly depression, are worsening.
- HADS score for depression over the cutoff, indicating the likely presence of a diagnosable mental disorder.
- Potential treatment failure identified via use of progress monitoring.

- More direct discussion and feedback of a "sense of meaninglessness" as a significant concern.
- More willing to consider participating in a group at this time.

Iterative Step 2: Accessing Best Available Research Evidence for a New PICO Question

Step 1 is to formulate a new PICO question, with revised interventions and outcomes.

> *For a 48-year-old male, currently undergoing chemotherapy for Stage IIIA colon cancer, is a group intervention or an individual intervention better for decreasing symptoms of depression and anxiety and a sense of meaninglessness?*

Steps 2 and 3 are to develop a search strategy by identifying key words and synonyms.

P—male, colon, colorectal, bowel, advanced cancer, neoplasm
I—individual intervention
C—group intervention
O—anxiety, depression, meaninglessness

Step 4 is to begin the search; in this instance, you again review the three major filtered literature resources previously accessed for initial background questions: *Psycho-Oncology* (Holland et al., 2010), the *Quick Reference for Oncology Clinicians* (Holland et al., 2006), and the *Handbook of Psychotherapy in Cancer Care* (Watson & Kissane, 2011). A quick review of the table of contents for the *Handbook of Psychotherapy in Cancer Care* indicates that Chapter 12 is titled *Meaning-Centered Group Psychotherapy*, which is clearly relevant, and thus you read it closely. Your review of this chapter indicates that this group psychotherapy is designed for those experiencing "despair, hopelessness, and desire for hastened death in advanced cancer patients" (p. 137). It is an 8-week group intervention consisting of various didactic presentation and experiential exercises with the goal of diminishing despair, demoralization, and hopelessness. Two RCTs have been completed, both of patients with advanced (Stages III or IV) cancers, including colorectal (13% and 16%) cancer patients. One of the studies provided the intervention in a group therapy modality (Breitbart et al., 2010), and the other provided a very similar intervention as an individual modality (Breitbart et al., 2012).

Iterative Step 3: Appraising the Evidence

You appraise these two RCTs by use of the modified Quality of Study Rating Form (see Appendix B; QSRF, Gibbs, 1998). The MCGP group was found to have statistically significant greater improvements in spiritual well-being and a sense of meaning than a control group. There were also some decreases in hopelessness, anxiety, and desire for hastened death from pretreatment to posttreatment and continuing through to follow-up, but these improvements were not found to be statistically different from the control group. This might be attributed to a relatively small sample size. Results for within-group, pre- to postintervention, show medium to large effect sizes ranging from 0.40 to 0.74 for primary outcomes of spiritual well-being, which includes faith and sense of meaning/peace, for the MCGP group. On the 100-point QSRF study rating scale, the group MCGP study scored 80, indicating reliable and valid results, despite a small sample size. The small sample was the result of a significant problem with dropouts. Only 51% (25/49) of the treatment group and 31% (13/49) of the control group completed treatment, indicating 49% and 69% dropouts. This was mostly the result of the serious health problems with this sample of patients experiencing advanced cancers with poor prognoses, and the resulting difficulties in scheduling and regularly attending a weekly group therapy session. Given the difficulties in doing an RCT with a sample of advanced cancer patients, MCGP was adapted to be used with individual cancer patients—individual meaning-centered psychotherapy (IMCP).

You also appraise this study (Breitbart et al., 2012) of the individual intervention (IMCP) by use of the QSRF. The IMCP study modified the original group intervention to an individual intervention consisting of seven 1-hour individual sessions provided by clinical psychologists (or psychology graduate students), compared to a control group of seven sessions of massage therapy. Results showed significantly greater improvement in spiritual well-being (faith and sense of meaning) and quality of life in those receiving IMCP compared to the massage therapy group, but no group differences in anxiety, depression, or hopelessness. Results for within-group, pre-post intervention comparisons on the primary outcomes of spiritual well-being, faith, and sense of meaning range from 0.35 to 0.68, considered medium to large effects. This study also scored 80 on the 100-point QSRF rating form indicating good reliability and validity of results. Of most importance, this individual intervention had much less attrition through patient dropouts with 66% of patients who began IMCP completing all seven sessions (only 34% dropouts). Given the relevance of these two studies to the concerns of KG, you do not complete a formal search strategy of unfiltered sources.

Appraisal Conclusions

- There is a well-developed and tested intervention for advanced cancer patients experiencing a loss of meaning/purpose and a sense of meaninglessness.
- Two RCTs have been completed of a meaning-centered psychotherapy intervention both finding improved spiritual well-being that includes enhanced faith and sense of meaning/peace.
- Both studies report medium to large effect sizes and thus both appear to be beneficial.
- A direct comparison of the individual intervention (IMCP) to the group intervention (MCGP) has not been done.

Iterative Step 4: Translating the Evidence

Once again, translating the accessed and appraised evidence involves considering degree of fit of these studies to your current patient, KG. Medical/disease-related variables that fit well include cancer stage (all Stages III or IV) and type (16% and 13% of participants had colorectal cancer). KG is a few years younger than the mean age of both studies (54 and 60 years), and a small majority of participants in both studies were female (60% and 51%). The vast majority (80% and 84%) of participants were Caucasian, as is KG. Thus, based upon medical/disease and demographic variables, this is a reasonably good fit. There is a good degree of fit with the focus of the therapy and patient-identified issues. KG is struggling with a sense of meaninglessness, and both of these studies showed improved spiritual well-being, which includes faith and a sense of meaning/peace, along with some other benefits. However, neither of these studies found any significant improvements in symptoms of depression. Regarding which modality—individual or group—is best, the two studies both found medium to large effects and were not designed to directly test this question. Thus, either format would be beneficial, indicating there is no definitive answers to the PICO-posed question of which is better.

Step 5: Integration—Pulling It All Together and Developing a Revised Treatment Plan

First, given reliable and valid results from two well-designed RCTs, the evidence seems strong that a meaning-centered psychotherapy should be beneficial for KG. Second, regarding clinical expertise and local resources, you recall that despite the recognized benefits of group interventions, many community cancer centers have difficulties initiating and maintaining group interventions in the busy oncology setting (Grande et al., 2006; Plass & Koch, 2001; Taylor, Falke, Shoptaw, & Lichtman, 1986). Fortunately, as a result of some recent training and the availability of a treatment manual (Breitbart & Poppito, 2014a), your cancer center is now offering MCGP that includes ongoing, long-distance supervision. You learn that a new group is starting in a few weeks and so you call KG to inform him.

Brief Telephone Contact With KG

In your phone call you inform him of the availability of the group, and you explain that it is for patients with various types of cancer, like him, who have interest in discussing how their cancer experiences have affected the meaning and purpose in their lives. It meets weekly, for 90 minutes, for 8 weeks. He sounds interested and asks some questions about how these group work, and you reassure him of the agreed-upon confidentiality of all of the members, the probable similarities of group members, and that it is normal to be apprehensive about meeting others, but most people find that it gets easier quickly, particularly when they realize everyone in the group has similar concerns. He agrees to try it, and you both agree that it is important to continue to complete the HADS and that the group members are also completing another questionnaire (FACIT Spiritual Well-Being) at the start and end of the 8 weeks. You make plans to call him monthly to complete the HADS over the telephone once per month, and remind him he can call and schedule to see you for individual counseling, in the future, if needed.

Revised Treatment Plan

- Provision of meaning-centered group psychotherapy
- Continued progress monitoring by monthly completion of HADS
- Supplemental augmentation of the treatment plan by use of the Functional Assessment of Chronic Illness Therapy (FACIT) Spiritual Well-Being Scale (SWB) to measure change in overall spiritual well-being, consisting of two subscales of faith and sense of meaning/peace, as used in the MCGP study.

Follow-Up

You remain in touch with KG with monthly phone calls and he completes the HADS each time; his scores on both anxiety and depression decline at both month 1 and 2 to scores of 5 and 3 for anxiety and 6 and 3 for depression—below the cut-off in month 2. In addition, he offers that he is enjoying the group and finds some improvement in accepting the reality of his disease and living with uncertainties. His scores on the FACIT-SP are also consistent with his self-report.

Step 6: Evaluation of Evidence-Based Practice

Evaluation occurs at two levels: monitoring of patient outcomes and monitoring of EBP of psycho-oncology.

Monitoring of Patient Outcomes

Monitor KG's outcomes by routine use of the HADS and by periodic use of the FACIT-SP. These self-report questionnaires measure four constructs relevant to KG's presenting problems: anxiety, depression, faith, and sense of meaning/peace. In fact, the use of the HADS allowed for feedback resulting in a change in the treatment plan, potentially avoiding a treatment failure. Thus, feedback from the HADS has already been used to manage and revise the overall treatment approach.

Monitoring of Evidence-Based Practice of Psycho-Oncology

At the level of the individual psycho-oncology practitioner, evaluation involves assessment of a variety of components of the EBP process. Examining the overall six-step process (AAA TIE) by use of a series of relevant questions (see Table 4.9) is the starting point. Next, archiving the critically appraised topics (CATs) from this case is also needed. As described in Chapter 4, a completed CAT includes a well-organized summary of the entire EBP process, including the clinical bottom-line results, the citation, clinical question, search terms, study description, and evidence summary as appraised. Develop a CAT for this case and save in your Dropbox folder.

In summary, this case example illustrates a number of important points when doing EBP. It shows the recursive EBP process—how changes in the clinical situation warrant repeated development of PICO questions that then guide multiple literature searches and their subsequent appraisal. It also shows the importance of the use of self-report questionnaires as a method for monitoring patient progress, and how close attention to changes in these outcome measures can result in important treatment modifications. Lastly, this example shows how a broader definition of *clinical expertise* to include the availability of local resources—as emphasized in some models of EBP (Council for Training in Evidence-Based Behavioral Practice [EBBP], 2009)—is most relevant to the ability to disseminate and implement an evidence-based group treatment.

CHAPTER SUMMARY

This chapter focused on group psychosocial health service interventions. The evidence-based practitioner needs general background knowledge from which to formulate relevant clinical questions. Thus, after some introductory information about group interventions, the best available research evidence was reviewed by organizing study characteristics (cancer type, stage, disease continuum) and their ease of dissemination (theoretical approaches, accessibility, patient acceptability, trainability) around a table of exemplars (Table 7.1). The best available evidence for group interventions is for women with either early- or late-stage breast cancer and for men with prostate cancer. A variety of psychological, psychosocial, and biobehavioral outcomes have been studied with improvements noted in overall quality of life, such as decreased distress/anxiety/depression and improved well-being. Cognitive-behavioral and existential approaches dominate the literature, while a few approaches emphasize practical, nontheoretical methods. Ease of dissemination is generally good as a result of availability of published manuals, treatments that average 2–3 months of weekly sessions, and the predominance of theoretical approaches that are familiar to most practitioners. Following this review, a detailed case example was provided to illustrate the sequential competencies and iterative process of EBP. This case demonstrated the recursive process of EBP as additional literature searches and appraisals evolve as new clinical questions arise. The importance of progress monitoring as supplemental augmentation of treatment was also emphasized as a process used to avoid patient harm and treatment failure. Finally, as the EBP steps are followed, the process of adapting the treatment plan was shown, given patient needs/preferences, clinical expertise, and the availability of local resources.

8

Couple-Focused Psychosocial Health Service Interventions

This chapter provides background knowledge about psychosocial health service interventions focused on the cancer patient and his or her partner and offers a detailed example of how to do evidence-based practice (EBP), where the best available evidence suggests a couple-focused intervention. Like the previous chapters, the evidence-based practitioner will often begin an encounter with a new patient with the need for general background knowledge about couple's interventions. Potential background questions may include the following:

- Are couple-focused interventions effective?
- Which theoretical approaches are most common?
- For whom (cancer site, stage) are couples approaches most commonly provided?
- Are these interventions described in treatment manuals that are available?
- Do they require specialized training?
- What types of outcomes are measured?
- How many sessions are usually provided?
- Who are the professionals typically offering these interventions?
- Do patients find these interventions acceptable?

The following summary of general background knowledge is designed to answer some of these background questions.

BACKGROUND KNOWLEDGE

Over the past 20 years, research on adaptation to cancer has grown as studies have emphasized the impact of the disease on families and couples (Northouse & McCorkle, 2010; Zaider & Kissane, 2010). Couple-focused interventions have emphasized the impact of the illness on relationships, particularly those of women with breast cancer and men with prostate cancer.

Research studying the effects of cancer on couples notes that the stressors of the illness affect both the cancer patient and the partner and that both influence each other's coping and support processes. A healthy relationship is seen as a resource from which one can draw support that serves to buffer cancer-related stressors, that provides needed emotional support, and that helps both partners process the impact of the cancer experience. Transactional processes (between partners) that serve to maintain a sense of closeness and intimacy have been emphasized (Manne et al., 2006). Couple-focused research in psycho-oncology is generally new and much of it is preliminary; thus, more research is needed to strengthen the evidence base (Jacobsen & Jim, 2008). However, since the mid-1990s, a body of research on couples and cancer has become available to guide EBP in psycho-oncology. This chapter focuses on exemplars of best available evidence for couple-focused research as identified, reviewed, and selected during 2010 to 2014 with publications from 2005 to 2012.

Research Evidence: Couple Focused

Literature reviews of couple-focused interventions in oncology have either been narrative summaries (e.g., Baik & Adams, 2011) or focused on specific issues such as sexuality/body image (Scott & Kayser, 2009) or couples' distress at end of life (McLean & Jones, 2007). Summaries suggest that there is some evidence of effectiveness (Baik & Adams, 2011), but no systematic or meta-analytic reviews have focused exclusively on couple-focused interventions for cancer patients. One large meta-analytic review did summarize results by intervention type (Faller et al., 2013). In this review, 10 randomized controlled trials (RCTs), involving 1,115 cancer patients examined the effectiveness of couples psychotherapy on emotional distress, anxiety, depression, and quality of life. A small but significant effect size ($d = .23$) was found for decreased emotional distress at posttreatment, but not for anxiety, depression, or quality of life. No significant effects were found for follow-up. Small effect sizes indicate that the patients receiving the treatments score between the 54th to 62nd percentile on treatment outcomes compared to those not receiving the treatment, and success rates are between 52% and 57%. The Faller and colleagues (2013) review was limited by only considering individual patient outcomes of distress, anxiety, depression, and quality of life, as many couples interventions also consider relational outcomes such as marital satisfaction, couples communication, and overall relationship quality. More detailed knowledge is available in the unfiltered primary literature.

Unfiltered Primary Literature

Table 8.1 includes 15 exemplars of best available evidence for couple-focused interventions in oncology. Ten RCTs of conjoint couple-focused interventions, one RCT of a couple-focused group intervention, and four quasi-experimental single-group pretest posttest studies are included. Sample sizes range from a large RCT of 235 couples coping with prostate cancer (Northouse et al., 2007) to

Table 8.1. Exemplars of Best Available Evidence for Couple-Focused Interventions, for Individual and Relational Outcomes, for Varied Cancer Types and Stages: Study Characteristics and Ease of Dissemination

	Study Characteristics		Ease of Dissemination[a]		
Citation/ Location	**N, Diagnosis, Stage/ No. of Groups**	**Results/Outcomes**	**Intervention Description, Theory, Accessibility**	**Therapist Characteristics**	**Patient Acceptability/ Trainability[b]**
RCTs—conjoint sessions, couple-focused interventions, individual and/or relational outcomes					
Northouse et al., 2007 *Midwest US*	235 couples prostate (65% early stage, 21% adv. stage), 2 groups (FOCUS, TAU)	No significant difference on any Pt QOL outcomes; significant difference on spouse outcomes—better physical, (*d* = .28) mental (*d* = .25), QOL; less negative appraisal of caregiving (*d* = .32), uncertainty, (*d* = .28), hopelessness (*d* = .27)	3, 90-minute home visits + 2, 30-minute phone sessions. Manualized L&F stress-appr High accessibility	Masters-prepared RNs training in FOCUS	69% (263/383) eligible couples agreed 88% (113/129) completed treatment High trainability
Porter et al., 2009, 2012 *N. Carolina US*	130 couples GI cancer (66% stage IV), 2 groups (PAED, AC.)	Significant difference in improved relationship quality in Pts who "held back" discussing cancer-related concerns. No significant difference in psychological distress, improvements maintained at 8 weeks	4 sessions (first 75 minutes, others 45 minutes) over 8 weeks. No manual CBCT No accessibility	Masters-prepared social worker or psychologist female	27% (150/559) of eligible couples agreed 45% (29/65) completed treatment Low trainability

(*Continued*)

Table 8.1. Continued

	Study Characteristics		Ease of Dissemination[a]		
Citation/ Location	**N, Diagnosis, Stage/ No. of Groups**	**Results/Outcomes**	**Intervention Description, Theory, Accessibility**	**Therapist Characteristics**	**Patient Acceptability/ Trainability[b]**
Scott et al., 2004 *Brisbane Australia*	97 couples, 57 breast, 37 gynecological, early stage, 3 groups (CanCOPE, MI, PC)	CanCOPE increased couple coping communication ($d = 1.23$), decreased Pt distress ($d = .22$) and avoidance of intrusive thoughts ($d = .34, .39$), more positive sexual self-schema ($d = .80$), perceived partner acceptance ($d = .44$), less decline in sexual intimacy ($d = .91$)	5, 2-hour sessions (pre-surgery, week 1, 6 and 6 months) In Pt home, + 2, 30-minute phone calls Manualized CSPT Medium accessibility	Female psychologists	94% (97/103) of eligible couples agreed 90% (85/94) completed treatment Moderate trainability
Canada et al., 2005 *Texas US*	84 couples, early-stage prostate, ED, 2 groups (couples, males alone)	No benefit to couples intervention vs. males alone. Improved sexual function and satisfaction for Pt and spouse at end of treatment, but not at 6 months Increased use of surgical or medical treatment for ED	4 sessions (first 60–90 minutes, others 45–60 minutes) CBT communication techniques, Manualized Low accessibility	1 PhD psychologist, 1 masters-prepared counselor	No data on % of eligible participating 61% (51/84) completed treatment High trainability
Manne et al., 2011 *Northeast US*	71 couples, early-stage prostate, 2 groups (IECT, TAU)	Marginal improvement in well-being in some couples; most effective with Pts with higher concerns at baseline. Some adverse effects noted	5, 90-minute sessions manualized CSPT Low accessibility	5 therapists 5-hour training, degree or profession unknown	21% (71/340) eligible enroll 70% (26/37) completed treatment Moderate trainability

Kayser et al., 2010 *Northeast US*	63 couples, breast early stage, 2 groups (PCIP, TAU)	No significant difference in overall QOL for Pts or partners; pre-post improvements in well-being noted (*d* = .26 to .55)	9 biweekly 1-hour sessions over 5 months Manualized L&F; STM Medium accessibility	Clinical social workers	13% (63/478) of screened participated 75% (27/36) completed treatment High trainability
Kuijer et al., 2004 *Rotterdam Netherlands*	59 couples, mixed types/stage (56% mets.), 2 groups (ET, WL)	Sig. decline in Pt and partner perception of underinvestment/overbenefit (*d* = .44), improved relationship quality (*d* = .43), decreased Pt distress (*d* = .55)	5, 90-minute biweekly ET sessions No manual CBCT No accessibility	Psychologist trained in ET	92% (59/64) eligible enroll 81% (26/32) completed treatment Low trainability
McLean et al., 2011 *Toronto Canada*	42 couples late stage mixed types, 2 groups (EFT, TAU)	Significant difference improved marital functioning (*d* = 1.00) and patient perceived caregiver empathy (*d* = 1.00); no significant difference in depression or hopelessness	8, 1-hour weekly sessions (most OPT, some INPT and in home) Manualized, EFT, Medium accessibility	One EFT trained psychologist	93% (42/25) eligible enroll 82% (18/22) completed treatment Moderate trainability
RCTs—conjoint sessions, couple-focused, small sample size (<40), individual and/or relational outcomes					
Campbell et al., 2007 *N. Carolina US*	30 couples, AA prostate cancer stage unknown 1.5-year posttreat (CST, TAU)	No significant group differences on self- efficacy, general health, mood, or caregiver strain; feasible study; no to small pre-post effects	6, 1-hour weekly telephone sessions of CST, No manual, BSCT No accessibility	AA doctoral psychologists; specialized training	25% (40/157) eligible couples agreed 75% (15/20) completed treatment Low trainability

(Continued)

Table 8.1. Continued

Study Characteristics			Ease of Dissemination[a]		
Citation/ Location	**N, Diagnosis, Stage/ No. of Groups**	**Results/Outcomes**	**Intervention Description, Theory, Accessibility**	**Therapist Characteristics**	**Patient Acceptability/ Trainability[b]**
Baucom et al., 2009 *N. Carolina US*	14 couples early-stage breast (RE, TAU)	Pilot study—promising results, no analysis of statistical significance, most effect sizes favor intervention over control group for women (d = .61) and male partners (d = .35)	6 biweekly 75-minute sessions Manualized CBCT Low accessibility	Doctoral students in clinical psychology Special training	13% (14/107) eligible couples agreed 87% (7/8) completed treatment High trainability
RCTs—group sessions, couple-focused interventions					
Manne et al., 2005 *Northeast US*	238 couples, early-stage breast, 2 groups (CG, TAU)	Significant group difference—lower depression. Pts with less supportive partners and more physical impairments benefited more. Small effects (d = .02–.07)	6, weekly, 90-minute sessions, Manualized CSPT Medium accessibility	20 "therapists" (degrees not reported) + 6-hour training	33% (238/710) couples agreed 65% (78/120) completed treatment High trainability
Quasi-experimental—single-group, pretest, posttest					
Birnie et al., 2009 *Calgary, Canada*	21 couples, stage unknown mixed types, MBSR	Within-group effects measured; improved mood states (d = .35), reduced stress symptoms (d = .16), improved mindfulness (d = .21)	6–8, weekly, 90-minute sessions + 1, 3–6 hr silent retreat, No manual, Mindfulness No accessibility	Not reported, specialized training in MBSR	51% (21/41) completed treatment Low trainability

Manne et al., 2008 *Northeast US*	16 couples, early-stage breast, IECT	Model supported, promising results; reduced Pt psychological distress, increased Pt perceived partner closeness and cancer-specific closeness	5, weekly 60-minute conjoint sessions Manualized CSPT Medium accessibility	Not reported, Special training	88% (14/16) completed treatment Moderate trainability
Donnelly et al., 2000 *Northeast US*	14 Pts, 10 partners, breast; Stage IV on high-dose chemotherapy IPT	Feasibility test—Pt program satisfaction good to excellent; recruitment, accrual successful	IPT by telephone, individual sessions Pt mean = 16, partner mean = 11, Manualized, IPT Medium accessibility	1 clinical psychologist 4-day workshop	82% (14/17) eligible agreed 86% (12/14) completed treatment Moderate trainability
Lewis et al., 2008 *Pacific NW US*	20 male partners, of 0–III stage breast HHH	Pilot study—promising results; within-group effects measured; improved self-efficacy, Pt self-care skills, expression of affection, anxiety, and depressed mood	5, 1-hour, biweekly individual sessions Session descriptions BSCT Medium accessibility	Not reported special training	77% (20/26) completed treatment Low trainability

[a]Ease of dissemination is operationally defined as an intervention <12 sessions, provided by one qualified provider such as a social worker, psychologist, or nurse (adapted from Jacobsen & Jim, 2008).
[b]Trainability is an estimate of how easy an intervention is to train to others—operationally defined as High = manual available + nondoctoral provider, Moderate = manual available OR treatment provided by nondoctoral provider, Low = no manual and treatment provided by doctoral-level provider (taken from Chorpita et al., 2011).

(*Continued*)

Table 8.1. Continued

[c]Accessibility of Manual—High = online, Medium = published manual/book/workbook, Low = from researcher only, None = no manual available.

AA, African American; AC, attention-control; BSCT, Bandura's social cognitive theory; CanCOPE, educational materials, coping skills training, supportive counseling, supportive communication, partner support, sexual counseling, partner validation/empathic listening training, explore existential meaning of illness; CBCT, cognitive-behavioral couples therapy; CBT, cognitive-behavioral therapy; CG, couple-focused group—session content focused on enhancing support exchanges and coping skills; CSPT, cognitive, social-processing theory; CST, coping skills training; *d*, *Cohen's d* = standardized mean difference scores as reported in original study; ED, erectile dysfunction defined as inability to achieve and/or maintain an erection sufficient for intercourse; EFT, emotionally focused couples therapy; ES, effect size; ET, equity theory (a CBT approach based on perceptions of balance in the relationship—therapists stimulate perspective taking, cognitive restructuring, and behavioral exercises including homework to restore perceived equity or relational balance); FOCUS is F = family involvement, O = optimistic attitude, C = coping effectiveness, U = uncertainty reduction, S = symptom management; HHH, helping her heal (educational counseling intervention for male partners of breast cancer patients); IECT, intimacy-enhancing couples therapy; IPT, interpersonal psychotherapy; MBSR, mindfulness-based stress reduction; MI, medical information education; INPT, inpatient; L&F, Lazarus & Folkman cognitive, stress-appraisal theory; OPT, outpatient, QOL, quality of life; PAED, partner-assisted emotional support; PC, patient coping training; PICP, Partners in Coping Program—a CBT structured intervention with nine themes (assessment of relationship/social support, integrating tasks of illness, caring for children, personal coping, new coping skills, enhancing couples communication, promoting supportive exchanges, intimacy/sexual functioning, living with cancer); Pt, patient; RE, relationship enhancement; STM, systemic-transactional coping model; TAU, treatment as usual; WL, wait list control.

a pilot study of 14 breast cancer patients and 10 of their partners being provided interpersonal psychotherapy via telephone (Donnelly et al., 2000). A variety of types of interventions are included, some specifically developed for cancer patients and others adapted from previously developed, evidence-based couples therapy approaches.

Study Characteristics

Cancer Type, Stage, and Disease Continuum

Of the 15 studies in Table 8.1, six are of couples in which the female partner has breast cancer (Baucom et al., 2009; Donnelly et al., 2000; Kayser et al., 2010; Lewis et al., 2008; Manne et al., 2005, 2008) and one is a mix of breast and gynecologic cancer (Scott et al., 2004), four are of males with prostate cancer (Campbell et al., 2007; Canada et al., 2005; Manne et al., 2011; Northouse et al., 2007), and four are of mixed types of cancers (Birnie et al., 2009; Kuijer et al., 2004; McLean et al., 2011; Porter et al., 2009). Of the 15 studies, nine are of patients with early-stage disease (Baucom et al., 2009; Canada et al., 2005; Kayser et al., 2010; Lewis et al., 2008; Manne et al., 2005, 2008, 2011; Northouse et al., 2007; Scott et al., 2004), three are of advanced stage (Donnelly et al., 2000; McLean et al., 2011; Porter et al., 2009), one is of mixed stage (Kuijer et al., 2004), and stage is not reported in two studies (Birnie et al., 2009; Campbell et al., 2007).

The early-stage disease studies typically focus on adaptation to the diagnosis, treatment course, and related lifestyle changes within the context of a good prognosis and eventual return to a "new normal" following treatment and recovery. In contrast, those focused on later stage disease typically focus on significantly heightened distress as the couple is now facing their worst fears of a shortened life span and potential separation via death, in addition to the demands of additional treatment. Related reviews (e.g., McLean & Jones, 2007) have highlighted important differences in the issues faced by early- or late-stage disease.

Results and Outcomes Measured—Individual and/or Relational

The studies in Table 8.1 report a variety of types of outcomes. Couple-focused interventions measure outcomes at the individual and/or couple relationship level. Individual-level outcomes have included measures of anxiety, depression, uncertainty, hopelessness, body image, sexual self-schema, appraisal of caregiving, quality of life, and other forms of psychological distress, as reported by each study participant, in *reference to her or his own individual reactions* as either a patient or a partner. Studies have also measured couple-, dyad-, or relationship-level outcomes. These are *focused on aspects of the relationship* such as communication skills, intimacy, quality of the relationship, perceived equity in the relationship or empathy, and marital satisfaction. All of these outcomes have been measured at the end of treatment, with some studies including follow-up from 3 to 12 months.

In general, the results of these interventions are mixed, with a trend toward some modest improvements for most participants. Seven of the 11 RCTs report significant differences between the intervention and control groups, while 4 studies (Campbell et al., 2007; Canada et al., 2005; Kayser et al., 2010; Northouse et al., 2007) report no statistically significant differences on primary outcomes, with significant small effects on within group pre-post outcomes. Three other studies noted stronger outcomes in certain subgroups such as patients who held back expressing their concerns to their partner (Porter et al., 2009); reported higher concerns at baseline (Manne et al., 2011); or had less supportive partners and more physical impairments at baseline (Manne et al., 2005). These findings indicate the importance of further study of moderators and mediators to these interventions. Regarding the strength of outcomes, most studies report small effect sizes (d = .22 to .34), particularly for individual-level outcomes. Two studies (McLean et al., 2011; Scott et al., 2004) report large effect sizes on relational-level outcomes of marital functioning (d = 1.00), use of coping communication (d = 1.23), and patient-perceived partner empathy (d = .91), suggesting maybe these interventions have stronger effects on relational-level outcomes. The RCTs with small sample sizes (<40 couples) and the quasi-experimental, pre-post studies were feasibility studies and pilot tests to investigate any evidence of positive benefit. Replications of these studies with larger samples are anticipated, and future studies need to investigate the clinical significance of reported outcomes. Finally, as with many brief psychosocial interventions, longer lasting positive outcomes are limited, and more research is needed to answer questions such as where along the clinical course couples interventions are most needed, or with which patients (cancer type, stage), and at what frequency, intensity, or duration interventions are best for most participants.

Ease of Dissemination of Couple-Focused Interventions

Included in Table 8.1 is information about ease of dissemination of these couple-focused interventions. Ease of dissemination of couple-focused interventions is influenced by the same variables as with individual and group interventions as previously summarized. However, training and expertise in couples therapy is an additional consideration. Most local community oncology settings may not have trained couples therapists already affiliated with their cancer care setting. Thus, the dissemination and implementation of these evidence-based interventions are likely to be more complicated and require either more detailed training of oncology-affiliated staff or collaboration with more generalist couples therapists who may then require training in psycho-oncology.

Intervention Descriptions

The studied interventions have varied in modality, duration, frequency, and location. The most common has been a 1-hour weekly conjoint couples intervention, offered by a single therapist, over a relatively short period of time (4–24 weeks), in the outpatient oncology setting. Nine of the RCTs and two of the quasi-experimental studies were offered as conjoint couple sessions (i.e., both partners present for all sessions). One of the RCTs (Manne et al., 2005) was of a group intervention (multiple couples present for all sessions). Two of the quasi-experimental studies were couple-focused interventions but were offered as individual sessions; in one study only the male spouses of breast cancer patients were involved (Lewis et al., 2008), and the other study was provided via individual telephone sessions offered to patients with metastatic breast cancer and their partners separately (Donnelly et al., 2000). All studied interventions have been short term ranging from the briefest of four sessions (one for 75 minutes and three for 45 minutes) totaling 210 minutes to the longest of eight weekly, 90-minute sessions, plus one 60-minute session, totaling 726 minutes. Most sessions occurred weekly or biweekly and were completed within 4 to 24 weeks. The majority of studies offered the treatment within the outpatient oncology setting, although two were offered in the patients' home and two were via telephone contact.

Theoretical Approaches

Interventions have been guided by a variety of psychological theories and psychotherapy approaches with similar techniques and varied hypotheses about mechanisms of change. Some form of cognitive-behavioral theory (CBT), originating either from Bandura's social cognitive theory (Bandura, 1986) or Lazarus and Folkman's cognitive model of stress (Lazarus & Folkman, 1984) have dominated this literature. Cognitive-behavioral couples therapy (Epstein & Baucom, 2002) and an intimacy-based cognitive-social processing model (Manne & Badr, 2008) have also been very influential. Other interventions are based on the empirical evidence of patient and partner psychosocial needs (Kayser et al., 2010; Scott, Halford, & Ward, 2004).

Two well-researched theories of psychotherapy, modified for use with cancer patients, include emotionally focused couples therapy (McLean et al., 2011) and interpersonal psychotherapy (Weissman et al., 2000), as modified for use via telephone (Donnelly et al., 2000). The theories and their proposed mechanisms of change are summarized next.

Cognitive Model of Stress

Lazarus and Folkman's cognitive model of stress (Lazarus & Folkman, 1984), along with more recent revisions and additions (Park & Folkman, 1997), is a widely used theoretical model for designing interventions to enhance coping skills. Two of the studies in Table 8.1 are based on this model (Kayser et al., 2010; Northouse et al., 2007). This model's more recent focus on processes of meaning-making make it particularly applicable to use with cancer patients and families. The model specifies cognitive processes in reaction to life stressors in which one *appraises* various components of the stressor and his or her own coping abilities. In *primary appraisal*, an individual first encounters and appraises the stressor for its likelihood of causing harm, threat, or danger. This is influenced by *secondary appraisal* in which one considers what coping skills, strategies, resources, or past experiences one has had with the stressor and how one can bring them to one's coping efforts. Secondary appraisal can serve to buffer and influence primary appraisal, such that distress is less likely if one *appraises* one's coping skills as sufficient to cope. Thus, this model suggests that when a cancer patient encounters a stressful event, the severity of the stress response is the result of these two opposing appraisal processes, such that when primary appraisal is high and secondary appraisal is low, one experiences a high degree of distress. Conversely, if a cancer patient's secondary appraisal is high (i.e., one perceives oneself to have sufficient coping skills and/or resources) relative to the primary appraisal, the patient is less likely to experience high distress. Thus, interventions have been designed to identify the nature of couples' stressors and to build resources and coping skills to result in enhanced secondary appraisal. Enhanced resources and coping skills, and the resulting impact on secondary appraisal (i.e., "I can manage/cope with this pretty well now") is thus hypothesized to result in reduced stress.

Cognitive-Behavioral Couples Therapy

Within the broader tradition of behavior therapy—and its focus on learned behaviors—cognitive-behavioral couples therapy (CBCT) (Epstein & Baucom, 2002) has focused on learning new relationship skills, such as improved communication and expression of emotion. Four of the studies in Table 8.1 used CBCT (Baucom et al., 2009; Canada, Neese, Sui, & Schover, 2005; Kuijer, Buunk, De Jong, Ybema, & Sanderman, 2004; Porter et al., 2009), with two others (Campbell et al., 2007; Lewis et al., 2008) using Bandura's closely related, social cognitive theory (Bandura, 1986).

Because private, written emotional expression by cancer patients has been shown to enhance an individual patient's quality of life (Stanton et al., 2002), it has been hypothesized that public, overt expression of emotions within the context of a couple's relationship might also help. Improved communication and expression of emotions might result in improved intimacy and relational satisfaction. A couple who can discuss cancer-related worries and concerns could benefit by joint problem solving, or improved partner support, or lessened distress by each partner, when fears and apprehensions are directly addressed. Thus, some (Porter et al., 2009, 2012) have tested a CBCT intervention with an enhanced focus on partner-assisted emotional disclosure, in which specific skills are learned, aimed at helping patients disclose feelings and concerns directly related to their experience of cancer.

Cognitive-Social Processing Model

A cognitive, social-processing model of couples communication has emphasized the central role of intimacy—as a mechanism of change—defined as "a process whereby an individual expresses important self-relevant feelings and information to another and, as a result of the other's response, comes to believe that they are understood, validated, and cared for" (Manne & Badr, 2008, p. 2546). Four of the studies in Table 8.1 are based on this model (Manne & Badr, 2008; Manne et al., 2005, 2011; Scott et al., 2004).

This model emphasizes the importance of self-disclosure and partner responsiveness. When either partner initiates self-disclosure, intimacy results from the perception that her or his partner has understood, validated, and communicated care and concern. In this model, when focused on adaptation to cancer, relational processes have been identified that either enhance or compromise intimacy and subsequent adaptation to the challenges of cancer. Relationship-enhancing behaviors include reciprocal self-disclosure, partner responsiveness, and relationship engagement. Openly disclosing one's feelings and concerns about the experience of cancer is an example of *reciprocal self-disclosure*. Feeling understood, validated, and cared for in the relationship is a consequence of *partner responsiveness*, and being aware of the impact of cancer on the relationship, while still remaining actively engaged in working on the relationship, is *relationship engagement*. In contrast to these helpful and adaptive processes, relationship-compromising behaviors include avoidance of relevant issues, excessive criticism of one another, and undo pressure by one partner toward the other, who then withdraws (i.e., pressure-withdraw), engaging the other to pursue.

This model has been pilot tested as an intimacy-enhancing couples' therapy (IECT) with couples experiencing early-stage breast cancer (Manne & Badr, 2008) and prostate cancer (Manne et al., 2011) and seems promising. The breast cancer couples were noted to report an improved sense of closeness and reduced distress, while those prostate cancer couples experiencing greater cancer-specific distress and lower overall marital satisfaction at the start of the intervention were shown to benefit.

Emotion-Focused Couples Therapy

Emotion-focused couples therapy (EFT) is an established treatment for couples and has a strong evidence base for its effectiveness with presenting problems such as depression and trauma (Johnson, 2002). It was developed from an integration of experiential therapies and systems theory and emphasizes an adult couple's relationship as reflective of attachment processes (Johnson, 2004). Issues of attachment such as loss and separation are particularly relevant to a couple's relationship when they are facing cancer (McLean & Nissim, 2007). In such relationships, distress is theorized to result from insecure bonds in which attachment needs are threatened by relational behaviors such as overly rigid or strict adherence to patterns of interacting that inhibit emotional engagement. The one intervention in Table 8.1 using EFT was designed to increase emotional engagement by increasing flexibility in patterns of interacting and ultimately strengthening attachment bonds and lessening fears of loss and separation (McLean et al., 2011).

Interpersonal Psychotherapy

Interpersonal psychotherapy (IPT) was developed as a psychological treatment for depression, designed to decrease depressive symptoms and improve relationships (Weissman et al., 2000). A time-limited, flexible intervention, IPT emphasizes depression as a medical disorder—rather than as a characterological disorder—associated with four primary life experiences: role transitions, interpersonal conflicts, grief, and/or interpersonal deficits. These domains are highlighted as the patient learns new coping skills within the context of a supportive, encouraging, and empathic therapeutic relationship. Change is hypothesized to occur as a result of new knowledge, coping strategies, insights, and awareness regarding how these domains influence one's mood. IPT has been adapted and modified for primary care medical patients and for use via telephone. Given that the experience of cancer is often associated with life transition, grief/loss, and interpersonal changes, IPT is hypothesized to be a helpful intervention for cancer patients. Most recently, a small feasibility study (Donnelly et al., 2000) tested the use of IPT by telephone with breast cancer patients receiving cancer chemotherapy and a partner. Good program satisfaction and reasonable accrual rates were noted.

Dissemination Conclusions

Ease of dissemination varies across the nine studies reported in Table 8.1.

Two stand out as the easiest to disseminate. The first is the Northouse and colleagues (2007) study of conjoint couples sessions of early-stage prostate cancer, in which masters-prepared RNs intervened with the FOCUS program in five conjoint couples sessions, three of which were in patients' homes. The second is the Canada and colleagues (2005) study of couples with early-stage prostate cancer and erectile dysfunction, in which a PhD psychologist and a masters-level counselor provided four sessions of cognitive-behavioral therapy (CBT) communication techniques. Both studies have many of the positive characteristics of studies more easily disseminated. Northouse and colleagues' (2007) study is easily accessible online and is an educational program with high trainability, yet providing the intervention in patients' homes makes it much less feasible for many settings. Canada and colleagues (2005), although not as accessible (manual available via study authors only), is based upon a theoretical approach (CBT) widely practiced by many mental health professionals; it is not provided in patient homes and is also highly trainable. Both studies are short-term interventions of either four or five sessions. The Canada and colleagues study had a 61% completion rate, suggesting only moderate acceptability, while the Northouse et al. study had a 90% completion rate, suggesting very high acceptability, although the in-home setting likely influenced this.

Next in ease of dissemination are four studies (Kayser et al., 2010; Manne et al., 2011; McLean et al., 2011; Scott et al., 2004), all with a number of positive dissemination characteristics, and a few negatives. Three of the four (Kayser et al., 2010; McLean & Jones, 2007; Scott et al., 2004) have moderate accessibility with manualized interventions that are guided by books from well-known publishers. All four interventions are provided within a reasonable number of sessions (5–9), yet the Scott and colleagues' study was provided in patients' homes, which is less feasible for many settings. Trainability may be problematic for three of the four studies since in only one study (Kayser et al., 2010) was the intervention provided by masters-level providers, the other three by doctoral-level providers. One of the studies (McLean et al., 2011) is guided by a theoretical approach that involves significant prior training, and thus there may be fewer qualified providers in many settings. However, two of the studies had very low percentages of eligible patients who agreed to participate (13%, 21%). In all four studies, treatment completion rates were good (82%–90%), suggesting good patient acceptance.

The remaining two studies (Kuijer et al., 2004; Porter et al., 2009) appear to be difficult to disseminate. Although both report treatment outlines or protocols, neither reports an intervention manual that is available from the authors; thus, neither is accessible nor trainable. One of the studies (Kuijer et al., 2004) is guided by a theoretical approach (equity theory) not widely translated into specific therapy techniques, and both have relatively low intervention completion rates (56% and 66%), suggesting low patient acceptance. Reference citations for manualized interventions and related resources are provided in Box 8.1.

Box 8.1

Accessibility of Manuals: Reference Citations for Manualized Interventions and Related Resources From Exemplars of Best Available Evidence for Couples-Focused Interventions

RCTs—Conjoint Sessions, Couples-Focused Interventions, Individual and/or Relational Outcomes

FOCUS Program manual available online via Research Tested Intervention Programs (RTIPs). Retrieved December 20, 2014 from http://rtips.cancer.gov/rtips/programDetails.do?programId=102766.
Northouse et al. (2007)—Manualized.
Porter et al. (2009)—No manual. "Treatment outlines." No indication of outlines available from authors.
Scott et al. (2004)—Manualized.

Related Resources

Canada et al. (2005)—Manual available from authors.
Kayser et al. (2010)—Manualized.
Kayser, K., & Scott, J.L. (2008). *Helping couples cope with women's cancers.* New York: Springer.
Manne et al. (2011)—Manual available from authors.

Kuijer et al. (2004)—No manual.
McLean et al. (2011)—Manualized.

Resources related to McLean et al.

Johnson, S. M. (2004). *The practice of emotionally focused marital therapy: Creating connection.* New York: Brunner-Routledge.
Johnson, S. M., Bradley, B., Furrow, J., Lee, A., Palmer, G., Tilley, D. et al. (2005). *Becoming an emotionally focused couple therapist: The workbook.* New York: Routledge Taylor & Francis.
McLean, L. M., & Nissim, R. (2007). Marital therapy for couples facing advanced cancer: case review. *Palliative Support Care, 5*(3): 303–313.

RCTs—Conjoint Sessions, Couples-Focused, Small Sample Size (<40), Individual and/or Relational Outcomes

Baucom et al. (2009)—Manual available from authors.
Campbell et al. (2007)—No manual, "detailed written outline for each session." No indication of availability of outlines from authors.

RCTs—Group Sessions, Couples-Focused Interventions
Manne et al. (2005)—Manual available from authors.

Related Resources

Manne, S. L., & Ostroff, J. S. (2008). *Coping with breast cancer: A couple-focused group intervention, therapist guide.* New York: Oxford University Press.
Manne, S. L., & Ostroff, J. S. (2008). *Coping with breast cancer: Workbook for couples.* New York: Oxford University Press.

Quasi-Experimental—Single-Group, Pretest, Posttest
Birnie et al. (2009)—No manual.

Related Resources

Donnelly et al. (2000)—Manual adapted from:
Klerman, G. L., Weissman, M. M., Rounsaville, B. J., & Chevron, E. S. (1984). *Interpersonal psychotherapy of depression.* New York: Basic Books.
Lewis et al. (2008). Manualized. No indication of manual availability.
Manne et al. (2008)—Manual available from authors.
Speca, M., Carlson, L. E., Goodey, E., & Angen, M. (2000). A randomized, wait-list controlled clinical trial: The effect of a mindfulness meditation-based stress reduction program on mood and symptoms of stress in cancer outpatients. *Psychosomatic Medicine, 62,* 613–622.

Summary of the Evidence Base for Couple-Focused Interventions

A number of brief couple-focused interventions have been shown to result in positive benefits for both individual and relational outcomes for couples facing a variety of types and stages of cancer (although 73% were of either breast [$n = 7$] or prostate [$n = 4$]). Cognitive-behavioral therapies dominate this literature, although other approaches are being developed (e.g., interpersonal therapy, emotionally focused couples therapy), as are some novel approaches to delivery (i.e., telephone). Of the eight RCTs of conjoint couple-focused interventions, two have very good dissemination potential, four interventions have moderate potential, and dissemination is not feasible for two. Finally, as evidence-based practitioners select from the best available evidence, as summarized eariler, they also need to attend closely to their particular expertise and consider the study characteristics in matching interventions with particular patient/couple variables and/or preferences.

CASE EXAMPLE: HOW TO DO EVIDENCE-BASED PRACTICE OF A COUPLE-FOCUSED INTERVENTION

In addition to the earlier overview of the evidence base for couple-focused interventions in psycho-oncology, the following case example provides a detailed illustration of how to do EBP where a couple-focused intervention is warranted. This case emphasizes the application of EBP when considering best available evidence, both first and second line; the need for referral to a therapist with appropriate clinical expertise; and augmentation of a primary treatment with a second-line intervention available to the patient's partner when the patient is unavailable due to chemotherapy treatments.

Case Example 4—BJ: Couples Communication Relapse Reactive to Breast Cancer Diagnosis

Referral Information

A medical assistant (MA) at the cancer center approaches you after completing a screening for psychosocial distress. During the screening a 44-year-old White married female reported a high level of distress (9 on a 10-point scale) on the distress thermometer screening tool. The screening took place just minutes prior to the patient's first appointment with the oncologist, and she appeared quite tense and nervous. The MA reported that she felt as if the patient "was expecting to hear all bad news." The patient's husband was with her, but he seemed a bit distant and uninvolved. The MA was particularly struck by the husband's lack of any attempt to comfort his wife when she became distraught and a bit tearful. He "just seemed cold and aloof." On the problem list that is part of the screening, the patient indicated distress related to insurance/financial fears, worry, and family problems. The patient is already scheduled to see you in 3 days for further assessment of overall psychosocial adaptation. Prior to this appointment you review some basic information about the patient's diagnosis and stage, and you learn that she is tentatively diagnosed with Stage IIIC breast cancer. Her tumor was found to have spread to the chest wall, and cancer cells were found to have spread to axillary (in the armpit region) lymph nodes. Surgery is an option, and chemotherapy is likely. The patient has some family history of breast cancer in an aunt and one grandmother; both were diagnosed prior to age 50.

You Begin the Evidence-Based Practice Process

Step 1: Ask Specific, Clinical Questions: Both Background and Foreground

Relevant *biomedical* background questions include the following:

- What forms of treatment might be involved in Stage IIIC breast cancer?
- What types of side effects might she experience?
- What is her likely prognosis?
- What type of surgery are they considering (i.e., mastectomy, lumpectomy, other)?
- If surgery is an option, is reconstructive surgery feasible?

You review the clinical decision support tool *UpToDate* (2014), available to you as a staff person at your hospital-based cancer center, for information on *Stage IIIC breast cancer treatment.* You learn that for Stage IIIC—also referred to as locally advanced breast cancer (LABC)—surgery is likely an option, but it is determined by other variables (e.g., tumor histology, morphology). More information, best obtained from the patient's oncologist, is needed. Stage IIIC prevalence is about 10% of diagnosed breast cancers; it is more common in populations who do not get regular mammograms and is higher among younger women and underserved populations. This may indicate that the referred patient had not been having regular mammograms. Regarding treatment options, neoadjuvant (treatment given to shrink a tumor as a first step, prior to surgery) chemotherapy is the current standard approach, particularly if the patient is interested in breast conservation. You decide that identifying the patient's desires regarding breast conservation during the psychosocial assessment interview will be important. Overall survival rates are variable (depending on a variety of other prognostic factors), but in general the long-term survival rates for patients with locally advanced disease are about 50%. *UpToDate* provides an overview of possible chemotherapy protocols, but again, you require more information to determine exactly which side effects may be most likely. You realize that you will eventually be able to get this information from the patient's oncologist.

Relevant *psychosocial* background questions include the following:

- What evidence exists regarding the importance of partner support, relative to other sources of support for breast cancer patients?

- What type of support is most important from a spouse?
- What psychosocial outcomes of cancer treatments such as surgery (e.g., body image, sexuality) are of importance to consider?
- What evidence for couples therapy in cancer patients exists?
- Is there much, and if so, how strong is the research evidence for couples therapy from specific theoretical approaches (e.g., behavioral couples therapy, emotionally focused couples therapy) for breast cancer patients?

You look to your psycho-oncology resources first, which include the APOS/IPOS *Quick Reference for Oncology Clinicians* (Holland et al., 2006), the second edition of *Psycho-Oncology* (Holland et al., 2010), and the *Handbook of Psychotherapy in Cancer Care* (Watson & Kissane, 2011). A quick review of these sources is a good first start. In doing so, of most help is a review chapter in *Psycho-Oncology* by Zaider and Kissane (2010). From this review you determine that there is a limited but growing literature on interventions for couples. Most studies have been done with either breast cancer or prostate cancer patients, and they have focused on either (1) early-stage disease and its accompanying life transitions such as coping with treatment, readjustment of daily routines, or caregiving by spouses, or (2) advanced, late-stage disease and accompanying existential end-of-life challenges. Many of the interventions have been developed specifically to the oncology setting for couples in which one member is a cancer patient (e.g., Northouse et al., 2007), while others have taken previously efficacious couples therapies and adapted them for use with cancer patients (e.g., McLean et al., 2011). Although most couples therapy is via conjoint couples sessions (both partners present, face-to-face with one therapist), some intervention programs have also been done in groups (multiple couples, one or two therapists) (Manne et al., 2005).

In review chapters (e.g., McLean & Jones, 2007) the importance of support, specifically from a spouse, is emphasized as a buffer against the stressors of cancer. In fact, the reviews seem to agree on the following:

1. A diagnosis of cancer is equally (if not more) distressing for a partner.
2. The intimacy and closeness of a partner can serve as a buffer against the many stressors of cancer.
3. Emotional support is more important than other forms of support, such as informational or instrumental.

PubMed (Medline) and PsycINFO are good sources and using their controlled vocabulary terms, you develop a search strategy using *breast cancer OR breast neoplasm AND couples therapy*, restricting results to review articles only by selecting "literature review" as the methodology for PsycINFO and "review articles" for Medline. You complete the search on EbscoHost. One traditional narrative review of couple-based interventions focused on enhancing women's sexual adjustment and body image (Scott & Kayser, 2009) is identified. In this review, 12 studies met selection criteria. They include eight RCTs, two pilot studies, and two quasi-experimental studies. After quickly reviewing the abstract, you conclude that couple-focused interventions, targeted at outcomes such as sexuality and body image, produce stronger effects than no treatment, or standard care, and should include components that educate partners about the women's disease/treatment, focus on the couples' coping and support needs, and include specific sex therapy techniques, if needed. You also learn that there are many limitations in this literature and that it has been recommended that future studies closely follow the CONSORT standards. You conclude that this review may or may not be helpful, since you don't know enough information yet about your client, but it is helpful to know the potential relevance of sexuality/body image for some women, possibly your client. It will be important to assess for any such concerns by this patient.

Some relevant *foreground* questions include the following:

- How severe is this patient's level of distress? Does it reach the level of meeting diagnostic criteria for any mental disorders such as major depression, any anxiety disorder, or even posttraumatic stress disorder?
- Does she have any prior history of mental health treatment? If so, when, for what symptoms, and by what treatment modality(ies)?
- How does she describe her marital relationship and the degree of social support she is receiving, both generally from a variety of sources, and specifically from her husband?
- Is she experiencing concern about body image or sexuality?
- If warranted, is she willing to participate in couples therapy? If yes, does she have any prior experience in couple's therapy, and if so, was it beneficial? In what ways was it helpful or not helpful? Does she have any preference(s) or opinions about the type of couples therapy received?
- If warranted, does she think her husband would be willing to participate? If so, how much distress is he experiencing? Is he reporting symptoms of anxiety and/or depression?

Session 1

The first individual clinical interview: Assessment of psychosocial adaptation, initial establishment of psychotherapy relationship with general elements of empathy, alliance, and collaboration on goals/tasks.

The procedure for the semistructured psychosocial assessment of a newly diagnosed cancer patient, as described in Chapter 5, should be used for this patient. *BJ—Brenda J—and her husband are in the waiting room. You ask if she would like him to accompany her to the interview and she says, "Not now, maybe later." He appears content to wait in the waiting room. The interview begins with a brief explanation of its purposes (i.e., to hear her story, understand her experience with cancer to date, assess severity of any psychological symptoms, set goals for future appointments if needed). You explain confidentiality and its limits, and Brenda signs the necessary consent forms. You begin by asking her to tell the story of her recent medical care and diagnosis.*

She begins, "Well, I am not sure where to start. I noticed a lump one morning while taking a shower and, I guess, I convinced myself it wasn't anything. I didn't tell anyone for a few weeks, and even sort of forgot about it myself, and then noticed it again and was kind of freaked out, because it seemed like it had gotten bigger. Since I didn't have any insurance, I wasn't sure what to do, but a friend told me about an agency in town that would help you pay for mammograms, so I called them and got an appointment set up. I had the mammogram and, like I was afraid, they told me it looked like cancer and immediately asked me if I had a surgeon that I preferred. I was surprised and just went to the one they recommended. He did a biopsy and set me up to see an oncologist here last week. It all seems like it has happened so quickly!" When you ask her about her appointment with the oncologist, she explains that she was "terrified" and could hardly remember anything she (the oncologist) said, but fortunately her husband was with her and took good notes. "They are saying I will need chemotherapy and maybe surgery later. They are waiting for some more test results, and I see her again tomorrow. It sounds like they are wanting to start chemotherapy very soon."

You are using a supportive patient-centered approach, wanting to allow Brenda the opportunity to feel comfortable to express her emotions. As the "telling of the story" section of the interview begins to end, you become more directive in asking specific questions, assessing particular symptoms (overall distress, depression, anxiety, any physical complaints), checking any past history of mental health services, evaluating her perception of social support, particularly that offered by her husband and others. She indicates the household includes her husband and two children, a boy age 12 and a daughter age 9.

Ultimately the assessment goal of this interview is to determine the presence or absence of specific symptoms of anxiety, depression, and overall distress, while also evaluating psychosocial adaptation—defined as consisting of three parts (continued involvement in daily life, minimizing disruptions to life roles, and managing expected emotional distress).

By the end of the interview, you determine that Brenda presents with heightened levels of anxiety and depression. She feels "off and on" both worried/scared and sad. However, on most days she is able to continue to do her usual routine of working and caring for her family. She reports that she has had trouble sleeping; waking up in the middle of the night with intrusive thoughts of all that has happened and can't get back to sleep. During the day she has had frequent episodes of uncontrollable crying and finds this to be excessive and occasionally embarrassing since it seems like "They come on for no reason, about any time or place!"

When you ask her about social support, she indicates that her parents have been good, and even her two young children understand something serious is happening and have tried to comfort her when they see her upset, yet she hasn't explained everything to them yet. ("Until I know more about what my treatment is going to be, I don't know what to tell them.") She also reports good support from two very close female friends. You directly ask, "How has this experience been for your husband?" She pauses briefly and then says, "To be honest, I don't think I really even know. He has been with me and pretty much at my side throughout this, but he hasn't said much and seems really distant emotionally. We haven't been doing very well lately, even before my diagnosis; things weren't very good between us. I know he's pretty tired of all of my crying!" You learn that this is her first marriage and her husband's second. She was 27 when they married and he was 32. His first marriage was to a "high school sweetheart" and only lasted about 2 years. He had no children with his first wife. Brenda and her husband dated for about 2 years before marrying and have now been married for about 15 years. Regarding past mental health treatment, she has never participated in any individual therapy, but she and her husband did "try marriage counseling" about 4 years ago. "It wasn't very helpful, but things did get better for a while."

You next ask about the problem list from the distress-screening tool and learn that although she and her husband are both employed, she has no insurance and she is worried about how much of the expenses her husband's insurance will cover. "Some of our problems have been about how we disagree about money. When we went for marriage counseling in the past, some of it was because we were in a lot of debt, but we worked really hard to get out of it, and now I don't want my cancer to cause us to get in debt again."

By the end of the interview, you determine that she is experiencing an adjustment disorder with anxiety and depression and that her perceived level of social support is mixed; good support from friends and extended family (including her parents and children), but fair to poor support from her husband. The marital relationship has been problematic in the past, and it seems as if the stressors of her diagnosis and upcoming treatments have either added to the marital distress and/or reactivated poor communication skills. She reports fair to poor marital satisfaction.

In regard to treatment goals, you and she mutually decide that the options are to focus on the worry, tearfulness, and sadness or the lack of support from her husband. She is uncertain and finds it difficult to make any decision at this time, since she is also waiting to hear back from her oncologist tomorrow about her cancer treatment plan. For now, she is to think about which she might prefer and to talk to her husband about his interest/willingness to participate. You conclude this first interview with the plan to contact her in a few days after she knows more about the treatment plan for her cancer and she has time to talk to her husband.

Post Psychosocial Assessment Interview: Summary of Key Patient Characteristics

- 44-year-old, married, White female
- Diagnosed with locally advanced breast cancer (Stage IIIC)
- Family history of breast cancer prior to age 50
- Cancer treatments likely to include chemotherapy and surgery, but details not certain yet
- Worried about financial impact of her cancer care

- Delayed seeking a mammogram based somewhat on financial worries
- Past history of marital conflict and couples counseling
- Not sure if prefers individual or couples counseling
- Not sure if husband willing to participate in counseling
- No information yet about husband's distress level

Step 2: Accessing the Best Available Research Evidence
To access the best available evidence, you proceed by following, once again, the sequential steps (Gibbs, 2003). *Step 1* is to formulate a PICO question.

For a 44-year-old, married female, recently diagnosed with locally advanced breast cancer, is there any evidence that conjoint (one couple, both partners present) couples counseling increases partner support and marital satisfaction, and reduces anxiety and depression?

Keywords/terms, their synonyms, or related terms from various controlled vocabulary databases (e.g., PsycINFO's thesaurus, PubMed's MeSH terms) that correspond with each of the four PICO components are listed in *Step 2*, and possible synonyms are listed in *Step 3*.

P—breast neoplasm, cancer
I—couples therapy, couples/spouse counseling, marriage counseling, family intervention
C—no treatment or treatment as usual (TAU)
O—spouse or partner support, marital satisfaction, anxiety, depression, distress

You begin to access available evidence, Step 4, by beginning the search. You access the reference section of the book chapter in *Psycho-Oncology* (Zaider & Kissane, 2010), and you identify seven references that appear to be RCTs of couple-focused interventions for breast cancer. You also develop a search strategy of RCTs in the unfiltered databases of Medline, CINAHL, and PsycINFO. You access all three databases via EBSCOhost. Search terms are *cancer OR neoplasm AND (couples therapy OR couples counseling OR marriage counseling OR spouse intervention).* This search identifies 12 studies. Four of the 12 are not studies of couples' interventions with a female cancer patient and are eliminated. However, one of these four is a pilot study of an individual intervention for husbands of women with breast cancer, designed to enhance spousal communication and support (Lewis et al., 2008). You hold on to this one. Of the remaining eight, all are studies that include female breast cancer patients and their partners; seven of the eight are studies of conjoint couples therapy (Baucom et al., 2009; Kayser et al., 2010; Kuijer et al., 2004; McLean et al., 2011; Northouse, Kershaw, Mood, & Schafenacker, 2005; Northouse et al., 2007; Scott et al., 2004), and two are group interventions (Katz, Bosch, & Herzog, 1998; Manne et al., 2005). Of the eight identified studies, five are exclusively of breast cancer patients, one is of breast and gynecologic cancers, and two are of mixed cancer types. Of the six conjoint couples therapy studies, three are of early-stage cancers (Baucom et al., 2009; Kayser et al., 2010; Scott et al., 2004), two are of late-stage cancer (McLean et al., 2011; Northouse et al., 2005), and one is of mixed stages (Kuijer et al., 2004). The two group studies are both of early-stage disease (Katz, Bosch, & Herzog, 1998; Manne et al., 2005). Another important factor to consider is whether, in these studies, participants were screened for identified distress, prior to inclusion in the study, or whether the study was designed for any breast cancer patient and partner, regardless of level of distress. You quickly review the inclusion criteria and find that only two studies included prior screening in which patients/partners were selected because of elevated levels of distress (Kuijer et al., 2004; McLean et al., 2011). You select four studies for more detailed appraisal: two conjoint studies of mixed cancer types that used prior screening of patients (Kuijer et al., 2004; McLean et al., 2011), one couple-focused study (Northouse et al., 2005) exclusively of late-stage breast cancer patients and their caregivers (62% of caregivers were spouses), and one couple-focused group (CG) intervention focused exclusively on early-stage breast cancer patients (Manne et al., 2005).

Step 3: Appraising the Research Evidence

You use a modified version of the Quality of Study Rating Form (QSRF) (Gibbs, 2003) to appraise these four studies. You modify the original QSRF by adding questions designed to evaluate ease of dissemination and quality of patient match (see Appendix). Three of the four studies were very comparable on strength of the evidence as determined by their score on the QSRF. The one study that did not score well is eliminated (Kuijer et al., 2004).

Of the remaining three studies, only the McLean et al. (2011) study measured both relational and individual outcomes and thus comes closest to answering the original PICO question. This study found significant improvement in marital functioning and in patient's perception of her partner's empathic behaviors at both posttreatment and at 3-month follow-up, with reported effect sizes in the high range (d = 1.00). Of importance to note from the other studies is the finding that in the group intervention by Manne and colleagues (2005), they found decreases in depression and overall distress in those participating in the intervention group, particularly among women who reported that their husbands were less supportive. Regarding theoretical approach and dissemination, the Manne and colleagues (2005) study developed a couple-focused group intervention based upon cognitive social-processing theory about how people process traumatic events. It is readily available via a therapist manual and couples workbook (Manne & Ostroff, 2008a, 2008b). The McLean and colleagues (2011) study modified emotionally focused couples therapy (EFT) for use with cancer patients of mixed type and late stage. A manual and information about the modification is also available (McLean et al., 2008). With this information available you are now ready for the second counseling session.

Session 2

Prior to this appointment, Brenda called to let you know that her husband, Paul, would be with her for the second session. He agreed it would be helpful and she wants him to join her. Further information from her oncologist indicated that the cancer treatment plan is to start with chemotherapy first to shrink the tumor prior to any surgery and that breast conservation should be feasible.

You begin the first conjoint session by confirming your understanding of the cancer treatment plan, and you come to realize that the patient and her husband's understanding is essentially the same as yours. You then direct your question to Paul, asking about his experience since the diagnosis, and he explains, "I don't know. . . . It's been difficult, but I have tried to remain positive . . . tried to be upbeat . . . and not let it get to us! I think the best thing I can do is to try to always look on the positive side and try to encourage her to do the same." You first summarize what Paul has said, and then ask if this strategy of trying to encourage Brenda to remain positive has been working. Paul looks at his wife before responding, and then offers, "She has always been more of a 'glass is half empty' type person than me." Brenda responds, "I just don't think he understands how difficult this has been . . . how scary this is for me . . . and how hard it has been for me to cope. He just sees the tears from me and thinks I should be able to 'shut them off' anytime I want, but I can't."

It becomes clear to you from this interaction that, as hypothesized, Brenda's perception of the adequacy of emotional support from her husband is very low. It seems that he has a rationale behind this that suggests that if they are both "negative" in their thought processes, things will only be worse and so he tries to remain positive. However, in the process, Brenda has felt unsupported and distant from Paul. Although he reports some general distress, he denies any specific symptoms of anxiety or depression.

Next, you confirm what you learned last time about their marital history, and they acknowledge that their relationship hasn't always been good, and that when they participated in marriage counseling in the past, it was mostly about difficulties in communicating about a variety of things, but mostly money. They both agree that during their prior marital counseling things got better, but after a while they fell back into their usual problems in communicating. Now, they both worry about the cost of her treatments and, as of late, have simply avoided talking at all about money. They both acknowledge feeling pretty "distant" from each other lately, and Brenda continues to report frequent episodes of uncontrolled crying that she wishes she could better control. She is also quite apprehensive about the upcoming chemotherapy, and she still has lots of questions about what to expect. She does have an appointment tomorrow with one of the nurses to learn more about her particular chemotherapy regimen, anticipated side effects, and so on. She has been told that once her chemotherapy starts, it will be scheduled every third week.

You ask if Brenda and Paul each think that couples counseling would be helpful at this time. They both agree that it is necessary, but they are unsure how or when to proceed, since her chemotherapy will be starting soon and she anticipates being very tired, and maybe nauseous. You offer that you can come back to issues of scheduling, but first you want to explain to them the research on couples therapy for breast cancer patients that you recently reviewed, emphasizing different treatment modalities. You offer, "Helpful forms of couples therapy do exist and have been adapted for use with couples facing cancer. Most involve the couple being seen together. One particular couples therapy seems to be very helpful and is available through some local counselors who specialize in couples therapy. There are also some treatments that are done in a group format with a number of couples, but such a group is not available locally." You also explain an educational program focused on improving husbands' communication skills to enhance the support a patient needs. They indicate they think the couples therapy would be best, but Brenda expresses concern about being able to participate regularly if she is not feeling well during chemotherapy.

A few general goals are agreed upon. Brenda and Paul agree that good outcomes will include feeling closer and more supported by one another, communicating better about how they each feel, and, particularly for Brenda, experiencing less distress as noted by less frequent crying and better overall control of emotions. She shares that she thinks her overall worry and distress will be better if they can function better as a couple. You explain the importance of tracking how they are doing with the counseling, and so you collect baseline self-report data from both of them that include the revised dyadic adjustment scale (RDAS) (Busby, Crane, Larson, & Christensen, 1995) and for Brenda, the FACIT-B (Cella et al., 1993), a measure of quality of life in cancer patients. Both also complete the Hospital Anxiety and Depression Scale (HADS) to assess levels of anxiety and depression.

On the RDAS at baseline Brenda scores a 74 and Paul a 97 (higher scores on this measure indicate "better" perceived marital functioning), indicating Paul perceives the relationship as better than does Brenda (Spanier & Filsinger, 1983). Their subscale scores indicate that they see the relationship in different ways: Brenda indicates less satisfaction with the expression of affection, and she indicates that they agree less on matters important to the relationship than does Paul. She also reports overall less marital satisfaction. Compared to other couples, their total dyadic adjustment scores range from the 27th (Brenda) to the 40th percentile (Paul) of all married couples, indicating that between 60% and 73% of all couples report higher marital adjustment. On the FACIT-B, Brenda's overall total score indicates a below-average quality of life (standard score of 46, given a 0 to 100 possible range), with her lowest score on the emotional (standard score of 38) and functional well-being (standard score of 28) subscales. On the HADS, Brenda's total score of 23 with subscale scores of 14 for anxiety and 9 for depression are considered above the cutoff for presence of anxiety and depressive symptoms, usually consistent with an adjustment disorder. Paul's HADS score (total = 6) indicates no significant symptoms.

Post First Conjoint Session: Summary of Key Couple Characteristics

- 44-year-old, White female, first marriage and 49-year-old, White male, second marriage
- Married 15 years
- Two children, ages 12 (boy), 9 (girl)
- Diagnosed with locally advanced breast cancer (Stage IIIC)
- Awaiting start of cancer treatments (neoadjuvant chemotherapy and surgery)
- Both worried about financial impact of her cancer care
- Past history of marital conflict and couples counseling
- Both willing to participate in therapy, but anticipate chemotherapy regimen may interfere with scheduling regular sessions
- Self-report scores indicate both reporting marital distress, with Brenda reporting more than Paul. Total scores indicate they report between the 27th and 40th percentile on overall marital adjustment.
- Self-report distress scores (HADS) indicate she is experiencing symptoms of anxiety and depression comparable to an adjustment disorder; he is not.
- Her self-reported quality of life is a little below the average breast cancer patient, with her lowest scores on emotional and functional well-being.

Step 4: Translating the Research to a Particular Patient/Couple

Your next step is to translate the best available evidence to the specific needs of this particular couple. Potential best available evidence includes the emotionally focused couples therapy (EFT), which was studied as eight, 1-hour weekly conjoint couples sessions, and the cognitive social-processing couple-focused group (CG) intervention, studied as six, 90-minute weekly group sessions. Both studies scored similarly on the QSRF and thus have equal strength of evidence. In addition, the EFT intervention is a modification of a couples therapy intervention previously identified as empirically supported (Johnson et al., 1999). The group intervention is not offered anywhere locally, but a few local couples therapists provide the EFT couples therapy. You have referred to them before and are familiar with the quality of their work.

Since the client has some concern that chemotherapy might interfere with regularly scheduled couples therapy, consideration of other options is important to attend to her preferences. You recall that in the previously accessed literature, one study (Lewis et al., 2008) of an individual intervention targeted exclusively to spouses of breast cancer patients, titled *Helping Her Heal* (HHH), was reviewed. This one group, pretest, posttest pilot study ($n = 20$ spouses) tested a five, 1-hour individual spouse educational intervention and found that, among other positive outcomes, spouses reported improved marital adjustment, some from a clinical range to a nonclinical range. With such a small sample and no control group, these results must be considered with caution and are not the best available evidence, but they do provide another intervention alternative, specifically for Paul, if his wife becomes unable to participate during her chemotherapy. You conclude that HHH is best considered as a second-line treatment to use to augment their primary EFT therapy, particularly during times Brenda may not be available during chemotherapy.

Before proceeding any further, you need to consider the quality of the match between these studies and this particular couple and their ease of implementation. First, the EFT study matches well because, like the current couple, it is of couples with later stage disease. It screened for greater than normal distress, mean age of 52 years (versus the 44-year-old patient), showed positive outcomes on both individual and relational outcomes (i.e., marital functioning), and a large percentage (85%–87%) of participants completed the study (i.e., good acceptability). Implementation within the cancer center is not possible since you are not trained in EFT, but there are viable local EFT therapists to whom you have previously referred.

Next, the CG intervention matches well because it is a study of couples with recently diagnosed breast cancer, 61% were receiving chemotherapy at the time of the intervention, their mean age was 49 years, and results showed decreases in depressive symptoms, particularly by patients who reported unsupportive spouses. It matches less well because it is of early-stage breast cancer, and there was a particularly large refusal to participate (77%) and a very low completion rate (35%), indicating either difficulty participating or low acceptability. The CG intervention has very good dissemination as a therapist treatment manual (Manne & Ostroff, 2008a) and couples workbook (Manne & Ostroff, 2008b), and both are commercially available and multiple (n = 20) therapists provided the intervention after a 6-hour training program. Ease of implementation as a group intervention is low as many oncology settings report difficulty organizing and developing group intervention programs. It is not available locally.

Finally, although as a nonrandomized small-sample pilot study, with a much lower strength of evidence, you realize that the HHH individual intervention for spouses of breast cancer patients has good ease of dissemination. It seems to be a good match for Paul, particularly during weeks when his wife may not be able to participate in couples therapy due to her chemotherapy. It is based on Bandura's social-cognitive theory, an approach you know well, and the study (Lewis et al., 2008) includes a description of the specific areas of emphasis for each of the five sessions. Thus, HHH seems relatively easy to learn and implement, particularly since it is administered as an individual, educational session which you feel qualified to provide.

Step 5: Integration—Pulling It All Together and Developing a Treatment Plan

Integration involves pulling together all three components of EBP: accessed and appraised best available evidence; clinical expertise; and patient characteristics, culture, and preferences. In the current case, the literature suggests the option of offering one of three treatments: EFT conjoint couples therapy, a couple-focused group intervention, or an individual intervention for the patient's spouse (HHH).

Best available evidence is either the EFT couples therapy or the couple-focused group intervention. The group intervention is not available locally, but the EFT therapy is available via referral. In regard to clinical expertise, you are not competent to provide EFT. You do feel competent to provide the second-line HHH intervention since it is based on a theoretical approach familiar to you and you have access to session-by-session descriptions of the content. It is offered as an individual therapy, which makes implementation feasible and flexible. Patient preferences are EFT and, if needed, flexibility in scheduling due to potential side effects of chemotherapy. You have concerns that Paul may not remain involved if sessions are not regular, and so you consider ways to incorporate the HHH intervention during occasions when Brenda may not feel well enough to attend their EFT sessions.

Thus, in this case, the integration of all three components of EBP is complex and influenced not only by the strength of the evidence but also by the quality of the match between the evidence and the preferences or unique needs of this couple and the available clinical expertise. You next meet with the couple to collaborate on a treatment plan.

Couples Session 2: Treatment Options, Collaboration on Goals and Treatment Tasks

This second conjoint session occurs 1 week after the first session on a day and time convenient for Brenda when she has to come to the cancer center for some preliminary blood work. Since your last appointment, Brenda has completed her "chemo teaching" appointment with the oncology nurse practitioner and now understands much more about her chemotherapy. She will have chemotherapy once every 3 weeks, and she will have somewhere between four and six of these cycles, depending on how well they are working. Her first treatment is scheduled to happen in 3 days. She has been told it will last about 5–6 hours and that she will be given medication for nausea and vomiting, and she will likely feel tired and fatigued for a few days after the treatment. Her employer has been helpful, and she reports that they are allowing her to try to work if she feels well enough, but they will be flexible. Although Brenda is apprehensive about chemotherapy, she feels a little less anxious simply because she now knows a bit more about what to expect. Paul sits quietly and listens as Brenda explains this to you.

You shift focus toward discussion of treatment options. They explain they have been considering the options as you explained them at the last session and are interested in the couple's therapy, but wish they didn't have to be referred elsewhere. You acknowledge that you also wish it was available here at the cancer center, but you also provide your opinion on the high quality of the couples therapy available and assure them you will pursue a referral. You also suggest that since you are located here at the cancer center you can check in on Brenda during her chemotherapy infusions to stay in touch. They are pleased to hear that. Finally, in regard to HHH, you suggest that, if Paul is interested, during some of the time while Brenda is receiving chemotherapy, you could meet with him to do the HHH educational program. Brenda likes this idea a lot; Paul is less enthusiastic but indicates his willingness to try it out and see how it goes.

Because these decisions are made rather quickly, this becomes an abbreviated session and Brenda moves on to have her blood drawn and to pick up some written materials about her chemotherapy. During her blood draw you are able to arrange for an initial appointment with the EFT therapist and, you explain, you will check in with them at her first chemotherapy.

Tentative Treatment Plan: Adaptation and Integration

- Referral for EFT couples therapy as first-line, evidence-based treatment
- Augmenting couples therapy with HHH, a second-line educational intervention to improve husband's communication skills specific to a spouse with breast cancer
- Adaptation of HHH from a five-session, every-other-week format to an every 3-week format, provided during his wife's chemotherapy sessions

Step 6: Evaluation of Evidence-Based Practice

Monitoring Patient Outcome: Repeat Administrations of RDAS and FACIT-B

In the final EBP step, the evidence-based practitioner evaluates the effectiveness of the entire EBP process. The emphasis here is on patient outcomes and an evaluation of varying degrees of emphasis on the three EBP components.

Patient outcome will be monitored by repeat administration of the two outcome measures, one focused on relational variables (i.e., RDAS—marital functioning) and the other on individual patient outcomes (i.e., FACIT-B—quality of life). As these outcome data are collected, modification of the treatment plan may be needed if progress is not noted and particularly if any deterioration, decline, or harm is evident.

Evaluation of Evidence-Based Practice Components

In evaluating the EBP components in this case example, it is important to consider the decision-making process and the process of adopting, adapting, or abandoning best available evidence (see Chapter 4 for more detail). In this case, the EBP integration process is influenced by (a) availability of local treatment options, (b) a lack of clinical expertise in the strongest intervention (EFT), (c) attention to patient treatment preferences and concerns about chemotherapy side effects, (d) augmentation of the first-line evidence (EFT) with a second-line intervention (HHH), and (f) adaptation of a second-line intervention (HHH) in frequency of sessions to align with patient preferences.

Finally, the intentional archiving of the literature searches from the this case as critically appraised topics (C.A.T.s) is needed. A completed CAT includes a well-organized summary of the entire EBP process, including the clinical bottom-line results, the citation, clinical question, search terms, study description, and evidence summary as appraised. Develop a CAT for this case and save in your Dropbox folder.

CHAPTER SUMMARY

This chapter was about psychosocial health service interventions for couples. It included information about both the needs of couples as a dyad facing cancer and couple-focused interventions as a treatment modality. As in prior chapters, evidence-based practitioners need background knowledge before they can formulate relevant, clinical questions. Thus, best available research evidence was reviewed and organized around Table 8.1, which summarized study characteristics and ease of dissemination of 15 exemplars. The best available evidence for couple-focused interventions indicates positive benefits for couples facing a variety of types and stages of cancer, with the majority of the evidence being for couples where one partner is either a breast or prostate cancer patient. Benefits have been found in both individual and relational outcomes. Cognitive-behavioral therapies dominate this literature, although other approaches are being developed such as emotionally focused couples therapy, as are some novel methods of delivery (i.e., telephone). Overall ease of dissemination varies, ranging from two that seem highly disseminable as short-term interventions, with easily accessible manuals, high trainability, and approaches well known by most psycho-oncologists. Four others have moderate ability to be disseminated, and two are very difficult. Following this review, a detailed case example illustrates the recursive process of the evidence-based competencies. The case highlights EBP where patient preferences, local availability of treatment options, and clinical expertise (lack of) are highlighted.

9

Family-Focused Psychosocial Health Service Interventions

In the often fragmented US health care system, as more and more care is being provided in freestanding outpatient oncology settings, family members, friends, and others close to the patient are assuming more and more responsibility for the care of their loved one (Glajchen, 2011). Families have been conceptualized as second-order patients (Rait & Lederberg, 1990) reacting to the stressors of cancer as interdependent emotional systems. With this in mind, this chapter provides background knowledge about psychosocial health service interventions focused on the family system and family members of the cancer patient. Also provided is a detailed case example of how to do evidence-based practice (EBP) where the best available evidence suggests an intervention focused on the family. Like the previous chapters, the evidence-based practitioner will often begin an encounter with a new patient with the need for general background knowledge about family-focused interventions. Potential background questions may include the following:

- Which family-focused interventions are most effective?
- Who (i.e., which cancer professionals) provides family-focused interventions?
- For which patient types/stage and which family members are effective interventions available?
- Which theoretical orientations are most prominent in these family-focused interventions?
- Are manuals available that describe the interventions?
- How are family-focused interventions provided (i.e., frequency, session length, location/setting)?
- What treatment modality (family, individual, or group) is most commonly used for these interventions?
- Is family systems theory used as a guiding theoretical framework for these interventions?

The following summary of general background knowledge is designed to answer some of these background questions.

BACKGROUND KNOWLEDGE

Family-focused psychosocial health service interventions have emphasized the impact of the illness on families of young children (Stehl et al., 2009), adolescent survivors (Kazak et al., 2004), and caregivers of the terminally ill (Candy et al., 2011). Evidence-based interventions in psycho-oncology targeted at family stressors have focused primarily on parents/families of children or adolescents diagnosed with cancer (Kazak et al., 2005) and the family caregivers of adults facing advanced disease, terminal illness, and death (Candy et al., 2011). In the pediatric psycho-oncology literature, research has targeted adolescent survivors of childhood cancers and their families and, in one example of a family-systems intervention, an integrative cognitive-behavioral and family-systems intervention aimed at reducing symptoms of posttraumatic distress (Kazak et al., 2004) has been tested. In an additional study, an intervention focused on parent/caregiver distress in families of children with newly diagnosed cancers has also been tested (Kazak et al., 2005). Despite a number of challenges in doing research with children and families, these studies report reasonable acceptance and feasibility, as well as encouraging preliminary results. In addition, they also demonstrate the ongoing need for family-focused interventions across the disease continuum. This line of research is likely to grow. However, given the focus of this book on the EBP of adult psycho-oncology, family-focused interventions directed at the adult family caregivers will be emphasized.

Some of the best available research evidence for EBP comes from interventions focused on informal caregivers and the multiple challenges in caring for a family member with a terminal illness (Candy et al., 2011; Higginson et al., 2003; Schildmann & Higginson, 2011). Much of this research follows efforts to improve the quality of palliative and hospice care (National Quality Forum, 2006). Some studies have used multidisciplinary health care teams, providing hospice and palliative care services (Harding & Higginson, 2003; Higginson et al., 2003) directed primarily at patients and only secondarily to caregivers. Others have directly targeted caregivers and have provided a variety of interventions designed to affect psychological and physical health (Candy et al., 2011; Schildmann & Higginson, 2011). In these studies, the needs of the family caregiver have been emphasized throughout.

Family Systems Theory and Cancer

Family systems theory, the application of principles of general systems theory (von Bertalanffy, 1968) to families, has been and is likely to continue to be the dominant theoretical approach to family therapy in more general family interventions. Few randomized controlled trials (RCTs) with cancer patients have used family systems theory. However, as the evidence base for psychosocial health service interventions targeted to families grows, studies are needed that utilize family systems theory. Thus, an understanding of systems principles and their application to families facing cancer (Jacobs, Ostroff, & Steinglass, 1998; Kazak, Simms, & Rourke, 2002; Rolland, 2005) has becoming increasingly important to appreciate the impact of cancer on families across the life cycle (Veach, Nicholas, & Barton, 2002).

In family systems theory, two primary forces—change and stability—guide the dynamic interaction between family members. *Change* is often conceptualized as that which comes from normal development over time. As families come to grow, change is inevitable. The young couple has children. The children grow and develop and are eventually launched from the family. As such change occurs, demands on the family, the couple, and the nature of relationships change. Conversely, *stability* is conceptualized as a regulatory function that serves to maintain order, predictability, and routine. Thus, there are family rules, rituals, and routines, and individual family members have generally predictable roles. Such stability helps to make family life stable, predictable, and more controllable. As families grow, normal developmental tasks are encountered as the family moves through time (Carter & McGoldrick, 1980). Normal family life cycle changes are managed with the order, predictability, and routine that come with stability. In healthy families, this dynamic interaction between change and stability is managed well. In unhealthy families, it is routinely mismanaged, and in families facing cancer, balancing inevitable change with stability is extremely challenging—particularly when cancer strikes the developing family unprepared or unable to manage the additional tasks of a chronic, often incurable disease (Veach et al., 2002). The unhealthy or dysfunctional family responds to the stressors of a serious illness with an overreliance on one or the other of these two forces (change or stability), resulting in imbalance between these competing forces. In the family where stability is overemphasized, change is slow to occur and families are described as *rigid, enmeshed*, or *fragile*. Conversely, families reacting with too little stability and control seem to always be in flux or in change and can be described as *disengaged, chaotic*, or *out of control*. The healthy and functional family finds a middle ground and reacts with resilience, finding a workable balance between its needs for change and stability (Walsh, 2003). The application of family systems theory to families facing cancer relies on an understanding of the impact that cancer can have on the family system. Despite the influence of family systems theory on family therapy in general mental health settings, interventions targeting family system principles (e.g., enmeshment, disengagement) in psycho-oncology are rare (e.g., Kissane et al., 2006). Such interventions are frequently recommended (Jacobs et al., 1998; Kazak et al., 2002; Rait & Lederberg, 1990; Wellisch, 1995, 2000), occasionally conceptualized (Jacobs et al., 1998; Veach et al., 2002; Wellisch, 1995, 2000), but only rarely incorporated into empirically based interventions (Kissane et al., 2006). However, as the family-focused evidence base in psycho-oncology grows, it will be important that interventions consider these important family system principles.

Research Evidence: Family Focused

The current chapter focuses on exemplars of best available evidence for family-focused interventions identified, reviewed, and selected during 2010 to 2014, with publication dates from 2005 to 2011.

Filtered, Secondary Literature: A Systematic Review

One systematic review of 11 RCTs totaling 1,836 participants investigated whether supportive interventions for informal caregivers of terminally ill patients would improve the psychological and physical health of the caregivers (Candy et al., 2011). This Cochrane review found modest research support for reduced psychological distress in the short term (d = .15), and only marginal benefits for improved coping skills and quality of life (d = .05). A summary of this important review is provided in Table 9.1.

Other than this one systematic review, the best available evidence of family-focused interventions is found in unfiltered, primary literature.

Unfiltered, Primary Literature

Nine exemplars of best available evidence for family-focused interventions, targeted primarily to family caregivers, are summarized in Table 9.2. Sample sizes range from 476 to 12 families, with seven of the nine having samples sizes larger than 100. All are RCTs.

Study Characteristics

Cancer Type, Stage, and Disease Continuum

Of the nine studies summarized, four (Hudson et al., 2005; Meyer et al., 2011; McMillan et al., 2006; Walsh et al., 2007) are focused on family caregivers (mostly spouses) of patients with various types of advanced cancers receiving palliative care *in the terminal phase* of disease. Three others (Budin et al., 2008; Given et al., 2006; Northouse et al., 2005) are focused on caregivers of patients *with advanced disease, but not in the terminal phase* (e.g., within first two cycles after being informed of disease progression). Two other studies are included because of some unique characteristics. One—family-focused grief therapy (FFGT)—describes a family-systems intervention for families of terminally ill patients with various types of cancers, focused on the family's grief and bereavement at the end of the patient's life (Kissane et al., 2006). This study is included as a good example of the creative use of family systems principles. The other describes a feasibility study of a culturally sensitive, family-focused intervention for Native Hawaiian families, in which a family member was recently diagnosed (3–12 months) with cancer (Mokuau et al., 2008). This is included because of its unique inclusion of multicultural adaptation.

Results and Outcomes Measured

In the majority of studies in Table 9.2, the results were focused on caregivers of patients with cancer. Caregiver quality of life is the most common outcome

Table 9.1. Cochrane Systematic Review of Randomized Controlled Trials of Interventions for Informal Caregivers of Patients in Terminal Phase

Study Characteristics				Feasibility/Ease of Dissemination	
Citation	**Studies/Location**	**Participants**	**Results**	**Intervention Descriptions (participants, content, duration, manual)**	**Provider Characteristics**
Candy et al. (2011)	11 RCTs 7 US 2 Australia 2 UK	1,836 caregivers	Short-term reduced caregiver distress ($d = .15$); marginally improved coping skills and QOL ($d = .05$)	9 directed at caregivers (2 spouse, 3 family, 4 caregiver); 2 at patient; 7 provided informational and emotional support to caregivers, 1 grief therapy, 1 family life review, 0 instrumental aide/practical support Duration from 2 to 720 hours 7 studies manualized	8 by nurses, 2 by social workers, 1 multidisciplinary team

QOL, quality of life; RCT, randomized controlled trial.
SOURCE: Data from Candy, B., Jones, L., Drake, R. E., Leurent, B., & King, M. (2011). Interventions for supporting informal caregivers of patients in the terminal phase of a disease. *Cochrane Database of Systematic Reviews (Online)*(6), CD007617.

Table 9.2. Exemplars of Best Available Evidence for Family-Focused Interventions, Various Caregiver Outcomes: Study Characteristics and Ease of Dissemination

	Study Characteristics		Ease of Dissemination[a]		
Citation/Location	**N, Diagnosis, Stage/ No. of Groups**	**Results/Outcomes**	**Intervention Description, Theory, Accessibility**	**Therapist Characteristics**	**Patient Acceptability/ Trainability[b]**
RCTs directed at families as caregivers with patients receiving palliative care or in the advanced disease/terminal phase of cancer					
Meyers et al. (2011) *US multiple sites*	476 pt/caregiver dyads (70% spouse), mixed, advanced cancers; participants in clinical trials, 2 groups (COPE, TAU)	QOL for caregivers declined at a significantly slower rate than controls (0.3 SD or about 60th percentile) no change in caregiver problem-solving skills	3 conjoint sessions during first month of a clinical trial for advanced cancer Manualized PST adaptation Medium Accessibility	Health educators + specialized training in COPE	55% (476/876) of dyads agreed 36% (162/446) of caregivers completed treatment and 6-month follow-up High trainability
McMillan et al. (2006) *Southeast US*	354 pt/caregiver dyads, all hospice patients w/mixed, advanced cancers; 3 groups (COPE, supportive care, TAU)	Significant improvement in QOL, burden of Pt. symptoms and caregiving tasks at 30 days in COPE group; small effect estimates (.16, .28, .01), no change in caregiver mastery or coping type	3 sessions at Pt. home integrated with hospice care Manualized PST adaptation Medium Accessibility	nurse + 4-day training in COPE	92% (329/354) of dyads agreed 28% (31/108) completed treatment and 30-day follow-up High trainability

(*Continued*)

Table 9.2. Continued

	Study Characteristics		Ease of Dissemination[a]		
Citation/Location	**N, Diagnosis, Stage/ No. of Groups**	**Results/Outcomes**	**Intervention Description, Theory, Accessibility**	**Therapist Characteristics**	**Patient Acceptability/ Trainability[b]**
Walsh et al. (2007) *London UK*	271 family caregivers (64% spouse) of mixed, advanced cancers; caregivers screened for distress; 2 groups (CARE ADVISOR, TAU)	No significant difference on caregiver distress, but mean of intervention group lower than control on all three assessments (4, 9, 12 weeks), small effect sizes (d = .22, .20, .05)	5 sessions over 6-week period; face-to-face and telephone, integrated with palliative care, clinic, home/work Manualized No theory cited, Low accessibility	Nurse, social work + 1 month training in palliative care and hospice	76% (271/356) of eligible participated 83% (99/118) completed 4 weeks 72% (72/100) completed 9 weeks 76% (69/90) completed 12 weeks High trainability
Hudson et al. (2005) *Melbourne Australia*	106 family; caregivers (67% spouse), mixed, advanced cancers; Pts. in palliative care; 2 groups (Intervention, TAU)	No significant group differences; small effect (d = .30) on increases in caregiver reported rewards	2 home visits + 1 phone call + written materials, relaxation audiotape No manual L&F Stress-appraisal Medium Accessibility	Palliative care nurses + focus groups w/ caregivers	29% (106/358) of eligible participated 74% (40–54) completed 5 weeks data collection, 37% (20/54) completed final data collection after patient death. Low trainability

RCTs directed at families as caregivers with patients in mixed stages of disease (both early and late stage)					
Budin et al. (2008) *NYC US*	249 Pt. and caregiver dyads (54% spouse), mixed stage breast cancer; 4 groups (SE, TC, SE+TC, TAU)	All groups improved over time; few significant differences between TAU and any intervention; No intervention effects for partners; Pts. who received any intervention reported less side effect distress/severity and higher well-being	4 disease trajectory specific interventions (dx, recov from surgery, adjuvant therapy, survival) SE via videos TC via telephone Manualized L&F Stress-appraisal, Crisis Intervention Medium accessibility	Nurses + specialized training	42% (249/588) of eligible Pts. participated 67% of Pts. and 49% of partners completed all interventions Medium trainability
Given et al. (2006) *Midwest US*	237 caregivers (65% spouse) mixed cancers (74% breast or lung) mixed stage (66% late stage); 2 groups (CBT, TAU)	Less negative reaction to helping with symptom management by all caregivers; gender differences noted	10 contacts over 20 weeks; 5 face-to-face (while Pt. doing chemo), 5 telephone; focused on caregiver reactions to Pt. symptoms No manual Social learning No accessibility	RN with oncology experience	43% (263/609) of eligible Pts. and carers participated 80% (191/237) completed all interventions Low trainability

(Continued)

Table 9.2. Continued

	Study Characteristics		Ease of Dissemination[a]		
Citation/Location	**N, Diagnosis, Stage/ No. of Groups**	**Results/Outcomes**	**Intervention Description, Theory, Accessibility**	**Therapist Characteristics**	**Patient Acceptability/ Trainability[b]**
Northouse et al. (2005) *Midwest US*	182 Pt. and caregiver dyads (62% spouse), late-stage breast; 2 groups (FOCUS, TAU)	Significant difference at 3 months—less hopelessness ($d = .53$), less negative appraisal of illness ($d = .37$); differences not maintained at 6 months; no sig difference in uncertainty, coping, or QOL at 3 or 6 months	3, 90-minute home visits + 2, 30-minute phone sessions Manualized L&F Stress-appraisal High accessibility	Masters-prepared RNs + training in FOCUS	73% (182/250) agreed 74% completed 3, 6-month follow-up High trainability
RCT directed at bereavement of families of patients in terminal illness phase of disease					
Kissane et al. (2006) *Australia*	81 families (Pt, partner, at least 1 child over 12), prescreened w/ FRI or risk of poor psychosocial outcome, mixed cancer types, Pt. dying from cancer; 2 groups (FFGT, control)	Moderate reduction in distress at 13 months ($d = .26$) most decreased depression and distress in those most highly distressed. No change in family functioning. "Sullen" and "Intermediate" families showed most change in distress ($d = .32, .19$) and in depression ($d = .44, .30$)	4–8, 90-minute sessions over 9–18 months Manualized, Family systems, Medium accessibility	16 social workers, all were family therapists + 2, ½ day workshops in FFGT	71% (183/257) of families screened eligible 44% (81/183) agreed to participate 88% (40/45) completed FFGT High trainability

RCT, family intervention, feasibility study of a culturally sensitive approach, small-sample size (<40)					
Mokuau et al. (2008) *US Hawaii*	12 families (Pt. and 1–3 family members), Pts. all Native Hawaiian women with mixed cancer types, 3–12 months post diagnosis	Significant difference in improved family coping—spiritual support and mobilizing family to accept help. Pts. showed decreased psychological distress; lengthy recruitment, but otherwise feasible; cultural adaptation highly appreciated	6 sessions over 3 months in homes, libraries, business offices. No manual No theory cited No accessibility	4 social workers in teams of two. 3 natives of Hawaii, 1 lifelong resident & NCI cancer-info specialist	Accrual difficult (18 months for 12 participants) 100% (12/12) completed treatment Low trainability

[a]Ease of Dissemination is operationally defined as an intervention <12 sessions, provided by one qualified provider such as social worker, psychologist, or nurse (adapted from Jacobsen & Jim, 2008).
[b]Trainability = an estimate of how easy an intervention is to train to others—defined as High = manual available + nondoctoral provider, Moderate = manual available OR treatment provided by nondoctoral provider, Low = no manual and treatment provided by doctoral-level provider (taken from Chorpita et al, 2011).
[c]Accessibility of Manual—High = online, Medium = published manual/book/workbook, Low = from researcher only, None = no manual available.
CARE ADVISOR = intervention focused on caregiver needs across seven domains: patient care, physical health needs, time away, future plans, psych health/relationships/support network, relationship/communication with health care providers, finances; COPE = a cognitive/behavioral problem-solving approach summarized by the acronym COPE (Creativity, Optimism, Planning and Expert information); d = *Cohen's* d = standardized mean difference scores as reported or calculated using Wilson, D.B. online effect size calculator; FRI, family relationship index, a self-report measure of an individual's perception of their family cohesiveness, expressiveness, and capacity to deal with conflict; FFGT, family-focused grief therapy; FOCUS is a support/educational intervention with core components of F = family involvement, O = optimistic attitude, C = coping effectiveness, U = uncertainty reduction, S = symptom management; L&F, Lazarus & Folkman cognitive, stress-appraisal theory; PST = problem-solving therapy; Pt, patient; QOL, quality of life; RCT, randomized controlled trial; SE, standardized psychoeducation, four disease continuum-specific video interventions (diagnosis, recovery from surgery, adjuvant therapy, ongoing recovery); TAU, treatment as usual; TC, telephone counseling.

measured. Modest short-term improvements are noted. Most effect sizes are small (*d* = .05 to .30). Where significant group differences were found, results show better quality of life (McMillan et al., 2006; Meyers et al., 2011), decreased burden (McMillan et al, 2006), and less negative appraisal of caregiving (Northouse et al., 2005). Three studies (Budin et al., 2008; Hudson et al., 2005; Walsh et al., 2007) reported within-group improvements in hypothesized directions but failed to show between-group differences; thus, any positive outcomes cannot be attributed to the intervention. Studies tried to identify mechanisms of change, such as improved problem solving (McMillan et al., 2006; Meyer et al., 2011) or increased self-efficacy (Hudson et al., 2005) but failed to identify them.

In a study (Kissane et al., 2006) measuring family system constructs, family members in greatest distress at baseline reported significant declines in distress and depression at 6 and 13 months. Overall family functioning did not change, but in families classified as mildly or moderately dysfunctional (i.e., "sullen" or "intermediate") overall distress showed more and longer lasting change than those classified as "hostile." Effect sizes for decreased distress at 13 months were small (*d* = .18 to .32).

Ease of Dissemination of Family-Focused Interventions

As in previous chapters, Table 9.2 includes information about ease of dissemination. Ease of dissemination considers treatment length, its theoretical approach and techniques used, how easy or difficult it is to access a treatment manual, the characteristics of the therapist, patient acceptance, and how easy or difficult it is to train health care professionals. Dissemination of family-focused interventions in local cancer care settings is more complicated than the dissemination of individual or group interventions, given the need for specific training in family therapy. It is unlikely that many cancer care settings will have competent family therapists routinely affiliated with their setting. Dissemination of family-focused interventions will thus require either training of oncology-affiliated staff in more general family systems therapy and/or training of already well-trained family therapists in the basics of psycho-oncology (Veach et al., 2002).

Intervention Descriptions

The nine RCTs vary in modality, location, frequency, and duration. The modality for four studies (Budin et al., 2008; Given et al., 2006; McMillan et al., 2006; Walsh et al., 2007) was *individual* sessions to caregivers. The modality for two studies (Meyers et al., 2011; Northouse et al., 2005) was *conjoint* sessions to both patient and caregiver. Two studies (Kissane et al., 2006; Mokuau, Braun, Wong, Higuchi, & Gotay, 2008) used *family* sessions to a patient and one or two family members; and one study (Hudson, Aranda, & Hayman-White, 2005) consisted of both individual and conjoint sessions. Of the four with an individual modality, their locations varied. One was provided exclusively in participants' homes (McMillan et al., 2006), one in a clinic setting (Given et al., 2006), one via telephone contact (Budin et al., 2008), and one (Walsh et al., 2007) used multiple settings (home, clinic, caregiver work setting). Of the two studies with conjoint sessions, one was in patient homes (Northouse et al., 2005) and one in a clinic setting (Meyers et al., 2011). Of the two studies with family sessions, most sessions were held in patients' homes or other settings (e.g., clinic, public library, or business offices) guided by family convenience. Two studies (Hudson et al., 2005; Northouse et al., 2005) used telephone contacts to patients and caregivers as ways of following up earlier face-to-face sessions, and one study (Budin et al., 2008) used telephone contacts to follow up on patients' and caregivers' viewing of educational videos.

All nine studies were provided as brief interventions, ranging from three sessions (Hudson et al., 2005; McMillan et al., 2006; Meyers et al., 2011; O'Hara et al., 2010) of about 160–180 minutes to eight sessions totaling 720 minutes (Kissane et al., 2006). Although not all studies reported duration, the frequency and duration of interventions suggests that most studies range between 1 and 3 months of intervention, consisting of three to six sessions. One exception is the FFGT study (Kissane et al., 2006), which was considerably longer ranging from four to eight family sessions over 9 to 18 months. These nine family-focused interventions have been guided by various theoretical approaches.

Theoretical Approaches

The family-focused interventions in Table 9.2 include interventions from different theoretical orientations, including a cognitive model of stress, problem-solving therapy, and cognitive-behavioral therapy. Despite the fact that family systems theory is the predominant theoretical approach to family therapy, only one study (Kissane et al., 2006) used family system principles.

Cognitive Model of Stress

Lazarus and Folkman's (1984) cognitive model of stress is the theoretical approach used in three studies (Budin et al., 2008; Hudson et al., 2005; Northouse et al., 2005). As previously described (see Chapters 6 and 8), this model emphasizes primary and secondary appraisal in which one's perception of the degree of harm, threat, or danger is buffered by one's perception of the availability of coping skills, resources, or strategies one has to bring to the stressful situations. Thus, interventions are designed to identify the family stressors and to build additional resources, skills, and strategies to cope. As new resources and coping strategies are acquired, a family member's secondary appraisal of his or her own skills is improved and, it is hypothesized, the overall stress is thus reduced.

Problem-Solving Therapy

Two other studies were guided by the adaptation of problem-solving therapy (PST) to use with cancer patients (Nezu, Nezu, Friedman, Faddis, & Houts, 1999; Nezu et al., 2003). As described in Chapter 6, PST has been shown to be an effective cognitive-behavioral treatment for depression in the general adult population (Cuijpers, van Straten, & Warmerdam, 2007). PST includes a series of steps—problem orientation, problem definition/formulation, generation of alternatives, decision making, solution implementation, and verification—designed to enhance a person's ability to solve problems. In training of caregivers, these steps have been adapted to an educational model to be offered to cancer patients and their caregiving family members titled COPE (Houts et al., 1996), an acronym taken from its four major components of Creativity, Optimism, Planning, and Expert Information (COPE). Caregivers are taught how to use this model to more effectively solve cancer-related problems. In its most recent form (Bucher & Zabora, 2010), family caregivers are encouraged to follow the COPE model, which includes understanding types of problems that might arise, knowing what family caregivers can do to help or prevent the problems, being aware of possible obstacles to problem solution, knowing when and how to get expert professional help, and knowing how to carry out and adjust a plan of action. These newly developed problem-solving skills are hypothesized to reduce family caregiver distress and enhance quality of life.

Family Systems Theory

One study (Kissane et al., 2006) was guided by family systems theory and the family lifecycle (Carter & McGoldrick, 1980; Rolland, 2005) embedded within culturally influenced experiences of grief. Three key dimensions of family functioning were evaluated: cohesiveness, conflict, and expressiveness. *Cohesiveness*, the degree to which family members function together, can be significantly challenged during the experience of family grief and serves as a critical variable in family functioning. High cohesiveness can serve as a buffer against the stressors inherent in loss. How a family responds to *conflict* is also important. The ability of a family to resolve conflict indicates good adaptability and vice versa. Finally, *expressiveness*, or the degree to which family members freely express their thoughts and feelings within the family, is the third dimension used in this study. High expressiveness is associated with high adaptability, and low expressiveness is associated with family dysfunction. Kissane and colleagues (1998) used an assessment of these three family dimensions to classify families into five types: two well-functioning, two dysfunctional, and one intermediate. The two well-functioning types include those scoring very *high on cohesion* and those exhibiting *tolerance for differences* of opinion and good conflict resolution. The two dysfunctional types include those *hostile* families exhibiting high conflict, low cohesion, and poor expressiveness, and *sullen* families who also show low cohesion, poor conflict resolution, and poor communication. Lastly, there is an *intermediate* group who shows moderate cohesion and is negatively affected by the family strain of grief and bereavement. Key to this study was the notion that service provision should be directed at those families at greatest risk of poor psychosocial outcomes. Thus, services were provided only to those families assessed to be hostile, sullen, or intermediate.

The family therapy intervention consisted of the use of standard family therapy principles and techniques (e.g., a collaborative therapeutic alliance, use of a family genogram, fostering family assets and strengths, identifying explicit family patterns of functioning), with a strong emphasis on exploring patterns of family communication as they reflect family cohesion, conflict resolution, and expressiveness. Common themes of grief, loss, and family/cultural rituals were frequently encountered as a part of the family bereavement process. As families encounter the death of a family member, the hypothesized mechanism of change in family systems therapy is that with the help of family therapy sessions, explicit patterns of communication can be recognized and, when found to be dysfunctional, intentionally changed, and/or when found to be fostering of family strengths, encouraged and affirmed as helpful. When family therapy is effective, it has its impact on the family system patterns of communication indicative of increased cohesions, improved resolution of conflict, and openness/acceptance of family expressiveness.

Cognitive-Behavioral Therapy

One study (Given et al., 2006) was based upon social learning theory (Bandura, 1986) and utilized cognitive-behavioral techniques. Social learning theory emphasizes the acquisition of various self-management strategies as acquired via observation of others, skills training, and a variety of mastery experiences that enhance self-efficacy (i.e., perceived self-competence). In this study, as caregivers learned by observing or discussing coping strategies with others and developed new and effective coping skills by practice and eventual success or mastery, it is hypothesized that they then became better able to manage their own stress reactions with improved skill and self-confidence.

Cultural Adaptation

One study (Mokuau et al., 2008) was of a culturally sensitive intervention incorporating key characteristics of Native Hawaiian culture, such as its emphasis on family (*'ohana)* and the individual's responsibility (*kuleana*) to family, spirituality, and the use of proverbs (*'olelo no 'eau)*; and one study (Walsh et al., 2007) provided no theory-specific citations.

Dissemination Conclusions

Ease of dissemination varies across the 9 studies in Table 9.2. The Northouse et al. (2005) study of late-stage breast cancer patient–caregiver dyads, where the supportive and educational intervention FOCUS was provided by masters-prepared nurses, and patient acceptability rates are in the 70%–80% range, appears to be the most easily disseminated. The manual is highly accessible online via the Cancer Control P.L.A.N.E.T. Web site for research-tested intervention programs (RTIPs) that describes the three, 90-minute face-to-face sessions followed by two, 30-minute telephone contacts. This ease of access via an online Web site makes this study unique among the studies cited in Table 9.2. However, detracting from its ease of dissemination is the need for highly trained nurses and in-home interventions. The ability of highly trained nurses to be able to make home visits seems unlikely in most community cancer centers.

Three additional studies (Kissane et al., 2006; McMillan et al., 2006; Meyers et al., 2011) also have good dissemination potential with high trainability and moderate access to a manualized intervention. Two studies (McMillan et al., 2006; Meyers et al., 2011) are adaptations of a very effective therapy approach—problem-solving therapy—that reported very high effect sizes (d = 2.04 to 4.49) as an individual intervention (Nezu et al., 2003). These two studies are for family caregivers and patients with mixed types of cancer, all receiving end-of-life, palliative care. Both interventions have manuals available either via a published book (Nezu, Nezu, Friedman, Faddis, & Houts, 1999) or directly from the researchers. Despite good accessibility to a manual, these two studies report low patient acceptability, with difficulties in recruiting study participants and completion rates in the 20%–30% range. The third study is with bereaved families of terminally ill patients receiving a family systems therapy targeted to families at increased risk for negative outcomes (Kissane et al., 2006). This intervention has a manual available via a published book (Kissane & Bloch, 2002), and although less than half (44%) of identified eligible families participated, 75% completed the intervention.

The remaining four studies (Budin et al., 2008; Given et al., 2006; Hudson et al., 2005; Walsh et al., 2007) from Table 9.2 all have intermediate or moderate ease of dissemination. Two of them (Budin et al., 2008; Hudson et al., 2005; Walsh et al., 2007) require nurses with specialized training or prior experience in palliative care, which may be problematic in many community cancer centers. In contrast, another study (Given et al., 2006) requires nurses with oncology experience, which is more likely to be feasible in most oncology settings. However, this same study does not report the availability of a manual. These four studies varied in patient acceptability with 30%–76% of eligible participants agreeing to participate and intervention completion rates ranging between 50% and 76%. Finally, one study (Mokuau et al., 2008) reported no manual and low trainability due to the need for specific ethnic characteristics of the providers, and although 100% of participants completed the trial, it took 18 months to accrue only 12 participant families. Reference citations for manualized interventions and related resources are provided in Box 9.1.

Summary of the Evidence Base for Family-Focused Interventions

The majority of family-focused health service interventions for adult cancer patients are directed at family caregivers of patients with advanced disease or terminal illness. Caregiver quality of life is the most common outcome measured, with modest, short-term improvements noted. Although family systems theory is the predominant theoretical model for family therapy, only one of

Box 9.1

Accessibility of Manuals: Reference Citations for Manualized Interventions and Related Resources From Exemplars of Best Available Evidence, for Family-Focused Interventions

Randomized Controlled Trials Directed at Families as Caregivers With Patients Receiving Palliative Care or in the Advanced Disease/Terminal Phase of Cancer

Meyers et al. (2011)—Manual as published book.

Nezu, A. M., Nezu, A. M., Friedman, S. H., Faddis, S., Houts, P. S. (1999). *Helping cancer patients cope: A problem-solving approach.* Washington, DC: American Psychological Association.

Related Patient/Caregiver Resources

Bucher, J., Houts, P. D., Eds. *American Cancer Society complete guide to family caregiving.* 2nd ed. Atlanta, GA: ACS.

Houts, P. S. (1994). *American College of Physicians home care guide for cancer: How to care for family and friends at home.* Philadelphia, PA: The College.

McMillan et al. (2006)—The COPE intervention has been written into manual form and is available from the authors on request. Retrieved December 20, 2014 at http://health.usf.edu/nocms/nursing/CaregiverInterventionManualB.pdf

Hudson et al. (2005)—No intervention manual available.

Walsh et al. (2007)—Copies of the manual are available from the authors upon request.

Related Caregiver Resource

Caregiver guidebook is available from the authors at the following URL. Retrieved on December 10, 2014 from https://www.pcvlibrary.asn.au/

Randomized Controlled Trials Directed at Families as Caregivers With Patients in Mixed Stages of Disease (Both Early and Late Stage)

Budin et al. (2008)—No intervention manual.

Nurse Interventionist Training Manual

Haber, J. (2002). *Standardized psycho-education and telephone counseling training manual.* New York: NYU.

Related Intervention Description

Given et al. (2006)—No intervention manual available and no related resources available.

Hoskins, C. N., Haber, J., Budin, W. C., Cartwright-Alcarese, F., Kowalski, M. O., Panke, J., & Maislin, G. (2001). Breast cancer education, counseling, and adjustment: A pilot study. *Psychological Reports, 89*(3), 677–704. doi: 10.2466/pr0.89.7.677-704

Northouse et al. (2005)—Related manual available.

FOCUS Program manual for similar intervention with different population (prostate) available online via Research Tested Intervention Programs (RTIPs). Retrieved December 20, 2014 from http://rtips.cancer.gov/rtips/programDetails.do?programId=102766

Northouse, L. L., Walker, J., Schafenacker, A., Mood, D., Mellon, S., Galvin, E., . . . Freeman-Gibb, L. (2002). A family-based program of care for women with recurrent breast cancer and their family members. *Oncology Nursing Forum, 29*(10), 1411–1419. doi: 10.1188/02.ONF.1411-1419

Randomized Controlled Trial Directed at Bereavement of Families of Patients in Terminal Illness Phase of Disease

Kissane et al. (2006)—Manualized.

Kissane, D. W. Bloch. S. (2002). Family focused grief therapy: A model of family-centered care during palliative care and bereavement. Philadelphia, PA: Open University Press.

Related Intervention Description

Kissane, D., & Zaider, I. Z. (2011). Focused family therapy in palliative care and bereavement. In M. Watson & D. Kissane (Eds.), *Handbook of psychotherapy in cancer care* (pp. 185–197). Oxford, UK: Wiley.

Randomized Controlled Trial, Family Intervention, Feasibility Study of a Culturally Sensitive Approach, Small Sample Size (<40)

Mokuau et al. (2008)—No manual available.

the identified studies incorporated family systems theory into the intervention (Kissane et al., 2006). Instead, the cognitive stress model (Lazarus & Folkman, 1984) and the adaptation of problem-solving therapy (Houts et al., 1996) for use with caregivers (COPE) have been the predominant theoretical approaches used. The ease with which these studies can be disseminated for use in the local community cancer setting varies, with some showing good potential, particularly when manualized interventions are available via either the Internet or published books, the health care professionals who provide the study intervention are similar to those in community cancer settings making training feasible, and patients are receptive and willing to participate in the intervention.

CASE EXAMPLE: HOW TO DO EVIDENCE-BASED PRACTICE OF A FAMILY-FOCUSED INTERVENTION

In addition to the earlier overview of the evidence base for family-focused interventions, the following case example provides a detailed illustration of how to do EBP where a family-focused intervention is warranted. This case emphasizes the adaptation of best available evidence from a group treatment modality for caregiver dyads to an individual intervention; the important role of supportive counseling; how to augment supportive counseling with a structured caregiver education program; and ultimately how, when, and with whom to implement family-focused grief therapy after a patient dies.

Case Example 5—NM/AM Family: 50-Year-Old Male With Brain Tumor

Referral Information

About 3 weeks ago while attending a case conference, you heard a new patient presentation of a 50-year-old, local businessman who was diagnosed with a brain tumor. Yesterday, one of the radiation therapy staff members contacted you, explaining that the wife of this patient would like to talk to you. You were able to meet with her immediately after her husband's radiation appointment, and she explained that she would like to "have someone to talk to" while she and her family are "going through all of this." You agreed and set up an initial psychosocial assessment interview for next week, with her and her husband. In the meantime, you look over his medical record and learn that he has been diagnosed with a glioblastoma multiforme, and that the family consists of his wife of 30 years, two adult sons, and one adult daughter, ranging in age from the mid-20s to the early 30s, and a few grandchildren.

You Begin the Evidence-Based Practice Process

Step 1: Ask Specific, Clinical Questions: Both Background and Foreground

Relevant *biomedical* background questions include the following:

- What is glioblastoma multiforme and what are its treatment options, side effects, and prognosis?

You quickly look at the National Cancer Institute's Web site for general background information about brain tumors. When searching for "brain tumors," you at first find it a bit confusing until you notice a link to "neurologic" cancers, and there you look further under "brain tumor, adult." You learn that primary (not metastatic) malignant brain tumors occur in about 6.4 per 100,000 persons per year in the United States and that there are a number of different types of brain tumors related to the variety of different cell types within the brain, but that a glioblastoma is a type that forms from glial cells (nonneuronal cells in the brain that serve a variety of functions to protect and support neurons) and that glial cell tumors account for about 38% of primary brain tumors. You read that brain tumors are classified by the World Health Organization's (WHO) grading system from Grade I to Grade IV, based upon the histologic grade, which is a microscopic look at the cell structure that determines how abnormal the cancer cells look, relative to normal cells. The higher the grade, the higher the likelihood of cell growth and spread. Gliobastomas are Grade IV, the highest level.

Treatment of gliobastomas is influenced by the grade and the location of the tumor in the brain, but in general treatment includes surgery, radiation, and chemotherapy. Surgery's primary goal is to reduce intracranial pressure and conserve as much neurological function as possible. With many high-grade tumors, surgically implanting polymer wafers that contain the chemotherapy agent carmustine is another important goal of surgery. You also note that total removal of the malignant cells can only rarely be achieved, thus the need for further treatment. External beam radiation therapy (EBRT) for high-grade tumors is an important part of postsurgical treatment. The National Cancer Institute (NCI) site describes a systematic review and meta-analysis of five randomized trials (Laperriere, Zuraw, & Cairncross, 2002), finding a statistically significant advantage for the patients receiving radiation therapy. Overall survival in the experimental group was about 3 months longer than in the control group—from a median survival of 9 months to 12 months.

Chemotherapy, in the form of a daily oral pill (temozolomide), is also very likely. You notice that rather than a lot having been written about treatment side effects, instead there is more information about related problems such as seizures and/or rehabilitation of any functional limitations (speech, motor, etc.) that might occur as a result of the surgery. You anticipate that your patient will be taking additional medications (steroids, anticonvulsants) to control overall swelling in the brain and seizures, and you wonder if he has any residual physical, sensory, or other dysfunction as a result of the surgery.

Thus, the prognosis for your patient is not good, and you anticipate that he and his family are likely to experience his death sometime within the next year or even sooner.

Relevant *psychosocial* background questions include the following:

- What types of specific psychosocial concerns/issues are likely with primary brain tumors?
- Are there any specific family issues/concerns to be aware of that might complicate or be predictive of better or worse family adaptation?
- What is the general background knowledge about psychosocial interventions for families facing cancer, particularly cancers with a poor prognosis?

You begin by looking at a chapter in *Psycho-Oncology* (Holland et al., 2010) about the psychosocial issues related to central nervous system tumors (Valentine, 2010) and find that, in addition to a poor prognosis and significant stress on the patient, family, and caregivers, the types of patient dysfunction can include changes in cognitive function, personality, and behavior. The cognitive dysfunctions can include problems with memory, attention, arousal, perception, and other dementia-related symptoms, as well as other possible problems/limitations depending on the specific location of the tumor. Personality changes can also occur; sometimes these are very subtle exaggerations of premorbid traits, and at other times, they are more dramatic changes such as behavior that is very atypical of the patient but occurs as a result of less cognitive inhibition of behaviors. This book also has a special section on psychological issues of the family, with two specific chapters on spouse caregivers (Bucher & Zabora, 2010; Northouse & McCorkle, 2010). Common needs of spouse caregivers include accurate medical information, social support, effective communication with spouse/partner, specific caregiving coping strategies, and self-efficacy in performing caregiver tasks. Types of interventions designed to help both the patient and the spouse caregivers are also summarized.

Although the literature on psychosocial interventions is relatively limited, various psychoeducational interventions that provide support and education have found positive outcomes of less distress and improved quality of life for both patients and spouses, as well as enhanced caregiver self-efficacy, increased rewards of caregiving, and better caregiver coping. Other interventions have focused on enhancing caregiver skills and preparedness for the role of caregiver, emphasizing both general skills and specific skills focused on particular patient symptoms (e.g., pain). These interventions also reported positive results such as enhanced knowledge, better symptom management, and decreased caregiver depression. The Bucher and Zabora (2010) chapter provides some detail about the adaptation of problem-solving therapy for cancer patients (Nezu et al., 2003) to an educational format titled COPE—Creativity, Optimism, Planning, and Expert Information—for family caregivers. The detail and specificity of this intervention seems very relevant, and you note that the chapter provides a number of relevant references.

You search the National Guidelines Clearinghouse (http://www.guideline.gov) using the terms *cancer caregivers*, to look for any practice guidelines of relevance. You identify two, titled *Clinical Practice Guidelines for Quality Palliative Care* (National Consensus Project for Quality Palliative Care, 2009) and *Putting Evidence Into Practice: Evidence Based Interventions to Reduce Family Caregiver Strain and Burden* (Honea et al., 2008). The first one is an expert consensus, updated in 2009 from the original version of 2004 as developed by the National Consensus Project for Quality Palliative Care—a project overseen by four major national palliative care organizations (American Academy of Hospice and Palliative Medicine, Center to Advance Palliative Care, Hospice and Palliative Nurses Association, National Hospice and Palliative Care Organization). Its stated objectives are (1) to develop a comprehensive description of what constitutes high-quality palliative care and (2) to serve as a resource for health care professionals providing palliative care. It is not exclusively focused on cancer, but rather "chronic, debilitating, and life-threatening illnesses." You find that the recommendations are very broad and mostly administrative, consisting of eight domains of care, one of which seems most relevant—Psychological and Psychiatric Aspects of Care—and so you check those. These domain recommendations are also very broad, essentially recommending that competent psychological and psychiatric services be available and appropriately and competently provided when needed. You can take from these recommendations that health care systems should have in place a broad multidisciplinary and well-coordinated palliative care service, but there is not much of direct, immediate relevance to your family. The second guideline is more helpful. It is an expert consensus guideline of studies published between 1995 and 2006 to provide recommendations to reduce family caregiver strain and burden. Three levels of recommendations are provided, based upon the strength of the evidence: (1) recommended for practice, (2) likely to be effective, and (3) benefits balanced with harm. Cognitive-behavioral interventions are recommended for practice, and psychoeducational, psychotherapy, supportive, and multicomponent interventions are classified as likely to be effective.

Lastly, you review the *Handbook of Psychotherapy in Cancer Care* (Watson & Kissane, 2011) and note the relevance of two chapters. First, the initial chapter in this edited book (Lederberg & Holland, 2011) is titled *Supportive Psychotherapy in Cancer Care: An Essential Ingredient of All Therapy.* As the title implies, it outlines the core components, ingredients, and processes essential to the use of supportive therapy in a wide variety of cancer care contexts. Of most importance is the recognition that supportive therapy is "the single most important tool of the psycho-oncologist" (p. 3), which reminds you that you have always utilized a common-factors-style supportive therapy (see Chapter 3 for more detail), with emphasis on the importance of the therapeutic alliance as your primary approach, particularly early in the therapy process, and any time when there is insufficient empirical evidence. With complicated family situations like this client, you are likely to need to utilize this essential approach.

Second, a chapter on family therapy in palliative care—family-focused grief therapy (FFGT) (Kissane & Zaider, 2011) is relevant. You learn that this intervention uses various family system principles such as cohesion, adaptability, and communication to first assess family characteristics and to consider their relevance to how families cope during the loss of a loved one.

Noting that family systems theory is the predominant theoretical approach to family therapy, you also review some literature on family systems principles and cancer. This source (Veach et al., 2002) presents theoretical and conceptual ideas organized by crossing the clinical course of the disease (diagnosis, treatment, rehabilitation, survival, recurrence/advanced disease, and terminal illness) with the family life cycle (newly forming couple, family with young children, family with adolescents, family launching children, and family in later life) resulting in a series of chapters for each disease course, within which there are details of each family life cycle. A table in the introduction summarizes key issues in this clinical course–life cycle framework. Another helpful table provides a list of family system principles and their definitions. This list includes the concepts of cohesion, adaptability/flexibility, communication, and family structure, types of change, movement, and patterns of adjustment. Reviewing these principles and their definitions should help in the assessment of the family's overall adaptation.

Relevant *foreground* questions prior to Session 1 include the following:

- How much and how accurate is the information that the patient and his spouse have about his disease (e.g., treatment options, side effects, treatment related risks, prognosis)?
- Does he have any functional limitations following surgery?
- In addition to temozolomide, what other medications is he taking (anticonvulsants, steroids, etc.)?
- How are he, his wife, and family coping with his disease?
- What is the quality of the family's social support (emotional, instrumental, and informational)?
- How much home care, as his primary caregiver, is his wife currently contributing?
- Does the patient, spouse, or any family member have any past experience with mental health services, and if so, what were they and how did they go? Do those past experiences influence any current treatment preferences (individual, couples, family)?
- Are there any demographic, cultural, disease, developmental, or treatment-related factors that might influence treatment preferences?

Session 1

The first clinical interview: Assessment of psychosocial adaptation, both individually and family.

You plan to follow the psychosocial assessment interview process as detailed in Chapter 5, modified to focus on both partners as individuals and to attend to relevant family system principles.

You meet the patient Neil M. and his spouse, Alice M., in the waiting room and accompany them as they walk to your office. As usual, you begin by explaining confidentiality and its limits and the purpose of this first interview. They understand and provide written consent before beginning by telling you their story. You learn that Neil had a couple incidents of headaches and dizziness, accompanied by numbness in his left hand. This frightened Alice, more than he, so she urged him to go to their family doctor, who ordered a CT scan and MRI. A few days later, their family doctor called and insisted they see him as soon as possible in his office. They were scared with the urgency of it all, and yet weren't certain what to expect. He told them there was "some type of mass" in Neil's brain and referred them to a neurosurgeon. They saw the neurosurgeon who explained the need for surgery as soon as possible, offering, "This could be a serious brain tumor," but explained that they wouldn't know exactly "what they were dealing with" until after surgery.

Just 5 days later, Neil had surgery. Alice explains that she was "prepared that he might not live through the surgery." However, he did, and despite some significant pain during the first 24 hours, has done well, and presently is in the midst of radiation therapy and takes "some oral drug" once each day as his chemotherapy. He is also taking a steroid to control swelling in the brain and an anticonvulsant to control any seizures—fortunately, he has not had any seizures, but the possibly of such worries his wife a lot. He explains that he doesn't like the steroid as his face is getting pretty puffy/swollen (he is a bit self-conscious), and at times he gets a little nauseous, but it has helped with his appetite. His doctors aren't allowing him to drive, which "although you would think that is no big deal," his wife indicates that the lack of independence is really getting to him lately as he has always been very busy and active and finds the "nothing to do" sometimes the hardest thing to deal with. When asking about prognosis, you note that the patient is less interested in discussing this compared to his wife, who does seem to want to talk some about the future. You learn that they do have a pretty accurate understanding of the poor prognosis ("Yes, the doctors told us this cannot be cured, and that long-term survival is not likely"), yet they also have hope "for a miracle."

When focusing your assessment on Alice, you learn that she is experiencing many of the concerns detailed in the literature. These include:

- *some significant anxiety and worry,*
- *fears of the unknown future that they may be facing, and*
- *a lack of confidence in her abilities to take care of him, if needed, as he gets sicker.*

At present, however, Neil is surprising his doctors as his recovery from surgery and his ongoing radiation and chemotherapy treatments have not slowed him as much as expected; he is even continuing to do some work from home on those days he feels strong enough. He has no notable motor, sensory, cognitive, or any other functional limitations at present.

When asked about their relationship, they respond that "It is good/better now," implying that it hasn't always been so. You learn that Alice has always felt distant and unaccepted by Neil's family, which she attributes to being Hispanic ("I don't look much like the rest of them") and having been raised as an adopted child. You also sense neither of them wants to elaborate much more on their relationship, so you shift to further assessment of their family.

You learn that they have three adult-aged children (the two oldest are boys, and the youngest is a daughter), ranging in age from mid 20s to early 30s. All three are married and have children. Neil and Alice have a total of five grandchildren. In addition, Neil's mother lives in the same neighborhood as he and his wife, as does a sister of Neil, and they see them frequently, particularly since Neil has been sick. Alice reports that she is not pleased that Neil's mother visits so often, as they frequently disagree about his care. Alice explains that she has essentially no extended family as her mother died when she was very young, and she was placed in foster care before being adopted as an adolescent. She knows where her adoptive parents live but doesn't see them regularly. The current household is Neil and Alice, but their three children and grandchildren are frequently visiting, on nearly a daily basis, particularly since his diagnosis. When asked about how their children are coping with his disease, they both express concern, particularly for their two sons who they believe, "just don't understand how serious" this is and are acting as if Neil will eventually be back to normal and back to work. They indicate they don't know what to do about their children, but they are concerned. Alice says she has tried to talk to her sons, but they just seem to get mad whenever she brings it up, so she now avoids it. Her daughter is a bit easier to talk to and seems more realistic about the prognosis.

As you begin to end the interview and ask them about goals, you learn that they spoke about this before the appointment and agreed that the patient, Neil, is not interested in ongoing services as he feels like he is "doing so well he is surprising his doctors," but Alice would like to meet "just to have someone, outside of the family, to talk to." You ask about any prior mental health services and they indicate none, and therefore, they deny any specific preferences for types of therapy other than Alice who indicates, "I think I just need someone to talk to about all that has happened and might happen in the future—I'm not sure I can handle all of this on my own; it all has happened so fast."

You suggest that maybe a reasonable goal would be to focus on her needs as a caregiver for her husband and additional support for herself. She agrees, saying, "I need help trying to control this disease," by which she means learning more about how to do a good job at being his caregiver, while also coping with all of the changes impacting the entire family. She also indicates a desire to "not lose myself" in the midst of all of these stressors. You ask for clarification, and she indicates that she just knows she needs more support, or she could become so focused on caring for others that she won't take good care of herself. You agree and suggest that you search the literature for information on caregiving and that the two of you meet individually to provide supportive counseling and focus on her self-care. You and she schedule another appointment in 1 week, but before ending you ask them both to complete some questionnaires.

They both complete the HADS (Holland, Greenberg, & Hughes, 2006; Zigmond & Snaith, 1983) and Neil completes the FACIT-G (Cella et al., 1993). On the HADS, Alice scores a total score of 16 (5 on depression and 11 on anxiety), indicating a total score above the cutoff, suggesting the likelihood of a diagnosable mental disorder such as adjustment disorder with anxiety. Neil's total score is 9 (4 on depression and 5 on anxiety), indicating he is not experiencing a significant amount of anxiety or depression. On the FACIT, he reports a fair quality of life in most all domains (total score of 49 is at 47th percentile). He scores the lowest on physical well-being, where his score of 8 is at 39th percentile and functional well-being where his score of 11 is at 45th percentile. His social/family well-being score of 13 is at the 46th percentile, and his emotional well-being score of 17 is at the 58th percentile. His primary concern is that he can't yet go back to work and finds it hard to not drive or be as active as usual.

Post–Psychosocial Assessment Interview: Summary of Key Patient/Family Characteristics

Patient

- 50-year-old, White, married male, first and only marriage, diagnosed with glioblastoma multiforme
- Not experiencing any significant symptoms of anxiety or depression
- No significant postsurgical functional limitations
- Not interested in ongoing psychosocial health services
- Reports a close to average (47th percentile) overall quality of life on FACIT
- Primary complaint is inability to drive and be as independent as usual
- No prior mental health services
- Not interested in further services

Spouse

- 48-year-old, Hispanic female, wife of 30 years, first and only marriage
- Primary caregiver, supportive of husband and trying to "control this disease"
- Endorses mild to moderate overall distress, with more symptoms of anxiety than depression on HADS
- Interested in supportive counseling and learning more about how to provide for her husband's care
- Recognizes need for additional support for herself and need to focus on self-care
- No prior mental health services
- Prefers individual supportive psychotherapy with psychoeducational information regarding caregiving

Family

- Three adult-aged children, all married
- Five grandchildren
- Children live nearby, visit almost daily
- Extended family (paternal mother and sister) also live nearby and visit regularly
- Some conflict between spouse and her mother-in-law
- Some apparent past history of marital problems

Step 2: Accessing the Best Available Research Evidence

You structure your literature search around the steps outlined by Gibbs (2003), with *step 1* being to formulate a PICO question. In this case you are focusing your PICO question as an individual intervention for now (anticipating that future interventions may involve the family), focused on the request of the spouse caregiver for additional support and knowledge to help "control this disease."

For a 48-year-old, married, Hispanic female caregiver of a spouse with glioblastoma, experiencing mild to moderate anxiety, what is the best available evidence for an individual intervention that will increase knowledge and skills about caregiving, provide additional support and motivation for self-care, and decrease anxiety?

Step 2 involves listing the keywords from the PICO question, and *step 3* is to list synonyms. To help with step 3 you review the subject terms of three databases by looking at the PsycINFO Thesaurus, the Medline MeSH terms, and the CINAHL headings.

P—carer, family caregiver, caregiver burden, neurologic tumors, brain cancer, glioblastoma, advanced cancer, neoplasm
I—psychosocial, psychoeducation, palliative, counseling, psychotherapy, treatment, problem-solving, cognitive behavioral
C—no treatment or no comparator
O—knowledge, skills, anxiety, depression, distress, self-care

Step 4 is to begin the search, initially with unfiltered databases (PsycINFO, CINAHL, Medline), looking for recent systematic reviews or meta-analyses of the psychosocial intervention literature for family caregivers of cancer patients. Thus, you formulate a search strategy that is limited to recent (after 2005) literature reviews and includes the following search terms: *caregiver AND palliative AND cancer.* This search returns six review articles; three are either of older literature (published after 2005 but studies reviewed from 1990s) or appear not relevant (e.g., exclusively about prostate cancer patients), while the remaining three appear relevant, and so you review their abstracts. One is primarily a review of research methodology with no reporting of intervention effectiveness (Schildmann & Higginson, 2011); another is a review of 26 published studies (nonrandomized, observational, and qualitative) focused on the practical informational needs of caregivers providing in-home, end-of-life care to persons with cancer (Bee, Barnes, & Luker, 2009) and looks relevant; and a third (Harding, List, Epiphaniou, & Jones, 2012) is a follow-up (published in 2012) of an earlier review (Harding & Higginson, 2003) of intervention studies focused on the needs of the informal caregiver. You more closely review these latter two.

In this first review article (Bee et al., 2009) data are reported from 26 studies using various structured/unstructured interviews, surveys, and validated self-report questionnaires regarding what types of information or skills informal caregivers of in-home, end-of-life care of cancer patients believe they need. Results showed eight categories of informational needs:

- medication and pain management
- physical symptoms and comfort
- nutrition
- personal hygiene/elimination
- positioning
- technical equipment
- professional/local support
- emergency measures

These categories seem reasonable and potentially relevant to your client, particularly if needed in the future, if her husband's disease progresses as anticipated. The study provides a table with general examples of these categories of unmet practical needs of in-home caregivers that proves to be a helpful overview, but you will want a more detailed and specific resource guide in the future.

The final relevant review (Harding et al., 2012) is a follow-up, published in 2012, of an earlier review completed in 2003 (Harding & Higginson, 2003). The more recent review reports an encouraging trend of an increasing number of peer-reviewed published intervention studies focused on the needs of the informal caregiver, with improved methodology (i.e., more RCTs, quasi-experimental designs, more collecting pre-post data) and promising positive outcomes. Group psychoeducational interventions were the most common (2 of 10 were RCTs) with individual, psychological interventions second most common (2 of 8 were RCTs). Although there are mixed results in both treatment modalities, both modalities do report positive outcomes, such as improved quality of life, decreased care burden, more positive affect, and improved positive rewards of caregiving.

In summary, you have accessed evidence that synthesized the informational needs of caregivers when providing in-home care, and you recognize that this may prove helpful for your client, Alice. Providing this information seems premature because her husband is presently functioning quite well. This information might be helpful later. You have also learned that both group psychoeducational interventions and individual psychological interventions have some supportive evidence of positive outcomes when provided to informal, family caregivers.

To identify possible interventions, you need a more tailored search of *unfiltered literature*, trying to identify RCTs for informal/family caregivers of patients with advanced-stage cancer. Returning to *Step 4*, you design a search strategy from the PIC-identified terms and synonyms, restricting this search to RCTs published between 2005 and 2013. You develop a search via EbscoHost of PsycINFO, CINAHL, and Medline using the following search terms:

SU (glioblastoma OR brain tumor OR neoplasm OR advanced cancer) AND SU (Caregivers OR family) AND SU (treatment OR Psychosocial OR psychoeducational OR problem-solving OR cognitive behavioral) AND SU (caregiver burden OR distress OR anxiety OR quality of life)

This search returns two studies (Meyers et al., 2011; Northouse et al., 2005), both of which appear relevant and which you will further appraise, but first you will appraise the study on the practical informational needs of caregivers providing in-home, end-of-life care (Bee et al., 2009).

Step 3: Appraising the Research Evidence

The Bee and colleagues study (2009) has a number of limitations, acknowledged by the authors, that include potential selection bias, nonrepresentativeness of the samples, and little information about internal validity of study procedures. The majority of studies were one-time investigations by local groups or individuals interested in the practical needs of their particular sample of informal caregivers. The review simply synthesized these results and noted similar themes of informational needs. They appear to have reasonable face validity and provide a general overview of types of practical information that your client Alice may need in the near future. However, you will need to be careful in not assuming the information fits your client's needs, but rather tailor it, in collaboration with her own reactions to the benefit of the information for her particular local context.

The Meyers and colleagues (2011) study tested the effect of a cognitive-behavioral, problem-solving intervention, provided by specially trained health educators with 348 patient and caregiver (70% spouses) dyads enrolled in various clinical trials for treatment of their advanced cancers against a control group of patients and caregivers receiving the usual care inherent in participating in a clinical trial. The intervention consisted of three conjoint (therapist met with the patient/caregiver dyad) sessions in which participants learned to use the Creativity, Optimism, Planning, and Expert information (COPE) problem-solving model. Patients were diagnosed with mixed types of cancer, with the largest percentages being gastrointestinal, genitourinary, thoracic, and breast. Reported results for the primary outcome of quality of life of the cancer patients indicate that there were no differences between the two groups. However, for quality of life of the caregivers, those who received the problem-solving intervention showed a slower rate of decline (less than half) in quality of life than in the control group over a

6-month follow-up. There were no differences in problem-solving skills for either group. Thus, although the results for the cancer patients showed no benefits, for caregivers it appears that what might be an inevitable decline in quality of life in caregivers of terminally ill patients happens at a slower pace than for those not receiving the COPE intervention.

The Meyers and colleagues (2011) study is appraised by use of the CONSORT checklist and the QSRF-adapted (Gibbs, 1989) form (see Appendix B). Eighteen of the 25 items on the CONSORT checklist are identified, and on the QSRF the total quality score is 75 of a possible 100. These combined scores indicate that the study results can be trusted as being reliable and valid. The strengths of the study include its overall design as a randomized controlled study, with a well-described, manualized intervention, a good sample size (n = 348), good power to detect an effect for both patient and caregiver participants, and an accompanying participant workbook titled *The Home Care Guide for Cancer* (Bucher & Zabora, 2010). Some weaknesses were also noted. Reliability data for the primary outcome measure were not provided, only about half (55%) of screened dyads agreed to participate in the study, and a small percent (36%) of participants completed the intervention and the 6-month follow-up. This small completion percentage may be due to the nature of the sample as advanced cancer patients participating in a cancer-treatment clinical trial, or it may indicate low acceptability by participants.

The Northouse and colleagues (2005) study tested the effects of a family intervention (FOCUS) provided by masters-prepared nurses to a group of 134 patient–caregiver dyads of women with advanced breast cancer versus a treatment as usual control group on the primary outcome of quality of life. The FOCUS intervention includes components of educational information and support, organized around the acronym FOCUS—Family involvement, Optimistic attitude, Coping effectiveness, Uncertainty reduction, and Symptom management. It is based upon the Lazarus and Folkman (1984) cognitive model of stress. The manualized intervention consisted of three, 90-minute, once-per-month home visits with each dyad, plus two additional, 30- minute telephone booster sessions. Results found no significant differences in quality of life for either the patient or the caregiver participants. The secondary outcomes of negative appraisal of the illness and hopelessness (for patients) and negative appraisal of caregiving by caregivers did show some improvement at the 3-month follow-up, but none of the improvements were maintained at the 6-month follow-up.

The Northouse and colleagues (2005) study is appraised by use of the CONSORT checklist and the QSRF-adapted (see Appendix B; Gibbs, 1989) form. Thirteen of the 25 items on the CONSORT checklist are identified, with limitations noted in the reporting of detailed information about the randomization process and patient/caregiver participation (no participant flowchart). On the QSRF, the total quality score is 77. These combined scores indicate that the study results are reliable and valid, despite some difficulties in transparency of reporting detailed information, as indicated by some missing information on the CONSORT checklist. The strengths of the study are its overall design as a randomized trial, the availability of an online accessed treatment manual, and higher participation and completion rates than in the Meyers et al. (2011) study. Weaknesses are the lack of positive outcome for overall quality of life and the lack of any sustained positive effects at the 6-month follow-up.

Summary

The practical information from the Bee and colleagues (2009) study has reasonable face validity and thus is worth considering as helpful information that your client might need, particularly in the near future if her husband's health declines and she is doing more in-home care. In regard to the two other studies, although they are both well-designed RCTs with sufficient power and with clearly described manualized interventions, neither study had very impressive positive outcomes. The COPE intervention study (Meyer et. al., 2011) had stronger outcomes than the FOCUS study, finding slower rates of decline in quality of life than the control group, and these outcomes were maintained over a 6-month period. The COPE intervention study also seems more accessible. In a quick re-review of the Bucher and Zabora chapter in *Psycho-Oncology*, you learn that the most current edition of this guide—*The ACS Compete Guide to Family Caregiving*—is now available via the American Cancer Society Web site (http://www.acs.org), and that it has been used in individual sessions. Although both studies were of patients with advanced cancers, neither included patients with glioblastoma, or even other types of primary brain tumors. The COPE study had more varied types of cancers, while the FOCUS study was exclusively with advanced breast cancer patients/caregivers. Both studies were targeted and provided to couple dyads, not individual caregivers like your client Alice, whose preference is for individual sessions.

With this information in mind, you proceed to Session 2, where you plan to do further assessment of the marital relationship, provision of support, and a focus on treatment planning.

Session 2: Focus on Further Assessment of the Marital Relationship, Provision of Support, Treatment Planning, and Patient Collaboration

You meet Alice and accompany her to your office for this first individual session. You ask about how she and her husband are doing, and she replies, "He's about the same, but I am not doing so well." She then begins a long recounting of their marital relationship, and you learn that it has been marked by much conflict, very poor communication, and several incidents (a number of years ago) of physical violence when he was drinking alcohol. Alice explains that she married into a family in which arguments, alcohol use, and conflict were almost always ongoing. Over time she became used to this, but on occasion it would get worse, and these episodes of violence would occur. On several occasions, they caused her to consider leaving, but given the lack of any close family of her own, she always stayed, feeling she had no other realistic options. Prior to Neil getting sick, Alice seriously considered pursuing divorce, but never said anything to her husband or family, and now, Alice strongly reports she is "committed to seeing this out"—implying she plans to stay in the relationship throughout her husband's illness. When assessing the current status of their relationship, she indicates that since he has been sick, they have actually gotten along better. He seems to feel some remorse and guilt about the past and has made some initial efforts to discuss their relationship and even to provide some apologies. She appreciates this but feels "bittersweet" that it's "almost too late."

Throughout this part of the session, you are listening closely, providing general supportive counseling, and encouraging honest expression of emotion. Toward the end of this part of the session, Alice explains that her three children (now young adults) were aware of the fights, arguments, and abuse, but the two oldest (one son and one daughter) often blamed her, believing that she should just be quiet "and let dad have his way, you know he's never gonna change." In contrast, her youngest son has always been "her ally"—having even stayed living at home longer than the others, fearing if he left, the abuse by his dad might get worse. You recognize that all of this family systems information is helpful and may prove to be very important because this family is likely to struggle and may experience significant conflict as they face the terminal illness of their husband/father.

You now switch focus and explain to Alice your thoughts about goals and treatment plan. You remind her of the previously identified goals focused on her needs as a caregiver, while providing ongoing emotional support for her. She again agrees, and you explain what you found in reviewing the literature. You provide the general list of categories of information, taken from the Bee and colleagues (2009) review. She glances at the list and indicates that "Yes, I think this is the kind of information I will want to have as he gets worse." You then also explain about the COPE intervention (Meyers et al., *2011) and its emphasis on problem-solving skills and the findings that caregivers who participated maintained a little better quality of life than those who did not receive the intervention, throughout a 6-month period. You explain that is was initially developed for patients and their primary caregiver, who met together with a trained educator for three sessions, but that it is also adaptable to be used one-on-one in individual sessions. You also explain the other study you reviewed (Northouse* et al., *2005) and how its results weren't as strong as the COPE study, and that it was provided to the patient and her or his caregiver in home visits.*

Alice again indicated that her husband, Neil, isn't interested in participating—probably because he worries that the sessions might be more couples therapy and he doesn't "believe in counseling"—and she indicates that he wouldn't be comfortable with having someone visit their home. Thus, you collaboratively agree to proceed with a combination of (a) general supportive counseling focused on her individual needs to "not lose herself" in the midst of this stressful time, and (b) COPE educational sessions focused on learning problem-solving skills. She agrees and indicates that the problem-solving skills will be of particular help as her in-home caregiving responsibilities increase. You once again ask her to complete the HADS, and she scores a 4 on depression and an 8 on anxiety, indicating modest improvement overall with most of the change indicating less anxiety than at the first session. You schedule another appointment for next week.

Post Session 2: Additional Information of Key Family Characteristics

- History of marital conflict with a few incidents of domestic violence
- Husband from a high-conflict family of origin
- Adult children have formed alliances with one particular parent
- Alice agrees to participate in supportive counseling and individual, educational sessions on problem-solving skills via the COPE intervention plan.

Step 4: Translating the Research to a Particular Patient and Family

The primary question in translating the results of the accessed and appraised literature is *How well do the findings of these studies translate (generalize) to your family?* As usual, this is a question of transporting the nomothetic to the idiographic; taking the results of a study—reported as mean values of a group of participants who received an intervention and experienced, *on the average*, a certain degree of benefit—and applying these group results to your specific family, given its local context that could include multiple differences from the group studied. These are issues of the fit and fidelity in which you will try to maintain the fidelity of the intervention while making it fit the needs of each particular patient/family.

In comparing the case of the family of Neil and Alice with the COPE study (Meyers et al., 2011), there are similarities and differences to consider. Demographically, the COPE study seems to be a good fit as it was provided to patients and their caregivers with mixed types of advanced cancer. Although patients with glioblastoma do not appear to have been in the study, your search did not identify any family caregiver intervention designed specifically for patients with glioblastoma, probably because of its relatively small prevalence rate. Like your family, 70% of caregivers in the COPE study were the patient's spouse. Although, the COPE intervention was provided conjointly to patient–caregiver dyads, you will be adapting it for individual sessions, and there is some reference to the feasibility of this form of adaptation (Bucher & Zabora, 2010). Improvements in quality of life in the COPE study are relevant to Alice's presenting concerns.

Finally, your earlier review highlighting the importance of supportive psychotherapy (Lederberg & Holland, 2011) continues to be highly relevant. It is likely to serve as the foundational approach, with a focus on provision of effective support through the use of a variety of "common factors" such as warmth, positive regard, and genuineness with attention to the importance of the therapeutic alliance, throughout what is likely to be a family ordeal.

Step 5: Integration—Pulling It All Together and Developing a Treatment Plan

Integration involves the process of pulling together all three components of EBP: best available evidence; clinical expertise; and patient characteristics, culture, and preferences. In this case example, the decision to proceed with an individual intervention comes from the patient/family preferences and requires some adaptation of the accessed/appraised intervention that was initially provided to patient–caregiver dyads. No data were found supporting this adaptation to an individual intervention, but reference was made to its feasibility (Bucher & Zabora, 2010).

Regarding clinical expertise, the problem-solving therapy model (Nezu, Nezu, Friedman, Faddis, & Houts, 1999) on which the COPE intervention is based is a well-known cognitive-behavioral form of psychotherapy, and any provider can have online access to the patient guide, *The ACS Complete Guide to Family Caregiving*—via the American Cancer Society Web site (http://www.acs.org). You feel confident with your general clinical expertise, and you have specific experience with cognitive-behavioral interventions so you will be capable of competently incorporating the COPE intervention.

Lastly, regarding patient characteristics and preferences, Alice (the spouse-caregiver) agrees to participate in this intervention, and although English is her primary language, as an Hispanic female it is helpful to know that there is a Spanish version of the patient guide, if needed.

This leads to an initial treatment plan based upon a broad foundation of supportive psychotherapy (Lederberg & Holland, 2011) as an important component of many psycho-oncology interventions. In this case, supportive psychotherapy is augmented with the COPE problem-solving educational intervention and the availability of a variety of practical information for in-home family caregivers as identified in the Bee and colleagues (2009) review. It is anticipated that individual sessions with Alice will begin with the provision of supportive therapy and augmented, within each session, when the client is receptive, with the problem-solving educational intervention as guided by use of *The ACS Compete Guide to Family Caregiving*. When Alice's overall mood and affect are relatively stable, sessions will be more structured in educating her on the problem-solving components, and when her mood and affect are more anxious, apprehensive, afraid, or depressed and discouraged—as anticipated given the poor prognosis—sessions will be more supportive.

Beginning with the COPE problem-solving intervention relatively early in the treatment process is consistent with the recommendation that such skills are best developed prior to their routine use in real-life, in-home caregiving situations. Lastly, it is anticipated that this tentative treatment plan may be modified as the patient status changes and, in the future, may involve more family members. Regarding the relative contribution of the three EBP components in this individual treatment plan, patient characteristics and preferences, and clinical expertise are highlighted as most relevant to this plan.

Sessions 3–8: Provision of Supportive Counseling, Augmented With COPE Problem-Solving Intervention

Over the next five weekly individual sessions, Alice is actively involved in treatment, discussing her husband's medical status, family relationships, and her own coping throughout his ongoing treatments. Neil has now completed a course of external beam radiation therapy (EBRT) and continues on his daily oral medication of Temodor. During these sessions you have been able to complete the three-session COPE educational intervention and find that, in general, Alice has learned improved problem-solving strategies, although given her husband's stable status, few new problems have developed.

She cancels her appointment for Session 8, and you speak with her by phone later that week. You learn that her husband had a repeat brain scan following some headaches and despite his lack of any new symptoms, the scan indicates that treatments are not working and his disease is progressing. It is recommended that he undergo another surgery to remove some additional necrotic brain cells. Alice is very discouraged and quite tearful over the phone, and she is beginning to worry more about her children and her own ability to provide the in-home care that seems likely after his surgery. She is preparing for the surgery, which is scheduled in just 2 days, so you postpone another appointment for now until after the surgery. Soon after the surgery, you talk again with Alice by phone and learn that the surgery, overall, went well, but Neil was left with some moderate weakness on his right side and is now undergoing inpatient rehabilitation and physical therapy. However, Alice realizes that her husband will be coming home soon, and the realities of additional in-home care are coming true. You remind her of the COPE skills she has been learning, and this seems to help somewhat, but she continues to be anxious.

You arrange an appointment for the next day, following her visit to her husband.

Session 8

As usual, most of this session is supportive, augmented by use of the COPE strategies. Alice is worried about how she will care for her husband when he returns home in a few days. Although she has been able to get some additional rest while he has been hospitalized, as soon as she thinks about his coming home, she gets scared. You remind her of the COPE strategies for maintaining an optimistic, hopeful attitude and together you brainstorm some ideas about what she can do to be less worried. She begins to identify the need for more help at home, and with some creativity she generates a list of 10 different friends and family members who have offered to help. Together you formulate a plan for how to ask and assign various tasks to some of the people. For instance, with her worries about positioning and transporting her husband around the house and onto their front porch, you remind her that the physical therapists he is working with have expert information and can train her how to safely position and move him; plus she identifies that this is a task well suited to her two sons, both of whom she wants to be more active in their father's care. She comments, "Maybe if they see how hard it is for him to even get around, they will begin to get the message that this is very serious." She reports that she finds this active problem solving helpful and recognizes how it alleviates some of her worries to have a plan in place. The session ends with a bit more hopefulness about the family's ability to provide Neil's in-home care.

Disease Progression, End-of-Life Care, Death, and Bereavement Services

Over the course of the next 2–3 months, Neil's disease progresses. As a family, Alice and her three children find ways to share the in-home caregiving responsibilities, and even her mother-in-law and sister-in-law (Neil's sister) make time to be present in the home and are helpful. There are pretty regular and routine arguments and conflict among many in the family, as they often don't agree on what is best for Neil. However, Neil and Alice have some very supportive, loving close times when he apologizes and she accepts his apologies for all of the past abuse. She is touched by this, is genuinely forgiving, yet realizes others in the family don't know about these conversations, and she believes, "The kids wouldn't believe me anyways, so I keep them to myself."

One telling incident of significant conflict arises when the oldest son gets mad when trying to help his father through an old, worn-out front door that doesn't open well. The door breaks and, in anger, the son tears it off the hinges, which scares Alice. All three children get in an argument over this, and the youngest son—coming to Alice's rescue—gets into a physical fight with his brother. The police have to be called, and the two sons are told to "stay away from each other" for a while. This disrupts the caregiving plan for a couple of weeks, until Neil deteriorates further and is bedridden. During the last 2 weeks of his life, the family rallies and, according to Alice, "It surprised me how we got along better during that time than usual." Neil dies 9 months after diagnosis. The family is now facing a time of grief and bereavement, and Alice asks for your help. You indicate that you will look for a possible referral to a qualified family therapist who works with families in bereavement.

Step 2: Accessing the Literature (cont.)

You return to your initial review of the literature and reread the chapter by Kissane and Zaider (2011) in the *Handbook of Psychotherapy in Cancer Care,* realizing that their research on family-focused grief therapy (FFGT) (Kissane & Bloch, 2002) might be helpful for this family. FFGT is based upon commonly understood family system principles of cohesion, conflict resolution, and expressiveness.

- *Cohesion* is defined as the family's ability to work together as a team and to be together in a healthy and productive manner, where individual family members can be both independent and autonomous yet feel close and connected to others within the family.
- *Conflict and the ability to resolve differences* is a component of a family's adaptability and flexibility, usually defined as their ability to adjust to life changes (such as a diagnoses of cancer) in a constructive, cooperative way, such that the usual rules and roles can change as needed. High-conflict families are often described as rigid, unstructured, and chaotic.
- *Expressiveness of both thoughts and feelings* is a component of family communication. Healthy communication is marked by a family's ability to listen to one another, take into account and respect varying opinions and feelings, while trying to understand another's perspective. Poor

expressiveness is marked by misinterpretations, inaccurate assumptions, and family secrets that hinder communication and problem solving.

In the FFGT research, families were classified into five different family types, based upon these three family components of cohesion, conflict resolution, and expressiveness. The five types were further divided into two broad categories of functional or dysfunctional. The two functional family types were titled *supportive* and *conflict resolvers*, while two dysfunctional types were named *hostile* and *sullen*. The fifth type was named *intermediate* because it fell between the functional and dysfunctional types and was characterized as having moderate cohesiveness.

The FFGT intervention is a brief, time-limited, and focused intervention ranging from four to eight sessions, depending on family needs, over a 9- to 18-month period. It is organized into three phases of assessment, intervention, and termination, and a detailed treatment manual is available (Kissane & Bloch, 2002). Only families at risk of poor psychosocial outcomes (53 of 81 screened families) classified as hostile, sullen, or intermediate were selected for participation. The primary outcomes were measures of distress, depression, anxiety, and social functioning. Results found that for the top 10% of family members reporting the most distress at the beginning of the intervention, significant improvement in anxiety and depression—small effect sizes—was reported at 6 and 13 months. No changes in family functioning were found across any groups, but there were differing degrees of individual family members' change depending on the family types. Sullen families showed the most positive change, with intermediate families also showing some positive change, yet hostile families reported worse outcomes than their control group. These modest benefits for a brief intervention for some family types are noteworthy.

Step 3: Appraising This Newly Identified Literature

Two questions arise when appraising this literature. How accurate is the family classification system and how valid and reliable are the results of the FFGT intervention? Regarding the first question of the accuracy of the family classification system, the authors of the overview chapter (Kissane & Zaider, 2011) in the *Handbook of Psychotherapy in Cancer Care* cite two studies investigating the predictive validity, sensitivity, and specificity of the 12-item, short version of the Family Relationship Index (FRI). In the first study (Kissane, McKenzie, et al., 2003), 257 families in palliative care were screened with the FRI. The FRI, when compared to a valid and reliable "gold standard" for identifying dysfunctional families, was found to accurately "screen in" 86% of dysfunctional families, while correctly "screening out" only 45% of families. A second study by different researchers used the FRI for screening 48 families of *newly diagnosed* adult cancer patients. This study found the FRI effective in identifying 100% of families experiencing clinical levels of depression and/or anxiety. However, like the first study, while sensitivity was 1.00, specificity was quite low at .23, indicating that the FRI is very good at identifying families at risk of poor psychosocial outcomes, but it is not very good at accurately identifying families *not* at risk (i.e., identifies a lot of false positives). As a screening measure, high sensitivity is usually of more concern than low specificity so that any families at risk of poor psychosocial outcomes are not missed. However, as a screening measure, it is also very important that further family assessment, typically through a clinical interview, occurs so that the false-positive families can be further evaluated (and often noted to be not at risk).

Regarding the effectiveness of FFGT, it has been tested in one RCT (Kissane et al., 2006) and found to have modest benefits for the most highly distressed of those in sullen and intermediate families, and to be potentially harmful in worsening conflict for hostile families. The RCT was evaluated with use of the CONSORT checklist for nonpharmacologic trials (Boutron et al., 2008a) and 19 of the 22 recommended items were present, indicating that the results are trustworthy with good validity and reliability.

Ongoing Supportive Therapy and Referral for Family Therapy

At your next session with Alice, you explain about FFGT and she seems receptive, as she explains that her family "made it through the funeral" without any major conflict, but she feels as if now everyone is "walking on eggshells" for fear that they might say something wrong and an argument would arise. You also explain how the Cancer Center does not offer specialized services like family therapy, but you do have some good referral options to qualified family therapists in the area. She is interested in more information.

You contact your family therapist referral who is familiar with FFGT, and you offer to do a screening of this family with use of the FRI. The family therapist agrees that that information would be very helpful. You next arrange for Alice and her children to complete the family screening measure (12-item FRI). They do so and are classified as an Intermediate family, suggesting that FFGT may be beneficial for them. You make the referral and plan to check in with Alice in about 3 months.

Step 6: Evaluation of Evidence-Based Practice

In this case example, the evaluation of EBP will include a dual focus on both individual and family outcomes. Regarding the individual intervention with Alice—the caregiver—repeat administrations of the HADS for ongoing assessment of symptoms of depression and anxiety is needed and will provide you with direct patient feedback of progress. Regarding the family intervention of FFGT, ideally the family therapist will also collect routine outcome evaluating both individual- and family-system-level outcomes. Individual-level outcomes might include measures of overall distress such as the Brief Symptom Inventory (BSI)—an 18-item version takes only about 4 minutes to complete and is used as a measure of treatment progress. Other possibilities include the HADS, the Beck Depression Inventory (BDI), or some measure of family system variables such as the Family Relationship Index (FRI). However, it is important to note that the

FFGT randomized trial did not find any changes on family systems variables such as cohesion, expressiveness, or conflict, but rather found improvements on measures of individual family member changes, particularly those reporting high levels of distress and depression at baseline.

A final evaluation of the EBP steps includes the intentional archiving of the literature searches from the aforementioned case as critically appraised topics (CATs). A completed CAT includes a well-organized summary of the entire EBP process, including the clinical bottom-line results, the citation, clinical question, search terms, study description, and evidence summary as appraised. Develop a CAT for this case and save it in your Dropbox folder.

CHAPTER SUMMARY

This chapter has been about family-focused interventions—both as a treatment modality and a focus of clinical attention. After recognizing that much of the literature has been focused on the impact of cancer on particular family members (e.g., caregivers, parents of young children), the importance of family systems theory in family therapy is explained. Next, best available evidence is reviewed. As in other chapters, the review is organized around a table (see Table 9.2) of exemplars with information about study characteristics and ease of dissemination. The majority of family-focused interventions are for caregivers of patients with advanced disease or terminal illness. The quality of life of the caregiver is the most common outcome, and study results indicate modest, short-term improvements. Despite family systems theory's predominance in the general family therapy literature, only one of the nine exemplars incorporated family systems theory into the intervention. Instead, the cognitive stress model and the adaptation of problem-solving therapy for use with caregivers (COPE) have been the predominant theoretical approaches. Ease of dissemination varies, but it is generally good with four studies of short-term interventions having relatively easy to moderate access to manuals and high trainability. Unfortunately, a couple of studies indicated relatively poor patient acceptability. The detailed case example illustrates how to do EBP across the core competencies. It focuses on how to adapt best available evidence across treatment modalities from caregiver dyads to an individual intervention, while also highlighting the importance of supportive counseling and how to augment it with a structured caregiver education program. Ultimately, this case also shows how, when, and with whom to implement family-focused grief therapy after a patient dies.

10

Challenges and Future Directions in the Evidence-Based Practice of Psycho-Oncology

As noted throughout this volume, the evidence-based practice (EBP) of adult psycho-oncology involves the application of a series of key competencies:

- Ask and formulate clinically relevant questions.
- Access and critically appraise relevant scientific literature.
- Translate the evidence to the needs/preferences of a particular cancer patient, couple, family, or patient group.
- Integrate the three pillars of EBP: best available evidence; clinical expertise/resources; and patient values, preferences, culture, and needs.
- Evaluate the overall process.

As illustrated in the five detailed case examples, the highly complex, recursive process of EBP is not easy to do, nor is there evidence that EBP of psycho-oncology is being implemented in most clinical practice settings (Frueh et al., 2012). Time, training, and the lack of resources are barriers. Busy practitioners do not have the time to access and appraise the evidence. Training in doing literature searches, appraising the literature, and implementing evidence-based interventions is inadequate. Access to databases, search engines, treatment manuals, and other resources is sparse. Recognizing these problems, this book was written as a resource that explains how EBP in psycho-oncology could be done if barriers were removed—an aspirational goal for the future.

Having reached this final chapter, you are now familiar with EBP in psycho-oncology, have seen how it can be implemented, and hopefully recognize its potential to narrow the gap between science and practice. Yet much more remains to be done to make EBP feasible in everyday practice. This final chapter will highlight some of the work remaining by discussing the following:

- The limitations of EBP, both generally in mental health care and specifically in psycho-oncology

- The current challenges to the dissemination and implementation of EBP and explain the interdependence between EBP and the science of dissemination and implementation
- A vision for the future of EBP in psycho-oncology focused on interprofessional collaboration, increased use of technology, and an updated transdisciplinary model of EBP.

THE LIMITATIONS OF EVIDENCE-BASED PRACTICE

What Evidence-Based Practice Does Not Do Well

EBP *does not promote risk taking and clinical innovation*, and as a result, it does not generate testable hypotheses for future research. It is not a good practice strategy for guiding researchers to new discoveries. Because it is inherently retrospective by looking back in time to see what has previously worked, it is not likely to contribute to new, future discoveries (Maier, 2012).

EBP *does not answer many relevant clinical questions*. The empirical evidence base will never answer all clinical questions, particularly in psycho-oncology. This includes existential or philosophical questions:

- In the face of terminal illness, how do I now want to live my life?
- What is a quality life for me?
- What constitutes hope, and how can I be realistically hopeful?
- What is a dignified, "good" death?

In the book *Cancer as a Turning Point* (LeShan, 1989), the pioneering psychotherapist Lawrence LeShan directs patients to consider these large, existential questions by asking, "When do you feel most alive?" These questions encourage patients to begin to ponder issues of quality of life and personal dignity infused by their own unique life perspective, values, and beliefs.

EBP is also limited in its ability to answer the idiographic local questions of the busy oncology practice. Given the inherent complexity of human behavior, in combination with multiple minidecisions to be made within the context of daily practice, it is unrealistic to expect that all practitioner actions would flow from research that has answered specific questions. Many clinical decisions are influenced not only by evidence but also by the unique, idiosyncratic needs of a particular patient, being seen in a particular setting, by a particular practitioner, at a particular moment in time (Stricker & Trierweiler, 1995). The evidence-based practitioner will never have answers for all such questions.

Gaps in Evidence-Based Practice

EBP is limited by gaps in one or more of the three primary components: best available evidence; clinical expertise; or patient characteristics, culture, and preferences. At present, the primary limitation in psycho-oncology is the limited evidence base. Multiple gaps in the literature remain and, to a certain extent, always will. As previously noted, the evidence base will never be capable of answering all clinically relevant questions. The evidence base in psycho-oncology has matured from its infancy, through childhood, to its currently characterized adolescence. It is sufficiently developed to provide an empirical basis from which to guide current practice, and it still has considerable room to grow. As detailed in Chapter 3, the psycho-oncology evidence base needs

- stronger theoretical/conceptual models,
- research designs and hypotheses that include demographic (e.g., age, gender, ethnicity) and disease status (e.g., cancer type, stage, disease continuum) variables,
- more replications of promising interventions,
- routine selection of study participants by prescreening to select those who are experiencing heightened levels of distress,
- continued improvement in the quality of reporting of studies by following appropriate journal reporting standards (e.g., CONSORT), and
- closer attention to ease of dissemination and implementation to the local setting.

What More Is Needed in Evidence-Based Practice

In addition to the previous list, more training on how to answer a wide range of clinical questions is needed. Answering intervention questions has been the dominant focus of most of the EBP training literature (Huang et al., 2006). Relative to answering intervention questions, considerably less has been published about how to answer other questions (see Table 4.2) such as those of diagnosis, etiology, or progress monitoring.

More literature on *how best to adapt available evidence* is also needed. As explained in Chapter 4, the competent use of EBP leads to clinical decisions involving three options: adopt, abandon, or adapt (Norcross et al., 2008). Decisions to adopt or abandon are relatively straightforward. Adapting the evidence is much more complex, and little literature addresses the process. Norcross and colleagues' (2008) emphasis on the importance of translation and integration recognizes the complexity in adapting evidence, and it acknowledges the tension between efforts to administer a treatment in a manner consistent with research (i.e., fidelity) while also considering patient preferences and needs (i.e., fit). Such tension is inherent in the complexity of adaption given the current EBP evidence gaps (see Fig. 4.4). More theoretical and conceptual literature is needed that describes methods of adaptation such as Persons' mix-and-match strategy (Persons, 2005), Shapiro's theoretical-eclectic approach that uses hypotheses about etiology to guide adaptation (Shapiro, 2009), or Ruscio and Holohan's

(2006) forms of adaptation such as augmentation, sequential or concurrent application, or the use of a tiered approach.

More empirical evidence is also needed. The majority of the literature has focused on questions of the absolute or relative efficacy of treatment interventions. As noted in prior chapters, most randomized controlled trials (RCTs) report significant positive outcomes demonstrating small to medium effects. Psychosocial health service interventions in psycho-oncology are effective. This is an important and encouraging conclusion given required screening for psychosocial distress by 2015 in all settings accredited by the Commission on Cancer (CoC) of the American College of Surgeons (ACoS) (2012). As screening for distress increases, more patient are likely to be identified, and an increase in the need for psychosocial services is anticipated. As need for services increases, it becomes important to better understand how these interventions work and what are the mediators and/or moderators of change. New knowledge about treatment components or change processes responsible for patient change will help guide the processes of adaptation of best available evidence. Future dismantling research that tests specific treatment components to identify those most crucial to patient change will also help. At present, the skilled evidence-based practitioner relies on her or his clinical expertise to translate the evidence, in light of the unique needs of each patient.

More knowledge about effective strategies for disseminating and implementing effective psychosocial interventions is also needed. Like the EBP of psychology in general (Frueh et al., 2012), there is little evidence that the EBP of psycho-oncology is implemented in most practice settings. Many challenges to the dissemination and implementation of EBP remain.

CHALLENGES TO THE DISSEMINATION AND IMPLEMENTATION OF EVIDENCE-BASED PRACTICE

What has historically been referred to as the "science to practice gap" is now the domain of dissemination and implementation science (Brownson, Colditz, & Proctor, 2012). Spurred by the recognition that only a small percent of people who could benefit from an evidence-based intervention actually receive it (McGlynn et al., 2003), dissemination and implementation research attempts to understand how to narrow the gap between new knowledge and its application in everyday practice. Its focus is to move beyond passive diffusion of research findings to pushing evidence-based knowledge to the real world. Successful dissemination and implementation research narrows the science to practice gap. It continues to be a relatively new science with considerable interest and growing consensus on definitions of terms. Dissemination is defined as "the targeted distribution of information and intervention materials to a specific public health or clinical practice audience. The intent is to spread knowledge and the associated evidence-based interventions" (Glasgow et al., 2012, p. 1275). Implementation is defined as "the use of strategies to adopt and integrate evidence-based health interventions and change practice patterns within specific settings" (Glasgow et al., 2012, p. 1275). Both are distinct from the more passive process of diffusion of research. Diffusion is the process by which information is spread through the traditional method of publishing findings in research journals. Diffusion alone has rarely led to new innovation—thus, the need for dissemination and implementation science.

At present, dissemination and implementation research in psycho-oncology is limited to a few reviews (Ellis et al., 2005) and a few ongoing clinical trials. These trials provide training for licensed mental health professionals to learn how to implement previously identified empirically supported treatments such as cognitive-behavioral therapy (Clark et al., 2012) or Andersen's biobehavioral psychological treatment (Andersen et al., 2008). Following on-site, face-to-face training, collaborating cancer care settings are offered

- ongoing support such as regular consultations and supervision via conference calls or online conversations,
- the provision of recruitment materials targeted at both professional referral sources and patients, and
- treatment manuals and patient workbooks (e.g., Cancer to Health [C2H[, available at http://cancertohealth.osu.edu/index.php/for-trainees).

Results regarding outcomes of these studies are not yet available.

Broader dissemination and implementation research in general mental health settings has focused on large-scale national and state-based efforts such as (a) the United Kingdom's Improving Access to Psychological Therapies Program (IAPT) (Clark, 2012) and (b) the Veterans Health Administration's (VA) effort in the United States (Ruzek, Karlin, & Zeiss, 2012), (c) implementation of well-researched, empirically supported interventions such as dialectical behavior therapy (Landes & Linehan, 2012) and multisystemic family therapy (McHugh & Barlow, 2012d; Schoenwald, 2012), and (d) the provision of specialty mental health settings for the chronically mentally ill (Frueh, Grubaugh, Cusack, & Elhai, 2009). Information coming from these trials and other reviews (Frueh et al., 2012; McHugh & Barlow, 2012a) has identified a number of barriers to dissemination and implementation, typically organized into three categories: provider, training, and organizational/systems.

Provider Barriers

As with many new innovations, the movement to incorporate EBPs has been met by some resistance, as reflected in the *attitudes* of front-line providers (McHugh & Barlow, 2012a). Practitioners are often leery of new innovations developed and promoted by researchers who may be quite naïve to the realities of the busy day-to-day world of the practitioner. EBPs in psychotherapy have been criticized due to the limitations of RCTs, controversies about mechanisms of change, and the perception that manualized interventions are to be offered inflexibly in a "cookbook" fashion. These attitudinal barriers are difficult to overcome, and even when practitioners do hold positive attitudes toward EBPs, there are still provider barriers. Positive attitudes toward EBPs are not highly correlated with actual demonstration of EBP behaviors (Gray, Elhai, & Schmidt, 2012). Although there are no data specifically on attitudes of psycho-oncologists toward EBP, it can be assumed that they have many of the same attitudes and opinions.

Psycho-oncologists who are not trained in evidence-based interventions will encounter the barrier of *competence* to provide the EBP intervention. Effective dissemination practices emphasize the need for provider training in the form of both didactic learning of new interventions, and ongoing supervision accompanied by regular feedback of observed performance (Drake et al., 2001; Mueser, Torrey, Lynde, Singer, & Drake, 2003).

Training Barriers

Given the highly complex nature of EBPs, training to competently provide the best available evidence is essential, but it remains a significant barrier. Adequate training requires significant resources of time and money—resources not readily available, particularly in local, community cancer care settings. Most of the literature on training to EBP has been focused on licensed professionals such as psychologists, psychiatrists, social workers, and other health care providers. Historically, these groups have received training via periodic continuing education. Unfortunately, there is little evidence that continuing education, in its usual form of didactic presentations or 1-day workshops, results in any significant change in providers' behaviors (VandeCreek, Knapp, & Brace, 1990).

Research on the best training procedures for successful dissemination and implementation has only recently begun (McHugh & Barlow, 2012c). Reviews of training for successful dissemination (Beidas & Kendall, 2010; Herschell, Kolko, Baumann, & Davis, 2010; Rakovshik & McManus, 2010) have organized procedures into two groups: didactic training and competency training. Didactic training is designed to increase a practitioner's *knowledge* about an intervention, while competency training is designed to increase the *clinical skills* involved in the provision of the evidence-based intervention. To date, empirical evaluations of various dissemination and implementation procedures for training in EBP are limited (McHugh & Barlow, 2012d). There are only a few controlled trials. Reviews have concluded that didactic training alone improves knowledge of specific interventions and attitudes toward EBP, but competency training is needed to improve dissemination and implementation. Improved clinical outcomes are more likely with longer competency training (McHugh & Barlow, 2012c). Important competency training components include ongoing supervision by an advanced clinician, provision of regular feedback, and directive guidance on treatment implementation.

Training of Evidence-Based Practice in Psycho-oncology
As a relatively young subspecialty, psycho-oncology is a growing field that requires specialized training. Some training opportunities such as fellowships in psycho-oncology and online webinars, as well as education and training via the Web site of the American Psycho-Oncology Society (APOS) Web site (http://www.apos-society.org/professionals/meetings-ed/webcasts.aspx) are available.

In addition, memberships in national (APOS) and international organizations (IPOS) continue to grow, as do publications relevant to EBP in psycho-oncology. However, despite such growth and the provision of a variety of clinical practice guidelines and other standards of care (see Chapter 1), direct training in the core competencies of EBP and how to implement them in psycho-oncology is missing. It is hoped that this book will help fill that gap by educating psycho-oncologists on how to implement the EBP core competencies (AAA TIE, Norcross et al., 2008).

Health Care System Barriers

Organizational and health care system barriers are the most challenging barriers to dissemination and implementation of EBPs. The translation of an evidence-based intervention developed and tested in a controlled research setting to an already existing and established health care system with its specific organizational structure and sometimes unique local needs and preferences is challenging (McHugh & Barlow, 2012a). Limited resources, cost concerns, and inadequate supervision to monitor treatment fidelity are common problems. In addition, organizations with limited resources are not likely to provide adequate incentives to either providers or administrators for what is often perceived as additional work. Thus, the local community cancer care provider may view dissemination efforts as simply "more work to do" or work that is more highly valued by administrators and other nonprovider stakeholders.

EVIDENCE-BASED PRACTICE AND DISSEMINATION-IMPLEMENTATION RESEARCH

As noted earlier, EBP is a highly complex, recursive process that is not easy to do. Even with positive attitudes and necessary training, the processes of accessing and appraising best available evidence, translating the findings to the needs and preferences of a specific patient, and arriving at a collaborative decision are time consuming. At present, the front-line psycho-oncologist does not have sufficient time and will need additional resources. In addition to knowledge about how to critically appraise the evidence, easier and quicker access to relevant databases of both filtered and unfiltered literature is needed. A conceptual model that integrates the variety of tools for making clinical decisions has been proposed (Haynes, 2006) and can guide the development of needed organizational resources (see Figure 4.3 in Chapter 4). In this 5S model—studies, syntheses, synopses, summaries, and systems—original *studies* (i.e., primary literature) published in professional journals are *synthesized* via various *synopses* such as systematic reviews and meta-analyses. Synopses are then *summarized* in the form of brief clinical synopses of key findings (Haynes, 2006). Next, in the final and most important step, best available evidence is made readily accessible by being incorporated into computerized decision support *systems* (CDSS). A CDSS is a computerized system built into the electronic health record that links the reviewed literature, synopses, and summaries to a specific patient's clinical needs. When needed, or even when reminded by the system, the evidence-based practitioner is provided quick and easy access to this information whenever reviewing the patient's electronic health record (Haynes, 2001).

The ideas behind making EBP more feasible have been discussed over the past 10–12 years, and yet little progress is evident in the development of decision support systems for psycho-oncology. To become reality, cancer care settings are going to need to provide financial and training resources toward this goal. Without such resources and the accompanying training to use them competently, EBP in psycho-oncology will not occur. To facilitate progress, Appendix C describes an abbreviated EBP approach. It includes relevant resources, references, and suggestions for making EBP in psycho-oncology more feasible.

Without EBP skills, disseminating and implementing best available evidence is much more difficult. A competent evidence-based practitioner working in a local community health care setting is invaluable to dissemination and implementation. Thus, the future direction of research on dissemination and implementation will impact the future of EBP. The following suggestions for the future success of disseminating and implementing evidence-based interventions have been offered (Frueh et al., 2012; Kerner et al., 2005; McHugh & Barlow, 2012b):

- Give greater attention to dissemination and implementation science, from which will come more funding and enhanced collaboration across multiple disciplines.
- Develop standardized and consistent methods of measuring clinical outcomes.
- Develop and test treatments that extend across traditional diagnoses (i.e., transdisciplinary treatments). Practitioners will never be competent to provide every newly developed, empirically supported treatment; rather, key concepts and treatment techniques applicable across multiple diagnoses are needed.
- Use stepped-care models of delivery to match the level of intensity of care needed. This is an effective way to manage patient need with treatment availability while also better managing costs.
- Increase the use of information technology.
- Increase the use of targeted "direct-to-consumer" marketing efforts. These efforts may result in "increased pull" as patients request needed services.

Any local dissemination and implementation efforts to implement EBP in *clinical practice settings* (Frueh et al., 2012) will benefit from the following suggestions:

- Establish and nurture broad-based organizational commitment and maintain key stakeholder involvement.
- Establish clear goals that are specific, measurable, and realistic, and regularly communicated to all key stakeholders.
- Provide ongoing training of providers to increase clinical skills and change attitudes.
- Provide practitioners with supervision, regular peer review, and patient self-reported outcome feedback to enhance the likelihood of successful interventions.
- Regularly conduct fidelity checks—develop methods for monitoring how the intervention is provided, with the goal of maintaining a balance between fidelity and flexibility.

Finally, a number of online resources have been developed to encourage collaboration in dissemination and implementation research in cancer control and psycho-oncology. A couple of examples include the following:

- The *Research to Reality (R2R)* network site—an online community designed to link cancer control practitioners and researchers with the goal of moving evidence-based programs into local settings. It includes ongoing discussion groups organized around specific dissemination and implementation topics, periodic cyber-webinars, a mentorship program, and descriptions of featured R2R partners. It can be accessed either directly (https://researchtoreality.cancer.gov) or through the Cancer Control P.L.A.N.E.T. portal (http://www.cancercontrolplanet.org).
- *Make Research Matter* is another helpful online resource (http://www.makeresearchmatter.org) that consists of four main tools designed to help researchers increase the dissemination and implementation potential of their interventions. The first and primary tool is a planning tool that consists of an online survey and a tailored report to aid researchers with their dissemination plan. The other tools are a searchable database of dissemination and implementation articles that is updated monthly, a narrative library that includes video vignettes and transcripts by dissemination and implementation experts of "how to" knowledge for various dissemination and implementation research questions, and a glossary of over 100 definitions of dissemination- and implementation research-related terms.

THE FUTURE OF EVIDENCE-BASED PRACTICE IN PSYCHO-ONCOLOGY

The future of EBP in psycho-oncology will require greater collaboration (Glasgow et al., 2012). Cancer care settings are becoming increasingly diverse and multidisciplinary (Gagliardi et al., 2011). A report of an expert panel outlining core competencies for interprofessional collaboration across multiple health care professions (Interprofessional Education Collaborative Expert Panel, 2011) is relevant to the future of psycho-oncology.

Interprofessional Collaboration in Oncology

Collaborative or integrative care in oncology is predicted to become more prevalent (Gagliardi et al., 2011) and increasingly important. Interprofessional collaboration is care in which multiple health care professionals, representing various disciplines (e.g., medical, surgical, radiation oncology, pathology/radiology, nursing, psychology, social work, psychiatry, and chaplaincy) collaborate routinely and regularly, typically within the same settings, with a *shared sense of responsibility for all patients' care*. The need for such care has been widely recognized (Institute of Medicine, 2001, 2006, 2008, 2011; Institute of Medicine & National Research Council, 2006) and yet is more the exception than the rule. A few studies (e.g., Fann et al., 2012) investigating patient outcomes in collaborative psycho-oncology have been tested, but many more are needed. The integration of behavioral health/mental health in *primary care*, with nearly 40 years of research (Gilbody et al., 2006; Miller et al., 2011), will serve as a model for testing patient outcomes in well-controlled, randomized trials. Future generations of health care professionals will be better prepared to collaborate (Interprofessional Education Collaborative Expert Panel, 2011). As collaborative/integrated care expands, models of EBP will also need to expand.

The Transdisciplinary Model of Evidence-Based Practice

Given the increased need for greater interprofessional collaboration, the original three-component model of EBP (see Fig. 4.1; Sackett et al., 1996) has been revised (Satterfield et al., 2009). As evidence-based medicine (EBM) has expanded and been endorsed by other health care disciplines, unanswered questions, differences in emphases, and shortcomings to the three-component model have been noted. These include problems such as

- how "evidence" is defined,
- the role of the practitioner(s) and his or her clinical expertise in decision making,
- how and when context, in the form of both local resources and patient characteristics, affects clinical decision making, and
- how seriously the needs, characteristics, culture, and preferences of patients are considered.

The importance and value of a revised model is reflected in the need for improved multidisciplinary collaboration to enhance translational research with its aim to narrow the research-to-practice gap.

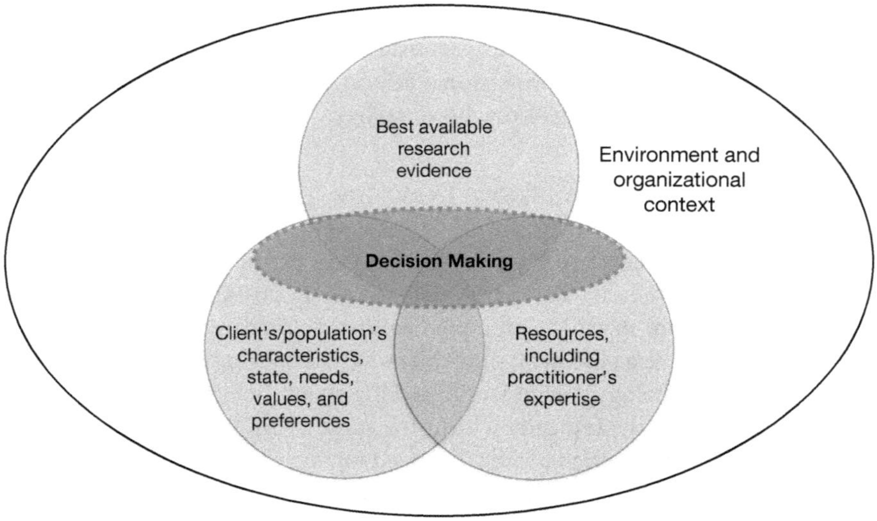

Figure 10.1 The transdisciplinary model of evidence-based practice.
SOURCE: Satterfield et al. (2009). Toward a transdisciplinary model of evidence-based practice. *The Milbank Quarterly, 87*(2), 368–390. Copyright 2009. Millbank Memorial Fund. Reproduced with permission of Wiley Periodicals Inc.

Figure 10.1 illustrates the transdisciplinary model of EBP (Satterfield et al., 2009).

This model maintains some of the characteristics of the original, three-circle model (see Fig. 4.1), while adding new components and rearranging others. The most obvious difference between the two models is the addition of a broader, ecological perspective. This broader framework incorporates the impact of environment and organizational context to settings where local knowledge is essential for successful implementation. A second change in the model is the addition of resources to the clinical expertise circle. From an ecological perspective, clinical expertise—albeit an important resource—is just one of many resources needed. This change acknowledges the importance of local resources for successful EBP. One important example, as discussed earlier, is the availability of clinical decision support systems (CDSS) that make EBP more feasible.

Another difference between the transdisciplinary and the traditional model of EBP is in the expansion of patient characteristics, culture, and preferences to include a broader perspective on patient populations, clinical state, needs, and values. This also emphasizes a broader ecological context consistent with disciplines such as public health and social work, where interventions are often offered at the group or population level. Given this difference, the transdisciplinary model more clearly distinguishes between a patient's state (e.g., cancer type, stage, treatment status, level of distress), the patient's values (e.g., incorporation of complementary treatment approaches), and the patient's needs (e.g., may not perceive a need for educational information, counseling services, or other supportive services, even if reporting psychosocial or symptom distress).

Although the illustration of best available research remains unchanged, the transdisciplinary or interprofessional collaboration will recognize differences in research types (qualitative or quantitative), designs/methodologies (RCTs, quasi-experimental, single-case designs, etc.), or data sources (e.g., patient satisfaction) and has noted that different disciplines will value and utilize different forms of evidence.

Increased Use of Technology

As with nearly all of modern medicine, the future of psycho-oncology will continue to be influenced by advances in information technology. Future collaboration between the fields of knowledge translation (Straus et al., 2009), information technologies, and implementation science (Eccles et al., 2009), with particular emphasis on "translational blocks" (Thornicroft et al., 2011) will have significant effects on EBP and its dissemination and implementation.

Newer technologies have and will continue to influence how cancer care professionals provide psychosocial health service interventions. Distress screening procedures have already been tested using problem-related touchscreen technology, located in the waiting room, for the identification of distress (Clark et al., 2009). This feasibility study found that use of touchscreen technology helped to narrow the gap between identification of distress and referral for psychosocial assessment and treatment. The use of technology may be particularly important in cancer settings where local support services are minimal or totally absent. The Cancer Support Community's *My Cancer Manager* is one such example allowing patients access to an online and/or iPad/iPhone version of an easily accessed means of screening for distress that then connects patients to related online resources (Cancer Support Community, 2012).

As the general public becomes increasingly comfortable and knowledgeable about the use of online resources, more turn to the Internet for information. Services that may have traditionally been offered via face-to-face contact have been adapted to be available online. An early study found an Internet-based patient support system was effective in increasing patients' comfort in participating in their own care, competence in seeking information, confidence in their doctors, and perceived social support. Findings suggested that these benefits were greatest for patients who have traditionally been underserved (Gustafson et al., 2001). Other trials have adapted interventions for administration via telephone. One such randomized trial of 405 mixed-cancer types prescreened patients with depression and cancer-related pain living in widely dispersed rural settings in Indiana, and found that telecare management, in concert with automated monitoring of symptoms, resulted in improved pain and depression outcomes at 1-year follow-up (Kroenke et al., 2010). Another RCT of telephone-administered cognitive-behavioral therapy for 89 patients who had undergone hematopoietic stem-cell transplantation 1–3 years earlier, reported fewer illness-related post-traumatic stress disorder symptoms, fewer intrusive thoughts, fewer symptoms of depression, and less overall distress than an assessment-only control group (DuHamel et al., 2010). Many more such studies and training opportunities are anticipated as the use of online technology for supportive services expands.

In conclusion, the future of psycho-oncology will involve the provision of cancer care to a diverse, growing population of survivors facing the challenges of cancer as a chronic illness. Interprofessional collaboration will expect health care professionals to provide services with a sense of shared responsibility for every patient. Care will be evidence based, and providers will be skilled at integrating (a) best available evidence with (b) clinical expertise and other resources, while (c) carefully considering the needs, values, preferences, and culture of each patient. Future success will depend on advances in overcoming barriers to EBP, improving strategies for disseminating and implementing best available evidence, and increasing availability of technology such as clinical decision support systems and Internet-based online or other forms of telehealth to reach all patients.

APPENDIX A

Meta-Analysis and Effect Size

Meta-analysis is a form of research in which reports of prior research are used to summarize the results of a particular area of study (e.g., couples therapy for cancer patients). The data used for the meta-analysis come from the statistical results as reported in prior studies (Lipsey & Wilson, 2001).

Effect size is a statistic that encodes statistical information from prior studies used in meta-analyses. Different types of study findings require different effect size statistics. For example, studies in which the statistical information is reported as correlation coefficients (*r*) use a different type of effect size statistic than studies in which the statistical information is reported as mean differences between groups (Cohen's *d* or Hedges' *g*) (Lipsey & Wilson, 2001).

Effect size benchmarks are used to interpret the meaning of effect sizes and, by convention, are labeled small, medium, and large effects as follows: small effects ($d = .20$ or $r = .10$), medium effects ($d = .50$ or $r = .30$), large effects ($d = .80$ or $r = .50$) (Cohen, 1988).

Interpretation of effect sizes involves translating effect size statistics to other more understandable/useful meanings and can be done in different ways. Effect sizes can be converted to the following:

- *Percentiles*, where a percentile indicates the relative standing of patients receiving an intervention (experimental group) compared to those not receiving the intervention (control group)
- *Success rates of treated patients*, where the percentage of those patients receiving a benefit of the intervention (treated group) is compared to those not receiving the intervention (control group).
- *Number needed to treat* (NNT), which refers to how many patients would need to receive the treatment, in comparison to those not receiving the treatment, before at least one patient would receive the benefits of the treatment

Effect Size Interpretations

Benchmark	d	r	Percentile	Success Rates	NNT
Large	.80	.50	79	69%	2.7
Medium	.50	.30	69	62%	4.1
Small	.20	.10	58	52%	10.0

APPENDIX B

Evidence-Based Practice in Psycho-Oncology:
The Quality of Study Rating Form (QSRF)

PRELIMINARY INFORMATION

Methods
Participants
Eligibility Criteria (inclusions/exclusion)

Settings/Locations from where recruited

Intervention Groups Descriptions (where, when in tx course, theory based)

Experimental intervention

Control/Comparison Group(s)

Outcome measure to compute ES1: ______________________________
Outcome measure to compute ES2: ______________________________
Outcome measure to compute ES3: ______________________________
Sample Size (attrition, participant flowchart?)

STRENGTH OF EVIDENCE (QUALITY OF STUDY RATING FORM)

Criteria for Rating Study

Clear Definition of Treatment					6. Subjects randomly assigned to treatment or control (10 pts.)	7. Analysis shows equal treatment and control groups before treatment (5 pts.)	8. Subjects blind to being in treatment or control group (5 pts.)
1. Who (4 pts.)	2. What (4 pts.)	3.Where (4 pts.)	4. When (4 pts.)	5. Why (4 pts.)			

Criteria for Rating Study (cont.)

9. Subjects randomly selected for study inclusion (4 pts.)	10.Control or nontreated group used (4 pts.)	11. Number of subjects in smallest treatment group exceeds 20 (4 pts.)	12. Outcome measure has face validity (4 pts.)	13. Treatment outcome measure was checked for reliability (5 pts.)	14. Reliability measure has value greater than .70 or percent of rater agreement greater than 70% (5 pts.)

Criteria for Rating Study (cont.)

15. Those rating outcome rated it blind (10 pts.)	16. Treatment outcome was measured after treatment was completed (4 pts.)	17. Test of statistical significance was made and $p < .05$ (10 pts.)	18. Follow-up was greater than 75% (10 pts.)	19. Total quality (add 1-18)	20. Effect size = (ES1) = SD units = (mean of treatment – mean of control or alternate treatment) ÷ (standard deviation of control or alternative treatment)

Criteria for Rating Effect Size

21. Effect size (ES2) = Absolute risk reduction = (percent improved in treatment) – (percent improved in control)	22. Effect size (ES3) = Number needed to treat = 100 ÷ ES2

EASE OF DISSEMINATION: CLINICAL UTILITY & CLINICAL EXPERTISE

Feasibility Criteria—an evaluation of transportability to the local setting

Intervention Provider?
Profession
Degree
Trainability—Ease of Training to Learn Intervention (High, Moderate, Low)
High = non-doctoral-level practitioner AND manual available
Moderate = manual available OR non-doctoral-level practitioner
Low = no manual available AND doctoral-level practitioner only

Length of the Intervention (time or number of sessions)
Acceptability by Patients

recruitment—% of eligible participants agreeing to participate
compliance—% completing treatment (Intent-to-treat) or % dropout

Study-Patient Matching: Translation to Local (rate strength of match—very good, good, fair, poor)

Study Participant vs. Patient Characteristics

Demographics	Disease Variables
Age Type	Gender Stage
Relational Status Prognosis	Disease Continuum/Treatment Status (recent dx, on tx, complete, survivorship, etc.)

Life Context (race/ethnicity/culture, explanatory model, developmental stage, etc.)
Idiosyncratic/Idiographic (unique individual patient characteristics of importance)

The QSRF Scoring Instructions

- Instructions for scoring.
  - Items 1 to 18 assess quality. These are summed in item 19. Item 19 ranges from 0 to 100. The closer to 100, the more confidence the rater can place in the study's findings.
  - Items 20, 21, and 22 are three relative indices of treatment effect size. These indices summarize the impact of treatment in standardized units.
- Explanation of criteria regarding study quality.
  - The first section of the QSRF states the identifying information regarding the client type (e.g., depressed, middle-aged men); intervention method (e.g., aerobic exercise four or more times a week); and the outcome measure(s)—preferably ones that can be used to calculate treatment effect size (e.g., score on Beck Depression Inventory).
  - Experience with the QSRF's reliability indicates that reliability will be highest for all-or-nothing points for each item; so give either

zero points or the particular point value indicated if the study meets the criterion, as numbered on the form and described in the following list:

1. *Who*: The authors describes who is treated by stating the subject(s)' average age *and* standard deviation of age, *and* sex or proportion of males and females, *and* clearly defines clients' presenting problem(s).
2. *What*: The authors tell what the treatment involves so specifically that you could apply the treatment with nothing more to go on than their description, *or* they refer you to a book, videotape, CD-ROM, article, or Web address that describes the treatment method.
3. *Where:* Authors state where the treatment occurred so specifically that you could contact people at the facility by phone, letter, or e-mail address.
4. *When:* Authors tell the *when* of treatment by stating how long subjects participated in the treatment in days, weeks, or months *or* tell how many treatment sessions were attended by subjects.
5. *Why:* Authors either discuss a specific theory that describes why they used one or more treatment methods, *or* they cite literature that supports the use of the treatment method.
6. *Subjects randomly assigned to treatment or control:* The author states specifically that subjects were *randomly assigned* to treatment groups or refers to the assignment of subjects on the basis of random numbers, computer algorithm, or accepted randomization procedures. This means that the procedure resulted in subject having an equal chance of being assigned to treatment or control groups.
7. *Analysis shows equal treatment and control groups before treatment:* Even though subjects have been randomly assigned, unequal treatment and control groups can occur by chance; so, to guard against this, the authors need to make comparisons across treatment and control groups on key client characteristics to see that they are similar prior to treatment (e.g., sex, race, age, economic status, condition, strengths).
8. *Subjects blind to being in treatment or control group:* Subjects who know they are in a control group can experience effects of being there, including demoralization or competition with experimentals. Subjects who know they are in a treatment group can experience powerful healing effects because they expect them. Give points for subjects blinded if two or more groups get some kind of treatment, if controls get some form of sham treatment that is not expected to have and effect but gives assurance to subjects that something is being done, if subjects serve in a delayed treatment control group where they serve as controls but get treatment later, or if subjects truly do not know whether they are in a treatment or control group.
9. *Subjects randomly selected for inclusion in study: Selection* of subjects is different from *random assignment. Random selection* means that subjects are taken from some potential pool of subjects for inclusion

in the study by using a table of random numbers or other statistically random procedures. For example, if subjects are chosen randomly from among all residents on a psychiatric ward, the results of the study can be generalized more confidently to all residents of that ward.

10. *Control (nontreated) group used:* Member of a *nontreated control group* do not receive a different kind of treatment; they receive *no* treatment. An example of a nontreated control group would be a group of subjects who are denied counseling while others are given group counseling. Subjects in a nontreated control group may receive treatment at a later date but do not receive treatment while experimental group subjects are receiving their treatment.
11. *Number of subjects in smallest treatment group exceeds 20:* Those in the treatment group or groups are those who receive some kind of special care intended to help them. It is this treatment that is being evaluated by those doing the study. To meet Criterion 11, *the number of subjects in the smallest treatment group must be at least 21.* Here, *number of subjects* means total number of individuals, not number of couples or number of groups.
12. *Outcome measure has face validity:* Face validity is present if the outcome measure used to determine the effectiveness of treatment makes sense to you. A good criterion for the sense of an outcome measure is whether the measure evaluates something that should logically be affected by the treatment. For example, drinking behavior has face validity as an outcome measure for treating alcoholism.
13. *Treatment outcome measure was checked for reliability:* For this criterion to be met, to merely say that the outcome of treatment was measured in some way is not enough. The outcome measure itself must be evaluated to check its reliability. *Reliability* refers to the consistency of measurement. The reliability criterion here is satisfied only if the author of the study affirms that *evaluations were made of the outcome measure's reliability (e.g., inter-rater agreement), and the author lists a numerical value of some kind for this measure of reliability.* Where multiple outcome criteria are used, reliability checks of any one of the major outcome criteria satisfy Criterion 13.
14. *Reliability measure has value greater than .70 or percent of rater agreement is greater than 70%:* The reliability coefficient in Criterion 13 is .70 or greater. Reliability coefficients typically range from –1 (perfect disagreement), through 0 (no pattern of agreement or disagreement), to 1 (perfect agreement).
15. *Those rating outcome rated it blind:* This criterion concerns the way bias can enter into measurement if the person measuring outcome knows whether the subject being measured is from a treatment or control group, or, worse, the person measuring outcome is in a position to determine the outcome measure. *Give the points for this criterion only if the person conducting the outcome measuring did not know which subjects were in treatment or control groups.*

16. *Treatment outcome was measured after treatment was completed: At least one outcome measure was obtained* after *treatment was completed.* Outcome measure both during treatment and after treatment is sufficient to meet this criterion.
17. *Test of statistical significance was made and $p < .05$:* Test of statistical significance are generally referred to by phrases such as "differences between treatment groups were significant at the .05 level" or "results show statistical significance for . . ." *Statistical significance* refers to the probability of obtaining an observed difference between treatment or control groups as great as or greater than by chance alone. Give credit for meeting this criterion only if the author refers to a test of statistical significance for a major outcome variable naming the statistical procedure (e.g., analysis of variance, chi-square, *t* test) *and* gives a *p* value, for example $p < .05$, *and* the *p* value is equal to or smaller than .05.
18. *Follow-up was greater than 75%:* The proportion of subjects successfully followed up refers to the number contracted to measure outcome compared with the number who began the study. Ideally, the two should be the same (100% followed up). To compare the proportion followed up for each group studies (i.e., treatment group(s), control group), determine the number of subjects who initially entered the study in the group and determine the number successfully followed up. (If there is more than one follow-up period, use the longest one). Then, for each group, divide the number successfully followed up by the number who began in each group and multiply each quotient by 100. If the *smallest* of these percentages exceeds 75%, then the study meets this criterion.
19. *Total quality point* (TQP) *(add 1–18):* Simply add the point values for Criteria 1–18 and record the value in Box 19. This value will range between 0 and 100.
20. *Effect size* (ES1) *or standardized mean difference* (magnitude of difference between groups in standard deviation units) calculated by the following:

$$\text{ES1} = \frac{\text{mean of treatment-mean of control or alternate treatment}}{\text{standard deviation of control or alternate treatment}}$$

This formula is for computing ES1 (standardized mean difference or difference in standard deviation units) when outcome means of treatment and control groups are given. To compute effect size from information presented in a study's report, select two means to compare; for example, outcome might be a mean of a treatment group compared with a mean of a nontreatment control group. Subtract the mean of the second group from the mean of the first group and divide this difference by the standard deviation of the second group. ES1 may be a negative or positive number. If the outcome measure's score gets greater as client outcome improves and ES1 is positive, then the treatment has had a positive effect, proportionate to the size of ES1. In this case, if ES1 is negative, then the treatment harms.

21. *Effect size* (ES2) *or absolute risk reduction:*

$$\text{ES2} = \left[(\text{number improved in treatment} \div \text{total number in treatment group}) \times 100\right]$$
$$- (\text{number improved in alternate treatment or control}$$
$$\div \text{total number in alternate treatment or control}) \times 100]$$

Absolute risk reduction (ES2) refers to the event rate in treatment relative to the event rate in the control group. Assume that you are comparing the proportion in a treatment group who are improved against the proportion in the control group who are improved.

22. *Effect size* (ES3) *or number needed to treat:*

$$\text{NNT} = \frac{100}{\text{ES2}}$$

NNT (ES3) is the number of clients that a clinician must treat with the experimental treatment in order to create a good outcome or to prevent one bad outcome in comparison to the control treatment. If controls do better, then this number is the number needed to harm.

Modified from Quality of Study Rating Form (QSRF) (Gibbs, 1989) and CONSORT statement for nonpharmacologic RCTs (Boutron et al., 2008a). Feasibility criteria taken from Jacobsen and Jim (2008) and concepts of translating to the local context from the Local Clinical Scientist model (Stricker & Trierweiler, 1995). QSRF and Scoring Instructions reprinted by permission of Taylor & Francis, Ltd. (http://www.tandf.co.uk/journals). The official citation that should be used in referencing the QSRF is Gibbs, L. E. (1989). Quality of study rating form: An instrument for synthesizing evaluation studies. *Journal of Social Work Education, 25(1),* 55–67 (http://www.informaworld.com).

APPENDIX C

An Abbreviated Approach to Evidence-Based Practice in Psycho-Oncology With Accessible Online Resources and References

Two Preliminary Steps: Acquire Background Knowledge and Check for Clinical Practice Guidelines

1. Background Knowledge: What more do I need to know regarding my patient?
   - Basic Cancer Knowledge (see *Three Online Resources—all references are at the end of this appendix*)
   - Psycho-Oncology Knowledge (see references for *Textbook, Quick Reference Guide, Handbook*)
2. Clinical Practice Guidelines: What guidelines already exist?
   - General Medical and Mental Health Guidelines (see *Three Online Resources*)
   - Research-Supported Psychological Treatments (see *One Online Resource*)
   - Psycho-Oncology Specific Guidelines (see *Two Online Resources*)

1. **Ask**: Write a good PICO (Patient, Intervention, Comparison, Outcomes) question
2. **Access**: Search for evidence
   - Secondary, Filtered Literature (see *Five Online Resources*)
   - Primary, Unfiltered Literature (use available local/organizational resources to create a hyperlink stored in a Word file on computer desktop for quick online access to databases; will need approved access)[a]
   - Use PICO terms and synonyms; check databases' controlled vocabulary (e.g., Medline MeSH; PsycINFO Thesaurus)
   - Select 1 or 2 most relevant RCTs to appraise

[a]Once the access link above is created, it should be stored on a Word file along with the other online resources listed. With this Word file stored on a local desktop or a remote server such as Dropbox, access to background knowledge, clinical practice guidelines, and primary/secondary literature becomes easier.

3. **Appraise**: Evaluate the quality of the evidence and strength of effect
   - Abbreviated evaluation strategy[b]: Evaluate study design and results of intervention
   - search study abstract and full article for following terms:
   - *random, intervention, control, primary outcomes/measures, statistical significance, effect size, mean difference, clinical significance, conclusions, limitations*
   - best quality comes from well-designed study with positive effects that are clinically significant
4. **Translate**: Which intervention best fits my patient? Quality of fit versus fidelity (see Fig. 4.4) Do I adopt, abandon, or adapt? If adapt, how (see Chapter 4)?
5. **Integrate**: Am I competent to provide the intervention and is my patient willing/interested/see the need?
6. **Evaluate**: What specific self-report outcome assessment measures will best evaluate patient progress?

---

[b]This abbreviated strategy for appraising the quality of a study and the strength of effects is recommended to be used as a time-saving strategy. It will provide a reasonably accurate overview of the study. However, it is important to note that it is inadequate to provide a detailed and comprehensive understanding of the quality of a study's results and could lead to inaccurate conclusions. When more time is available, use of the QSRF (see Appendix) or research reporting standards checklists (see Table 4.6) will provide a more detailed and accurate appraisal.

RESOURCES AND REFERENCES

Background Knowledge: What More Do I Need to Know Regarding My Patient?

Basic Cancer Knowledge: Three Online Resources

American Cancer Society (ACS). (2014). ACS. Retrieved February 8, 2014, from http://www.cancer.org/

American Psychosocial Oncology Society (APOS), online education resources. Accessed December 20, 2014, from http://www.apos-society.org/professionals/meetings-ed/webcasts.aspx

National Cancer Institute (NCI). Physicians Data Query (PDQ) Cancer Information Summaries. Retrieved February 9, 2014, from http://www.cancer.gov/cancertopics/pdq

Psycho-Oncology Knowledge: Textbook, Quick Reference Guide, Handbook

Holland, J. C., Breitbart, W. S., Jacobsen, P. B., Lederberg, M. S., Loscalzo, M. J., & McCorkle, R. (Eds.). (2010). *Psycho-Oncology* (2nd ed.). New York, NY: Oxford University Press.

Holland, J. C., Greenberg, D. B., & Hughes, M. K. (Eds.). (2006). *Quick reference for oncology clinicians: The psychiatric and psychological dimensions of cancer symptom management*. Charlottesville, VA: American Psychosocial Oncology Society (APOS).
Watson, M., & Kissane, D. (2011). *Handbook of psychotherapy in cancer care*. Chicester, West Sussex, UK: Wiley-Blackwell.

Clinical Practice Guidelines: What Guidelines Already Exist?

General Medical and Mental Health Guidelines: Three Online Resources

Agency for Health Care Research and Quality (AHRQ). (2014). National Guideline Clearinghouse. Retrieved February 8, 2014, from http://www.guideline.gov
American Psychiatric Association. (2009). Practice Guidelines. Retrieved December 20, 2014, from http://psychiatryonline.org/guidelines
National Institute for Clinical Excellence (NICE). (1999). Retrieved February 8, 2014, from http://www.nice.org.uk/

Research Supported Psychological Treatments: An Online Resource

American Psychological Association, Society of Clinical Psychology (2014). Website on research- supported psychological treatments. Retrieved December 20, 2014, from http://psychologicaltreatments.org/

Psycho-Oncology Specific Guidelines: Two Online Resources

National Cancer Institute Division of Cancer Control and Population Sciences. Cancer Control P.L.A.N.E.T. Retrieved February 9, 2014, from http://cancercontrolplanet.cancer.gov
National Comprehensive Cancer Network, Supportive Care (2014). Retrieved December 18, 2014, from http://www.nccn.org/professionals/physician_gls/f_guidelines.asp#supportive

Secondary, Filtered Literature: Five Online Resources

Campbell Collaboration—Review of Interventions and Policy Evaluations (C2-RIPE) http://www.campbellcollaboration.org
Cochrane Database of Systematic Reviews (CDSR) http://www.thecochranelibrary.com Database of abstracts of reviews of effects (DARE) http://www.crd.york.ac.uk/crdweb/
Evidence-based mental health. http://www.ebmh.bmj.com
PubMed (MEDLINE) http://www.pubmed.gov—*search Clinical Queries for reviews*

Primary, Unfiltered Literature: Author Sampleb

Ball State University's Access to Ebsco Information Services online research databases EBSCOhost https://login.proxy.bsu.edu/login?qurl=http%3a%2f%2fsearch.ebscohost.com%2flogin.aspx%3fauthtype%3dip%2cuid%26profile%3dehost%26defaultdb%3dpsyh

REFERENCES

Aaronson, N. K. (1991). Methodological issues in assessing the quality of life of cancer patients. *Cancer, 67*(3 Suppl), 844–850.

Adams, J. R., & Drake, R. E. (2006). Shared decision-making and evidence-based practice. *Community Mental Health Journal, 42*(1), 87–105.

Agency for Health Care Research and Quality (AHRQ). (2014). *National guideline clearinghouse.* Retrieved February 8, 2014, from http://www.guideline.gov

American Cancer Society (ACS). (2009). *Cancer facts & figures 2009.* Atlanta, GA: Author.

American Cancer Society (ACS). (2014). ACS. *Cancer facts & figures, 2014.* Retrieved May 5, 2015 from http://www.cancer.org/research/cancerfactsstatistics/cancerfactsfigures2014/index

American College of Surgeons (ACoS), Commission on Cancer (CoC). (2012). *Cancer program standards 2012: Ensuring patient-centered care.* Retrieved February 22, 2013, from www.facs.org/cancer/coc/programstandards2012.html

American Educational Research Association (AERA). (2006). Standards for reporting on empirical social science research in AERA publications. *Educational Researcher, 35*(6), 33–40.

American Psychiatric Association. (2009). *Practice guidelines.* Retrieved December 28, 2014, from http://psychiatryonline.org/guidelines

American Psychological Association. (2002). Ethical principles of psychologists and code of conduct. *American Psychologist, 57*(12), 1060–1073.

American Psychological Association. (2006). Evidence-based practice in psychology. *American Psychologist, 61*(4), 271–285.

American Psychological Association. (2014). *PsycINFO.* Retrieved February 8, 2014, from http://www.apa.org/pubs/databases/psycinfo/index.aspx

American Psychological Association JARS Working Group. (2008). Reporting standards for research in psychology: Why do we need them? What might they be? *American Psychologist, 63*(9), 839–851.

American Psychological Association, Society of Clinical Psychology. (2014). *Research-supported psychological treatments.* Retrieved December 20, 2014, from http://www.div12.org/psychological-treatments/

American Psychosocial Oncology Society (APOS). APOS Webinar Series. Retrieved May 6, 2015 from http://apos-society.org/APOS/Professionals/APOS_Webinar_Series/APOS/Professionals/Webinars.aspx?hkey=6c57ec9f-6375-4329-b6f4-d2d2420b1794

Andersen, B. L. (2002). Biobehavioral outcomes following psychological interventions for cancer patients. *Journal of Consulting and Clinical Psychology, 70*(3), 590–610.

Andersen, B. L., DeRubeis, R. J., Berman, B. S., Gruman, J., Champion, V. L., Massie, M. J., . . . Rowland, J. H. (2014). Screening, assessment, and care of anxiety and depressive symptoms in adults with cancer: An American Society of Clinical Oncology guideline adaptation. *Journal of Clinical Oncology, 32*(15), 1605–1619. doi: 10.1200/JCO.2013.52.4611

Andersen, B. L., Farrar, W. B., Golden-Kreutz, D. M., Emery, C. F., Glaser, R., Crespin, T. R., & Carson, W. E. (2007). Distress reduction from a psychological intervention contributes to improved health for cancer patients. *Brain, Behavior, and Immunity, 21*(7), 953–961. doi: 10.1016/j.bbi.2007.03.005

Andersen, B. L., Farrar, W. B., Golden-Kreutz, D. M., Glaser, R., Emery, C. F., Crespin, T. R., . . . Carson, W. E. (2004). Psychological, behavioral, and immune changes after a psychological intervention: A clinical trial. *Journal Of Clinical Oncology, 22*(17), 3570–3580.

Andersen, B. L., Kiecolt-Glaser, J. K., & Glaser, R. (1994). A biobehavioral model of cancer stress and disease course. *American Psychologist, 49*(5), 389–404.

Andersen, B. L., Yang, H. C., Farrar, W. B., Golden-Kreutz, D. M., Emery, C. F., Thornton, L. M., . . . Carson, W. E. (2008). Psychologic intervention improves survival for breast cancer patients: A randomized clinical trial. *Cancer, 113*(12), 3450–3458.

Andrykowski, M. A., & Manne, S. L. (2006). Are psychological interventions effective and accepted by cancer patients? I. Standards and levels of evidence. *Annals of Behavioral Medicine, 32*(2), 93–97. doi: 10.1207/s15324796abm3202_3

Antoni, M. H. (2003). *Stress management intervention for women with breast cancer.* Washington, DC: American Psychological Association.

Antoni, M. H., Lehman, J. M., Klibourn, K. M., Boyers, A. E., Culver, J. L., Alferi, S. M., . . . Carver, C. S. (2001). Cognitive-behavioral stress management intervention decreases the prevalence of depression and enhances benefit finding among women under treatment for early-stage breast cancer. *Health Psychology, 20*(1), 20–32. doi: 10.1037/0278-6133.20.1.20

Antoni, M. H., Wimberly, S. R., Lechner, S. C., Kazi, A., Sifre, T., Urcuyo, K. R., . . . Carver, C. S. (2006). Reduction of cancer-specific thought intrusions and anxiety symptoms with a stress management intervention among women undergoing treatment for breast cancer. *American Journal of Psychiatry, 163*(10), 1791–1797. doi: 10.1176/appi.ajp.163.10.1791

Baik, O. M., & Adams, K. B. (2011). Improving the well-being of couples facing cancer: A review of couples based psychosocial interventions. *Journal of Marital and Family Therapy, 37*(2), 250–266. doi: 10.1111/j.1752-0606.2010.00217.x

Bandura, A. (1986). *Social foundations of thought and action: A social cognitive theory.* Englewood Cliffs, NJ: Prentice-Hall.

Barlow, D. H. (2008). *Clinical handbook of psychological disorders: A step-by-step treatment manual.* New York, NY: Guilford Press.

Barratt, A. (2008). Evidence based medicine and shared decision making: The challenge of getting both evidence and preferences into health care. *Patient Education and Counseling, 73*(3), 407–412.

Baucom, D. H., Porter, L. S., Kirby, J. S., Gremore, T. M., Wiesenthal, N., Aldridge, W., . . . Keefe, F. J. (2009). A couple-based intervention for female breast cancer. *Psycho-Oncology, 18*(3), 276–283. doi: 10.1002/pon.1395

Beck, A. T., Rush, A. J., & Shaw, B. F. (1979). *Cogntive therapy of depression*. New York, NY: Guilford Press.

Bee, P. E., Barnes, P., & Luker, K. A. (2009). A systematic review of informal caregivers: Their needs in providing home-based end-of-life care to people with cancer. *Journal of Clinical Nursing, 18*(10), 1379–1393. doi: 10.1111/j.1365-2702.2008.02405.x

Beidas, R. S., & Kendall, P. C. (2010). Training therapists in evidence-based practice: A critical review of studies from a systems-contextual perspective. *Clinical Psychology: Science and Practice, 17*(1), 1–30. doi: 10.1111/j.1468-2850.2009.01187.x

Benson, H. (1975). *The relaxation response*. New York, NY: Harper Collins.

Bidstrup, P. E., Johansen, C., & Mitchell, A. J. (2011). Screening for cancer-related distress: Summary of evidence from tools to programmes. *Acta Oncologica, 50*(2), 194–204. doi: http://dx.doi.org/10.3109/0284186X.2010.533192

Birnie, K., Garland, S. N., & Carlson, L. E. (2009). Psychological benefits for cancer patients and their partners participating in mindfulness-based stress reduction (MBSR). *Psycho-Oncology, 19*(9), 1004–1009. doi: 10.1002/pon.1651

Boelen, P. A., de Keijser, J., van den Hout, M. A., & van den Bout, J. (2007). Treatment of complicated grief: A comparison between cognitive-behavioral therapy and supportive counseling. *Journal of Consulting and Clinical Psychology, 75*(2), 277–284. doi: 10.1037/0022-006x.75.2.277

Bossuyt, P. M., Reitsma, J. B., Bruns, D. E., Gatsonis, C. A., Glasziou, P. P., Irwig, L. M., . . . de Vet, H. C. (2003a). Towards complete and accurate reporting of studies of diagnostic accuracy: The STARD initiative. The Standards for Reporting of Diagnostic Accuracy Group. *Croatian Medical Journal, 44*(5), 635–638.

Bossuyt, P. M., Reitsma, J. B., Bruns, D. E., Gatsonis, C. A., Glasziou, P. P., Irwig, L. M., . . . Lijmer, J. G. (2003b). The STARD statement for reporting studies of diagnostic accuracy: Explanation and elaboration. The Standards for Reporting of Diagnostic Accuracy Group. *Croatian Medical Journal, 44*(5), 639–650.

Boutron, I., Moher, D., Altman, D. G., Schulz, K. F., & Ravaud, P. (2008a). Extending the CONSORT statement to randomized trials of nonpharmacologic treatment: Explanation and elaboration. *Annals of Internal Medicine, 148*(4), 295–309. doi: 148/4/295 [pii]

Boutron, I., Moher, D., Altman, D. G., Schulz, K. F., & Ravaud, P. (2008b). Methods and processes of the CONSORT Group: Example of an extension for trials assessing nonpharmacologic treatments. *Annals of Internal Medicine, 148*(4), W60–66. doi: 148/4/W-60 [pii]

Breitbart, W., & Applebaum, A. (2011). Meaning-centered group psychotherapy. In M. Watson & D. (Eds.), *Handbook of psychotherapy in cancer care* (pp. 137–148). Chicester, UK: Wiley-Blackwell.

Breitbart, W., Poppito, S., Rosenfeld, B., Vickers, A. J., Li, Y., Abbey, J., . . . Cassileth, B. R. (2012). Pilot randomized controlled trial of individual meaning-centered psychotherapy for patients with advanced cancer. *Journal Of Clinical Oncology, 30*(12), 1304–1309.

Breitbart, W., Rosenfeld, B., Gibson, C., Pessin, H., Poppito, S., Nelson, C., . . . Olden, M. (2010). Meaning-centered group psychotherapy for patients with advanced cancer: A pilot randomized controlled trial. *Psycho-Oncology, 19*(1), 21–28. doi: 10.1002/pon.1556

Breitbart, W. S., & Poppito, S. R. (2014a). *Meaning-centered group psychotherapy for patients with advanced cancer: A treatment manual*. New York, NY: Oxford University Press.

Breitbart, W. S., & Poppito, S. R. (2014b). *Individual meaning-centered psychotherapy for patients with advanced cancer: A Treatment manual.* New York, NY: Oxford University Press.

Brownson, R. C., Colditz, G. A., & Proctor, E. K. (2012). *Dissemination and implementation research in health: Translating science to practice.* New York, NY: Oxford University Press.

Bucher, J. A., & Zabora, J. R. (2010). Building problem-solving skills through COPE Education of family caregivers. In J. Holland, W. Breitbart, P. B. Jacobsen, M. Lederberg, M. Loscalzo, & R. McCorkle (Eds.), *Psycho-Oncology* (pp. 469–472). New York, NY: Oxford Press.

Budin, W. C., Hoskins, C. N., Haber, J., Sherman, D. W., Maislin, G., Cater, J. R., ... Shukla, S. (2008). Breast cancer: Education, counseling, and adjustment among patients and partners: A randomized clinical trial. *Nursing Research, 57*(3), 199–213.

Bultz, B. D., & Carlson, L. E. (2006). Emotional distress: The sixth vital sign-future directions in cancer care. *Psycho-Oncology, 15*(2), 93–95.

Burke, B. L., Arkowitz, H., & Menchola, M. (2003). The efficacy of motivational interviewing: A meta-analysis of controlled clinical trials. *Journal of Consulting and Clinical Psychology, 71*(5), 843–861. doi: 10.1037/0022-006x.71.5.843

Busby, D. M., Crane, D. R., Larson, J. H., & Christensen, C. (1995). A revision of the Dyadic Adjustment Scale for use with distressed and nondistressed couples: Construct hierarchy and multidimensional scales. *Journal of Marital and Family Therapy, 21*(3), 289–308. doi: 10.1111/j.1752-0606.1995.tb00163.x

Campbell Collaboration. (2014). Campbell systematic reviews. Retrieved Febraury 8, 2014, from http://www.campbellcollaboration.org

Campbell, L. C., Keefe, F. J., Scipio, C., McKee, D. C., Edwards, C. L., Herman, S. H., ... Donatucci, C. (2007). Facilitating research participation and improving quality of life for African American prostate cancer survivors and their intimate partners. A pilot study of telephone-based coping skills training. *Cancer, 109*(2 Suppl), 414–424.

Canada, A. L., Neese, L. E., Sui, D., & Schover, L. R. (2005). Pilot intervention to enhance sexual rehabilitation for couples after treatment for localized prostate carcinoma. *Cancer, 104*(12), 2689–2700.

Canadian Association of Psychosocial Oncology (CAPO). (2010). Standards of psychosocial health services for persons with cancer and their families: Canadian Association of Psychosocial Oncology retrieved May 6, 2015 from http://www.capo.ca/

Cancer Support Community. (2014). Cancer support helpline. Retrieved May 6, 2015 from http://www.cancersupportcommunity.org/MainMenu/Cancer-Support/Cancer-Support-Helpline.html

Candy, B., Jones, L., Drake, R. E., Leurent, B., & King, M. (2011). Interventions for supporting informal caregivers of patients in the terminal phase of a disease. *Cochrane Database Of Systematic Reviews, 6*, CD007617.

Carey, M. P., & Burish, T. G. (1988). Etiology and treatment of the psychological side effects associated with cancer chemotherapy: A critical review and discussion. *Psychological Bulletin, 104*(3), 307–325.

Carlson, L. E., Groff, S. L., Zhong, L., & Butz, B. D. (2012). Online screening for distress, the 6th vital sign, in newly diagnosed oncology outpatients: randomised controlled trial of computerised vs personalised triage. *British Journal of Cancer, 207*, 617–625.

Carlson, L. E., Angen, M., Cullum, J., Goodey, E., Koopmans, J., Lamont, L., ... Bultz, B. D. (2004). High levels of untreated distress and fatigue in cancer patients. *British Journal of Cancer, 90*(12), 2297–2304. doi: 10.1038/sj.bjc.6601887

Carlson, L. E., & Bultz, B. D. (2004). Efficacy and medical cost offset of psychosocial interventions in cancer care: Making the case for economic analyses. *Psycho-Oncology, 13*(12), 837.

Carlson, L. E., Clifford, S. K., Groff, S. L., Maciejewski, O., & Bultz, B. D. (2010). Screening for depression in cancer care. In A. J. Mitchell & J. C. Coyne (Eds.), *Screening for depression in clinical practice: An evidence-based guide.* (pp. 265–298). New York, NY: Oxford University Press.

Carlson, L. E., Groff, S. L., Maciejewski, O., & Bultz, B. D. (2010). Screening for distress in lung and breast cancer outpatients: A randomized controlled trial. *Journal of Clinical Oncology, 28*(33), 4884–4891. doi: JCO.2009.27.3698 [pii]10.1200/JCO.2009.27.3698

Carlson, L. E., Waller, A., Groff, S. L., & Bultz, B. D. (2013). Screening for distress, the sixth vital sign, in lung cancer patients: Effects on pain, fatigue, and common problems—Secondary outcomes of a randomized controlled trial. *Psycho-Oncology, 22*(8), 1880–1888.

Carter, E. A., & McGoldrick, M. (1980). *The family life cycle: A framework for family therapy.* New York, NY: Gardner Press.

Cella, D. F., Tulsky, D. S., Gray, G., Sarafian, B., Linn, E., Bonomi, A., . . . Brannon, J. (1993). The Functional Assessment of Cancer Therapy scale: Development and validation of the general measure. *Journal of Clinical Oncology, 11*(3), 570–579.

Chambless, D. L., & Crits-Christoph, P. (2005). The treatment method. In J.C. Norcross, L.E. Beutler & R. F. Levant (Eds.), *Evidence-based practices in mental health: Debate and dialogue on the fundamental questions.* Washington, DC: American Psychological Association.

Chambless, D. L., & Hollon, S. D. (1998). Defining empirically supported therapies. *Journal of Consulting and Clinical Psychology, 66*(1), 7–18.

Charles, C., Gafni, A., & Whelan, T. (1997). Shared decision-making in the medical encounter: What does it mean? (Or it takes at least two to tango). *Social Science and Medicine, 44*(5), 681–692.

Charles, K., Gafni, A., & Whelan, T. (1999). Decision-making in the physician-patient encounter: Revisiting the shared treatment decision-making model. *Social Science and Medicine, 49*(5), 651–661.

Chochinov, H. M., Kristjanson, L. J., Breitbart, W., McClement, S., Hack, T. F., Hassard, T., & Harlos, M. (2011). Effect of dignity therapy on distress and end-of-life experience in terminally ill patients: A randomised controlled trial. *Lancet Oncology, 12*(8), 753–762. doi: S1470-2045(11)70153-X [pii] 10.1016/S1470-2045(11)70153-X

Chochinov, H. M., & McKeen, N. A. (2011). Dignity therapy. In M. Watson & D. Kissane (Eds.), *Handbook of psychotherapy in cancer care* (pp. 79–88). Chichester, UK: Wiley-Blackwell.

Chorpita, B. F., Daleiden, E. L., Ebesutani, C., Young, J., Becker, K. D., Nakamura, B. J., . . . Starace, N. (2011). Evidence-based treatments for children and adolescents: An updated review of indicators of efficacy and effectiveness. *Clinical Psychology: Science and Practice, 18*(2), 154–172. doi: 10.1111/j.1468-2850.2011.01247.x

Clark, D. M. (2012). The English improving access to psychological therapies (IAPT) program: History and progress. In G. McHugh & D. H. Barlow (Eds.), *Dissemination and implementation of evidence-based psychological interventions.* New York: Oxford.

Clark, K., Bardwell, W. A., Arsenault, T., DeTeresa, R., & Loscalzo, M. (2009). Implementing touch-screen technology to enhance recognition of distress. *Psycho-Oncology, 18*(8), 822–830.

Clark, K., Greene, P., Duhamel, K., Loscalzo, M., Grant, M., Glazier, K., & Redd, W. (2012). A unique interactive cognitive behavioral training program for front-line cancer care professionals. *Journal of Cancer Education, 27*(4), 649–655. doi: 10.1007/s13187-012-0425-1

Classen, C., Butler, L. D., Koopman, C., Miller, E., DiMiceli, S., Giese-Davis, J., . . . Spiegel, D. (2001). Supportive-expressive group therapy and distress in patients with metastatic breast cancer: A randomized clinical intervention trial. *Archives of General Psychiatry, 58*(5), 494–501.

Classen, C. C., & Spiegel, D. (2011). Supportive-expressive group psychotherapy. In M. Watson & D. W. Kissane (Eds.), *Handbook of psychotherapy in cancer care* (pp. 107–117). Oxford, UK: Wiley.

Cochrane Collaboration. (2014). Cochrane Database of Systematic Reviews (CDSR). Retrieved February, 8, 2014, from http://www.cochrane.org/cochrane-reviews

Cohen, J. (1988). *Statistical power analysis for the behavioral sciences* (2nd ed.). Hillsdale, NJ: Erlbaum.

Collins, F. L., Leffingwell, T. R., & Belar, C. D. (2007). Teaching evidence-based practice: Implications for psychology. *Journal of Clinical Psychology, 63*(7), 657–670.

Compas, B. E., Haaga, D. A. F., Keefe, F. J., Leitenberg, H., & Williams, D. A. (1998). Sampling of empirically supported psychological treatments from health psychology: Smoking, chronic pain, cancer, and bulimia nervosa. *Journal of Consulting and Clinical Psychology, 66*(1), 89–112.

Conte, H. R. (1994). Review of research in supportive psychotherapy: An update. *American Journal of Psychotherapy, 48*(4), 494–504.

Conte, H. R., & Plutchik, R. (1986). Controlled research in supportive psychotherapy. *Psychiatric Annals, 16*(9), 530–533.

Council for Training in Evidence-Based Behavioral Practice (EBBP). (2015). Online training modules. Retrieved May 6, 2015,from http://www.ebbp.org/training.html

Coyne, J. C., Lepore, S. J., & Palmer, S. C. (2006). Efficacy of psychosocial interventions in cancer care: Evidence is weaker than it first looks. *Annals of Behavioral Medicine, 32*(2), 104–110. doi: 10.1207/s15324796abm3202_5

Crits-Christoph, P., Baranackie, K, Kurcias, J. S., Carroll, K., Luborsky, L. McLellan, T., et al. (1991). Meta-analysis of therapist effects in psychotherapy outcome studies. *Psychotherapy Research*, 1, 81–91.

Cuijpers, P., van Straten, A., & Warmerdam, L. (2007). Problem solving therapies for depression: A meta-analysis. *European Psychiatry, 22*(1), 9–15. doi: 10.1016/j.eurpsy.2006.11.001

Davidson, K. W., Trudeau, K. J., Ockene, J. K., Orleans, C. T., & Kaplan, R. M. (2004). A primer on current evidence-based review systems and their implications for behavioral medicine. *Annals of Behavioral Medicine, 28*(3), 226–238. doi: 10.1207/s15324796abm2803_11

Davidson, K. W., Goldstein, M., Kaplan, R. M., Kaufmann, P. G., Knatterud, G. L., Orleans, C. T., . . . Whitlock, E. P. (2003). Evidence-based behavioral medicine: What is it and how do we achieve it? *Annals Of Behavioral Medicine, 26*(3), 161–171.

Derogatis, L. R., Morrow, G. R., Fetting, J., Penman, D., Piasetsky, S., Schmale, A. M., . . . Carnicke, C. L., Jr. (1983). The prevalence of psychiatric disorders among cancer patients. *Journal of the American Medical Association, 249*(6), 751–757.

Des Jarlais, D. C., Lyles, C., & Crepaz, N. (2004). Improving the reporting quality of nonrandomized evaluations of behavioral and public health interventions: The TREND statement. *American Journal of Public Health, 94*(3), 361–366.

Devine, E. C., & Westlake, S. K. (1995). The effects of psychoeducational care provided to adults with cancer: Meta-analysis of 116 studies. *Oncology Nursing Forum, 22*(9), 1369–1381.

Devoto, E., & Kramer, B. S. (2006). Evidence-based approach to oncology. In A. E. Chang, P. A. Ganz, D. F. Hayes, T. J. Kinsella, H. I. Pass, J. H. Schiller, R. M. Stone & V. J. Strecher (Eds.), *Oncology: An evidence-based approach* (pp. 3–13). New York, NY: Springer.

Donnelly, J. M., Kornblith, A. B., Fleishman, S., Zuckerman, E., Raptis, G., Hudis, C. A., . . . Holland, J. C. (2000). A pilot study of interpersonal psychotherapy by telephone with cancer patients and their partners. *Psycho-Oncology, 9*(1), 44–56. doi: 10.1002/(SICI)1099-1611(200001/02)9:1<44::AID-PON431>3.0.CO;2-V [pii]

Drake, R. E., Goldman, H. H., Leff, H. S., Lehman, A. F., Dixon, L., & Mueser, K. T. (2001). Implementing evidence-based practices in routine mental health service settings. *Psychiatric Services, 52* (2) 179–182.

DuHamel, K. N., Mosher, C. E., Winkel, G., Labay, L. E., Rini, C., Meschian, Y. M., . . . Redd, W. H. (2010). Randomized clinical trial of telephone-administered cognitive-behavioral therapy to reduce post-traumatic stress disorder and distress symptoms after hematopoietic stem-cell transplantation. *Journal of Clinical Oncology, 28*(23), 3754–3761. doi: 10.1200/jco.2009.26.8722

Duncan, B. L., Miller, S. D., Wampold, B. E., & Hubble, M. A. (2010). *The heart and soul of change: Delivering what works in therapy* (2nd ed.). Washington, DC: American Psychological Association.

Eccles, M. P., Armstrong, D., Baker, R., Cleary, K., Davies, H., Davies, S., . . . Sibbald, B. (2009). An implementation research agenda. *Implementation Science, 4,* 18–18. doi: 10.1186/1748-5908-4-18

Edgar, L., Rosberger, Z., & Collet, J. P. (2001). Lessons learned: Outcomes and methodology of a coping skills intervention trial comparing individual and group formats for patients with cancer. *International Journal of Psychiatry in Medicine, 31*(3), 289–304.

Ellis, P., Robinson, P., Ciliska, D., Armour, T., Brouwers, M., O'Brien, M. A., . . . Raina, P. (2005). A systematic review of studies evaluating diffusion and dissemination of selected cancer control interventions. *Health Psychology, 24*(5), 488–500.

Elsevier Life Sciences Solutions. (2014). *EMBASE: Biomedical database*. Retrieved February 8, 2014, from http://www.elsevier.com/online-tools/embase

Epstein, N. B., & Baucom, D. H. (2002). *Enhanced cognitive-behavioral therapy for couples: A contextual approach*. Washington, DC: American Psychological Association.

Erikson, E. H. (1950). *Childhood and society*. New York, NY: Norton.

Faller, H., Schuler, M., Richard, M., Heckl, U., Weis, J., & Kaffner, R. (2013). Effects of psycho-oncologic interventions on emotional distress and quality of life in adult patients with cancer: Systematic review and meta-analysis. *Journal of Clinical Oncology, 31*(6), 782–793. doi: http://dx.doi.org/10.1200/JCO.2011.40.8922

Fann, J. R., Ell, K., & Sharpe, M. (2012). Integrating psychosocial care into cancer services. *Journal of Clinical Oncology, 30*(11), 1178–1186.

Fawzy, F. I. (1994). The benefits of a short term group intervention for cancer patients. *Advances: The Journal of Mind-Body Health, 10*(2), 17–19.

Fawzy, F. I., Fawzy, N. W., Arndt, L. A., & Pasnau, R. O. (1995). Critical review of psychosocial interventions in cancer care. *Archives of General Psychiatry, 52*(2), 100–113.

Fawzy, F. I., Fawzy, N. W., & Wheeler, J. G. (1996). A post-hoc comparison of the efficiency of a psychoeducational intervention for melanoma patients delivered in group versus individual formats: An analysis of data from two studies. *Psycho-Oncology, 5*(2), 81–89.

Feuerstein, M. (Ed.). (2007). *Handbook of cancer survivorship.* New York, NY: Springer.

Field, M. J., & Lohr, K. N. (1992). *Guidelines for clinical practice: From development to use.* Washington, DC: National Academy Press.

Fischer, E. P. (2006). Shared decision-making and evidence-based practice: A commentary. *Community Mental Health Journal, 42*(1), 107–111.

Forsythe, L. P., Kent, E. E., Weaver, K. E., Buchanan, N., Hawkins, N. A., Rodriguez, J. L., . . . Rowland, J. H. (2013). Receipt of psychosocial care among cancer survivors in the United States. *Journal of Clinical Oncology, 31*(16), 1961–1969. doi: 10.1200/JCO.2012.46.2101

Fouad, N. A., Grus, C. L., Hatcher, R. L., Kaslow, N. J., Smith Hutchings, P., Madson, M. B., . . . Crossman, R. E. (2009). Competency benchmarks: A model for understanding and measuring competence in professional psychology across training levels. *Training and Education in Professional Psychology, 3*(4, Suppl), S5–S26.

Fox, B. H. (1998). A hypothesis about Spiegel et al.'s 1989 paper on psychosocial intervention and breast cancer survival. *Psycho-Oncology, 7*(5), 361–370. doi: 10.1002/(SICI)1099-1611(1998090)7:5<361::AID-PON347>3.0.CO;2-U

Frueh, B. C., Ford, J. D., Elhal, J. D., & Grubaugh, A. L. (2012). Evidence-based practice in adult mental health. In P. Sturmey & M. Hersen (Eds.), *Handbook of evidence-based practice in clinical psychology* (Vol. 2, pp. 3–14). New York, NY: Wiley.

Frueh, B. C., Grubaugh, A. L., Cusack, K. J., & Elhai, J. D. (2009). Disseminating evidence-based practices for adults with PTSD and severe mental illness in public-sector mental health agencies. *Behavior Modification, 33*(1), 66–81. doi: 10.1177/0145445508322619

Fulcher, C. D., Badger, T., Gunter, A. K., Marrs, J. A., & Reese, J. M. (2008). Putting evidence into practice: Interventions for depression. *Clinical Journal of Oncology Nursing, 12*(1), 131–140.

Gagliardi, A. R., Dobrow, M. J., & Wright, F. C. (2011). How can we improve cancer care? A review of interprofessional collaboration models and their use in clinical management. *Surgical Oncology, 20*(3), 146–154. doi: 10.1016/j.suronc.2011.06.004

Gibbs, L. E. (1989). Quality of study rating form: An instrument for synthesizing evaluation studies. *Journal of Social Work Education, 25* (1), 55–67.

Gibbs, L. E. (2003). *Evidence-based practice for the helping professions: A practical guide with integrated multimedia.* Belmont, CA: Brooks/Cole.

Gilbody, S., Bower, P., Fletcher, J., Richards, D., & Sutton, A. J. (2006). Collaborative care for depression: A cumulative meta-analysis and review of longer-term outcomes. *Archives of Internal Medicine, 166*(21), 2314–2321. doi: 166/21/2314 [pii]10.1001/archinte.166.21.2314

Given, B., Given, C. W., Sikorskii, A., Jeon, S., Sherwood, P., & Rahbar, M. (2006). The impact of providing symptom management assistance on caregiver reaction: Results of a randomized trial. *Journal of Pain and Symptom Management, 32*(5), 433–443.

Glajchen, M. (2011). Caregivers in palliative care: Roles and responsibilities. In T. Altilio & S. Otis-Green (Eds.), *Oxford textbook of palliative social work* (pp. 223–233). New York, NY: Oxford University Press.

Glasgow, R. E., Davidson, K. W., Dobkin, P. L., Ockene, J., & Spring, B. (2006). Practical behavioral trials to advance evidence-based behavioral medicine. *Annals of Behavioral Medicine, 31*(1), 5–13. doi: 10.1207/s15324796abm3101_3

Glasgow, R. E., Klesges, L. M., Dzewaltowski, D. A., Bull, S. S., & Estabrooks, P. (2004). The future of health behavior change research: What is needed to improve translation of research into health promotion practice? *Annals of Behavioral Medicine, 27*(1), 3–12. doi: 10.1207/s15324796abm2701_2

Glasgow, R. E., Vinson, C., Chambers, D., Khoury, M. J., Kaplan, R. M., & Hunter, C. (2012). National Institutes of Health approaches to dissemination and implementation science: Current and future directions. *American Journal of Public Health, 102*(7), 1274–1281.

Goodwin, P. J., Leszcz, M., Ennis, M., Koopmans, J., Vincent, L., Guther, H., . . . Hunter, J. (2001). The effect of group psychosocial support on survival in metastatic breast cancer. *New England Journal Of Medicine, 345*(24), 1719–1726.

Grande, G. E., Myers, L. B., & Sutton, S. R. (2006). How do patients who participate in cancer support groups differ from those who do not? *Psycho-Oncology, 15*(4), 321–334.

Graves, K. D., Arnold, S. M., Love, C. L., Kirsh, K. L., Moore, P. G., & Passik, S. D. (2007). Distress screening in a multidisciplinary lung cancer clinic: prevalence and predictors of clinically significant distress. *Lung Cancer, 55*(2), 215–224. doi: S0169-5002(06)00535-6 [pii]10.1016/j.lungcan.2006.10.001

Gray, M. J., Elhai, J. D., & Schmidt, L. O. (2012). Trauma professionals' attitudes towards and utilization of evidence-based practices. *Behavior Modification, 31*, 732–748.

Greer, S. (1994). Psycho-Oncology: Its aims, achievements and future tasks. *Psycho-Oncology, 3*(2), 87–101.

Gustafson, D. H., Hawkins, R., Pingree, S., McTavish, F., Arora, N. K., Mendenhall, J., . . . Salner, A. (2001). Effect of computer support on younger women with breast cancer. *Journal of General Internal Medicine, 16*(7), 435–445.

Harding, R., & Higginson, I. J. (2003). What is the best way to help caregivers in cancer and palliative care? A systematic literature review of interventions and their effectiveness. *Palliative Medicine, 17*(1), 63–74.

Harding, R., List, S., Epiphaniou, E., & Jones, H. (2012). How can informal caregivers in cancer and palliative care be supported? An updated systematic literature review of interventions and their effectiveness. *Palliative Medicine, 26*(1), 7–22. doi: 10.1177/0269216311409613

Harmon, S. C., Lambert, M. J., Smart, D. M., Hawkins, E., Nielsen, S. L., . . . Lutz, W. (2007). Enhancing outcome for potential treatment failures: Therapist-client feedback and clinical support tools. *Psychotherapy Research, 17*(4), 379–392.

Haynes, R. B. (2001). Of studies, syntheses, syopses, and systems: The "4S" evolution of service for finding current best evidence. *EBM Notebook*, 6(March/April), 36–38.

Haynes, R. B. (2006). Of studies, syntheses, synopses, summaries, and systems: The "5S" evolution of information services for evidence-based healthcare decisions. *Evidince Based Medicine, 11*(6), 162–164. doi: 11/6/162-a [pii]10.1136/ebm.11.6.162-a

Heath, B., Wise Romero, P., & Reynolds, K. (2013). *A standard framework for levels of integrated healthcare.* Washington, DC: SAMHSA-HRSA Center for Integrated Health Solutions.

Helgeson, V. S., Cohen, S., Schulz, R., & Yasko, J. (2000). Group support interventions for women with breast cancer: Who benefits from what? *Health Psychology, 19*(2), 107–114. doi: 10.1037/0278-6133.19.2.107

Helgeson, V. S., Cohen, S., Schulz, R., & Yasko, J. (2001). Long-term effects of educational and peer discussion group interventions on adjustment to breast cancer. *Health Psychology, 20*(5), 387–392. doi: 10.1037/0278-6133.20.5.387

Helgeson, V. S., & McUmber, A. L. (2010). Social environment and cancer. In J. C. Holland, W. S. Breitbart, P. B. Jacobsen, M. S. Lederberg, M. J. Loscalzo & R. McCorkle (Eds.), *Psycho-Oncology* (2nd ed., pp. 62–68). New York, NY: Oxford Press.

Hellerstein, D. J., Pinsker, H., Rosenthal, R. N., & Klee, S. (1994). Supportive therapy as the treatment model of choice. *Journal of Psychotherapy Practice and Research, 3*(4), 300–306.

Hellerstein, D. J., Rosenthal, R. N., Pinsker, H., Samstag, L. W., Muran, J. C., & Winston, A. (1998). A randomized prospective study comparing supportive and dynamic therapies: Outcome and alliance. *Journal of Psychotherapy Practice and Research, 7*(4), 261–271.

Heneghan, C., & Badenoch, D. (2006). *Evidence-based medicine toolkit* (2nd ed.). Malden, MA: Blackwell.

Herschell, A. D., Kolko, D. J., Baumann, B. L., & Davis, A. C. (2010). The role of therapist training in the implementation of psychosocial treatments: A review and critique with recommendations. *Clinical Psychology Review, 30*(4), 448–466. doi: 10.1016/j.cpr.2010.02.005

Higginson, I. J., Finlay, I. G., Goodwin, D. M., Hood, K., Edwards, A. G. K., . . . Normand, C. E. (2003). Is there evidence that palliative care teams alter end-of-life experiences of patients and their caregivers? *Journal of Pain and Symptom Management, 25*(2), 150–168. doi: 10.1016/s0885-3924(02)00599-7

Hoffman, K. E., McCarthy, E. P., Recklitis, C. J., & Ng, A. K. (2009). Psychological distress in long-term survivors of adult-onset cancer: Results from a national survey. *Archives of Internal Medicine, 169*(14), 1274–1281. doi: 10.1001/archinternmed.2009.179

Hoffman, B. M., Zevon, M. A., D'Arrigo, M. C., & Cecchini, T. B. (2004). Screening for distress in cancer patients: The NCCN rapid-screening measure. *Psycho-Oncology, 13*(11), 792–799. doi: 10.1002/pon.796

Hogan, B. E., Linden, W., & Najarian, B. (2002). Social support interventions: Do they work? *Clinical Psychology Review, 22*(3), 381–440. doi: 10.1016/s0272-7358(01)00102-7

Holland, J. C. (1992). Psycho-oncology: Overview, obstacles and opportunities. *Psycho-Oncology, 1*, 1–13.

Holland, J. C. (1998). *Psycho-oncology*. New York, NY: Oxford University Press.

Holland, J. C., Andersen, B. L., Breitbart, W., Copas, B., Dudley, M. M., Fleishman, S., . . . Knight, S. J. (2010). Distress management: Clinical practice guidelines in oncology. *Journal of the National Comprehensive Cancer Network, 8*(4), 448–485.

Holland, J. C., Breitbart, W. S., Jacobsen, P. B., Lederberg, M. S., Loscalzo, M. J., & McCorkle, R. (Eds.). (2010). *Psycho-Oncology* (2nd ed.). New York, NY: Oxford University Press.

Holland, J. C., Greenberg, D. B., & Hughes, M. K. (Eds.). (2006). *Quick reference for oncology clinicians: The psychiatric and psychological dimensions of cancer symptom management*. Charlottesville, VA: American Psychosocial Oncology Society (APOS).

Holland, J. C., & Rowland, J. H. (1989). *Handbook of psychooncology: Psychological care of the patient with cancer.* New York, NY: Oxford University Press.

Holland, J. C., & Weiss, T. R. (2010). History of psycho-oncology. In J. C. Holland, W. S. Breitbart, P. B. Jacobsen, M. S. Lederberg, M. J. Loscalzo, & R. McCorkle (Eds.), *Psycho-Oncology* (pp. 3–12). New York, NY: Oxford University Press.

Honea, N. J., Brintnall, R., Given, B., Sherwood, P., Colao, D. B., Somers, S. C., & Northouse, L. L. (2008). Putting evidence into practice: Evidence based interventions to reduce family caregiver strain and burden. *Clinical Journal of Oncology Nursing, 12*(3), 507–516.

Houts, P. S., Nezu, A. M., Nezu, C. Maguth, & Bucher, J. A. (1996). The prepared family caregiver: A problem-solving approach to family caregiver education. *Patient Education and Counseling, 27*(1), 63–73. doi: 10.1016/0738-3991(95)00790-3

Howard, K. I., Moras, K., Brill, P. L., Martinovich, Z., & Lutz, W. (1996). Evaluation of psychotherapy: Efficacy, effectiveness, and patient progress. *American Psychologist, 51*(10), 1059–1064.

Howell, D., Currie, S., Mayo, S., Jones, G. W., Boyle, M., Hack, T., . . . Digout, C. (2009). *A pan-Canadian clinical practice guideline: Assessment of psychosocial health care needs of the adult cancer patient.* Toronto, ON: Canadian Partnership Against Cancer (Cancer Journey Action Group) and the Canadian Association of Psychosocial Oncology.

Howell, D., Keller-Olaman, S., Oliver, T., Hack, T., Broadfield, L., Biggs, K., . . . Syme, A. (2010). *A pan-Canadian practice guideline: Screening, assessment and care of psychosocial distress (depression, anxiety) in adults with cancer.* Toronto, ON: Canadian Partnership Against Cancer (Cancer Journey Action Group) and the Canadian Association of Psychosocial Oncology.

Huang, X., Lin, J., & Demner-Fishmen, D. (November, 2006). *Evaluation of PICO as a knowledge representation for clinical questions.* Paper presented at the Annual Symposium of the American Medical Informatics Association, Washington, DC.

Hubble, M. A., Duncan, B. L., Miller, S. D., & Wampold, B. E. (2010). Introduction. In *The heart and soul of change: Delivering what works in therapy* (2nd ed., pp. 23–46). Washington, DC: American Psychological Association.

Hudson, P. L., Aranda, S., & Hayman-White, K. (2005). A psycho-educational intervention for family caregivers of patients receiving palliative care: A randomized controlled trial. *Journal of Pain and Symptom Management, 30*(4), 329–341.

Institute of Medicine. (1999). *Ensuring quality cancer care.* Washington, DC: National Academy Press

Institute of Medicine. (2001). *Crossing the quality chasm: A new health system for the 21st century.* Washington, DC: National Academy Press.

Institute of Medicine. (2006). *Improving the quality of health care for mental and substance-use conditions.* Washington, DC: National Academy Press.

Institute of Medicine. (2011). *Patient-centered treatment planning: Improving the quality of oncology care: Workshop summary.* Washington, DC: National Academies Press.

Institute of Medicine. (2008). *Cancer care for the whole patient: Meeting psychosocial health needs.* Washington, DC: National Academies Press.

Institute of Medicine & National Research Council. (2004). *Meeting psychosocial needs of women with breast cancer.* Washington, DC: National Academies Press.

Institute of Medicine & National Research Council. (2006). *From cancer patient to cancer survivor: Lost in transition.* Washington, DC: National Academies Press.

Institute of Translational Health Sciences. (2013). *T-Phases of translational health research*. Retrieved May 18, 2013, from https://www.iths.org/about/translational

Interprofessional Education Collaborative Expert Panel. (2011). *Core competencies for interprofessional collaborative practice: Report of an expert panel*. Washington, DC: Interprofessional Education Collaborative.

Jacobs, J., Ostroff, J. S., & Steinglass, P. (1998). Family therapy: A systems approach to cancer care. *Psycho-Oncology* (pp. 994–1003). New York, NY: Oxford University Press.

Jacobsen, P. B. (2006). Lost in translation: The need for clinically relevant research on psychological interventions for distress in cancer patients. *Annals of Behavioral Medicine, 32*(2), 119–120.

Jacobsen, P. B. (2009). Promoting evidence-based psychosocial care for cancer patients. *Psycho-Oncology, 18*(1), 6–13. doi: 10.1002/pon.1468

Jacobsen, P. B. (2010). Translating psychosocial oncology research to clinical practice. In J. C. Holland, W. S. Breitbart, P. B. Jacobsen, M. S. Lederberg, M. J. Loscalzo, & R. McCorkle (Eds.), *Psycho-Oncology* (2nd. ed., pp. 642–647.). New York, NY: Oxford University Press.

Jacobsen, P. B. (March, 2013). *Promoting evidence-based psychosocial care of cancer patients: Current status and future prospects*. Paper presented at the Society of Behavioral Medicine, San Francisco, CA.

Jacobsen, P. B., Donovan, K. A., Swaine, Z. N., & Watson, I. S. (2006). Management of anxiety and depression in adult cancer patients: Toward an evidence-based approach. In A. E. Chang, P. A. Ganz, D. F. Hayes, T. J. Kinsella, H. I. Pass, J. H. Schiller, R. M. Stone, & V. J. Strecher (Eds.), *Oncology: An evidence-based approach*. New York, NY: Springer.

Jacobsen, P. B., & Jim, H. S. (2008). Psychosocial interventions for anxiety and depression in adult cancer patients: Achievements and challenges. *CA: A Cancer Journal for Clinicians, 58*(4), 214–230.

Jacobsen, P. B., Meade, C. D., Stein, K. D., Chirikos, T. N., Small, B. J., & Ruckdeschel, J. C. (2002). Efficacy and costs of two forms of stress management training for cancer patients undergoing chemotherapy. *Journal of Clinical Oncology, 20*(12), 2851–2862.

Jacobson, E. (1938). *Progressive relaxation*. Chicago: University of Chicago Press.

Jacobson, N. S., Roberts, L. J., Berns, S. B., & McGlinchey, J. B. (1999). Methods for defining and determining the clinical significance of treatment effects: Description, application, and alternatives. *Journal of Consulting and Clinical Psychology, 67*(3), 300–307.

Johnson, S. M. (2002). *Emotionally focused couple therapy with trauma survivors: Strengthening attachment bonds*. New York, NY: Guilford Press.

Johnson, S. M. (2004). *The practice of emotionally focused marital therapy: Creating connection*. New York, NY: Brunner-Routledge.

Johnson, S. M., Hunsley, J., Greenberg, L. S., & Schindler, D. (1999). Emotionally focused couples therapy: Status and challenges. *Clinical Psychology: Science and Practice, 6*(1), 67–79. doi: 10.1093/clipsy/6.1.67

Kabat-Zinn, J. (1990). *Full castastrophe living: Using the wisdom of your body and mind to face stress, pain and illness*. New York, NY: Random House.

Katz, C., Bosch, G., & Herzog, R. E. (1998). Group-therapy of couples after breast cancer diagnosis: Experimental pilot study. *Anticancer Research, 18*(3C), 2267–2269.

Kayser, K., Feldman, B. N., Borstelmann, N. A., & Daniels, A. A. (2010). Effects of a randomized couple-based intervention on quality of life of breast cancer patients and their partners. *Social Work Research*, *34*(1), 20–32.

Kazak, A. E., Alderfer, M. A., Streisand, R., Simms, S., Rourke, M. T., Barakat, L. P., . . . Cnaan, A. (2004). Treatment of posttraumatic stress symptoms in adolescent survivors of childhood cancer and their families: A randomized clinical trial. *Journal of Family Psychology*, *18*(3), 493–504.

Kazak, A. E., Simms, S., Alderfer, M. A., Rourke, M. T., Crump, T., McClure, K. S., . . . Reilly, A. (2005). Feasibility and preliminary outcomes from a pilot study of a brief psychological intervention for families of children newly diagnosed with cancer. *Journal of Pediatric Psychology*, *30*(8), 644–655. doi: 10.1093/jpepsy/jsi051

Kazak, A. E., Simms, S., & Rourke, M. T. (2002). Family systems practice in pediatric psychology. *Journal of Pediatric Psychology*, *27*(2), 133–143. doi: 10.1093/jpepsy/27.2.133

Kerner, J., Rimer, B., & Emmons, K. (2005). Introduction to the special section on dissemination: Dissemination research and research dissemination: How can we close the gap? *Health Psychology*, *24*(5), 443–446.

Khoury, M. J., Gwinn, M., Yoon, P. W., Dowling, N., Moore, C. A., & Bradley, L. (2007). The continuum of translation research in genomic medicine: How can we accelerate the appropriate integration of human genome discoveries into health care and disease prevention? *Genetics in Medicine*, *9*(10), 665–674.

King, D. A., Heisel, M. J., & Lyness, J. M. (2005). Assessment and psychological treatment of depression in older adults with terminal or life-threatening illness. *Clinical Psychology: Science and Practice*, *12*(3), 339–353.

Kissane, D. (2011). Survival following psychotherapy interventions. In J. C. Holland, W. S. Breitbart, P. B. Jacobsen, M. S. Lederberg, M. J. Loscalzo, & R. McCorkle (Eds.), *Psycho-Oncology* (pp. 479–482). New York, NY: Oxford University Press.

Kissane, D., & Zaider, I. Z. (2011). Focused family therapy in palliative care and bereavement. In M. Watson & D. Kissane (Eds.), *Handbook of psychotherapy in cancer care*. Oxford, UK: Wiley.

Kissane, D. W. & Bloch, S. (2002). *Family focused grief therapy: A model of family-centered care during palliative care and bereavement*. Philadelphia, PA: Open University Press.

Kissane, D. W., Bloch, S., McKenzie, M., McDowall, A. C., & Nitzan, R. (1998). Family grief therapy: A preliminary account of a new model to promote healthy family functioning during palliative care and bereavement. *Psycho-Oncology*, *7*(1), 14–25. doi: 10.1002/(SICI)1099-1611(199801/02)7:1<14::AID-PON313>3.0.CO;2-D

Kissane, D. W., Bloch, S., Miach, P., Smith, G. C., Seddon, A., & Keks, N. (1997). Cognitive-existential group therapy for patients with primary breast cancer—techniques and themes. *Psycho-Oncology*, *6*(1), 25–33. doi: 10.1002/(sici)1099-1611(199703)6:1<25::aid-pon240>3.0.co;2-n

Kissane, D. W., Bloch, S., Smith, G. C., Miach, P., Clarke, D. M., Ikin, J., . . . McKenzie, D. P. (2003). Cognitive-existential group psychotherapy for women with primary breast cancer: A randomized controlled trial. *Psycho-Oncology*, *12*(6), 532–546. doi: 10.1002/pon.683

Kissane, D. W., Grabsch, B., Clarke, D. M., Christie, G., Clifton, D., Gold, S., . . . Smith, G. C. (2004). Supportive-expressive group therapy: The transformation of existential ambivalence into creative living while enhancing adherence to anti-cancer therapies. *Psycho-Oncology, 13*(11), 755–768.

Kissane, D. W., Grabsch, B., Clarke, D. M., Smith, G. C., Love, A. W., Bloch, S., . . . Li, Y. (2007). Supportive-expressive group therapy for women with metastatic breast cancer: Survival and psychosocial outcome from a randomized controlled trial. *Psycho-Oncology, 16*(4), 277–286.

Kissane, D. W., Love, A., Hatton, A., Bloch, S., Smith, G., Clarke, D. M., . . . Snyder, R. D. (2004). Effect of cognitive-existential group therapy on survival in early-stage breast cancer. *Journal of Clinical Oncology, 22*(21), 4255–4260. doi: 10.1200/JCO.2004.12.129JCO.2004.12.129 [pii]

Kissane, D. W., McKenzie, M., Bloch, S., Moskowitz, C., McKenzie, D. P., & O'Neill, I. (2006). Family focused grief therapy: A randomized, controlled trial in palliative care and bereavement. *American Journal of Psychiatry, 163*(7), 1208–1218.

Kissane, D. W., McKenzie, M., McKenzie, D. P., Forbes, A., O'Neill, I., & Bloch, S. (2003). Psychosocial morbidity associated with patterns of family functioning in palliative care: Baseline data from the family focused grief therapy controlled trial. *Palliative Medicine, 17*(6), 527–537.

Kroenke, K., Theobald, D., Wu, J., Norton, K., Morrison, G., Carpenter, J., & Tu, W. (2010). Effect of telecare management on pain and depression in patients with cancer: A randomized trial. *Journal of the American Medical Association, 304*(2), 163–171. doi: 10.1001/jama.2010.944304/2/163 [pii]

Krouse, R. S. (2010). Gastrointestinal cancer. In J. M. Holland, W. S. Breitbart, P. B. Jacobsen, M. Lederberg, M. Loscalzo, & R. McCorkle (Eds.), *Psycho-Oncology* (pp. 140–145). New York, NY: Oxford University Press.

Kuijer, R. G., Buunk, B. P., De Jong, G. M., Ybema, J. F., & Sanderman, R. (2004). Effects of a brief intervention program for patients with cancer and their partners on feelings of inequity, relationship quality and psychological distress. *Psycho-Oncology, 13*(5), 321–334.

Lambert, M. J. (2001). Psychotherapy outcome and quality improvement: Introduction to the special section on patient-focused research. *Journal of Consulting and Clinical Psychology, 69*(2), 147–149.

Lambert, M. J. (Ed.). (2004). *Begin and Garfield's handbook of psychotherapy and behavior change* (5th ed.). New York, NY: Wiley.

Lambert, M. J. (2010). *Prevention of treatment failure*. Washington, DC: American Psychological Association.

Lambert, M. J. (2011a). Psychotherapy research and its achievements. In J. C. Norcross, G. R. Vandenbos, & D. K. Freedheim (Eds.), *History of psychotherapy: Continuity and change*. (2nd ed., pp. 299–332). Washington, DC: American Psychological Association.

Lambert, M. J. (2011b). Collecting client feedback. In J. C. Norcross (Ed.), *Psychotherapy relationships that work* (2nd ed., pp. 203–223). New York, NY: Oxford University Press.

Lambert, M. J., Duncan, B. L., Miller, S. D., Wampold, B. E., & Hubble, M. A. (2010). Yes, it is time for clinicians to routinely monitor treatment outcome. In B. L. Duncan, S. D. Miller, B. E. Wampold and M. A. Hubble (Eds.), *The heart and soul of change: Delivering what works in therapy* (2nd ed., pp. 239–266). Washington, DC: American Psychological Association.

Lambert, M. J., Morton, J. J., Hatfield, D. R., Harmon, C., Hamilton, S., Reid, R. C., & Burlingame, G. M. (2004). *Administration and scoring manual for the OQ-45.2 (Outcome Questionnaire)*. Orem, UT: American Professional Credentialing Services.

Lambert, M. J., & Ogles, B. M. (2004). The efficacy and effectiveness of psychotherapy. In M. J. Lambert (Ed.), *Bergin and Garfiels's handbook of psychotherapy and behavior change* (5th ed., pp. 139–193). New York, NY: Wiley.

Lambert, M. J., Vermeersch, D. A., Brown, S. D., & Lent, R. W. (2008). Measuring and improving psychotherapy outcome in routine practice. In S. D. Brown and R. W. Lent (Eds.), *Handbook of counseling psychology* (4th ed., pp. 233–248). Hoboken, NJ: Wiley.

Landes, S. A., & Linehan, M. M. (2012). Dissemination and implementation of dialectical behavior therapy: An intensive training model. In G. McHugh & D. H. Barlow (Eds.), *Dissemination and implementation of evidence-based psychological interventions*. New York, NY: Oxford University Press.

Landrine, H., & Klonoff, E. A. (1992). Culture and health-related schemas: A review and proposal for interdisciplinary integration. *Health Psychology, 11*(4), 267–276.

Laperriere, N., Zuraw, L., & Cairncross, G. (2002). Radiotherapy for newly diagnosed malignant glioma in adults: A systematic review. *Radiotherapy and Oncology, 64*(3), 259–273.

Lazarus, R. S. & Folkman, S. (1984). *Stress, appraisal, and coping*. New York, NY: Springer.

Lederberg, M. S., & Holland, J. C. (2011). Supportive psychotherapy in cancer care: An essential ingredient of all therapy. In M. Watson & D. Kissane (Eds.), *Handbook of psychotherapy in cancer care* (pp. 3–14.). Hoboken, NJ: Wiley.

LeMay, K., & Wilson, K. G. (2008). Treatment of existential distress in life threatening illness: A review of manualized interventions. *Clinical Psychology Review, 28*(3), 472–493. doi: 10.1016/j.cpr.2007.07.013

Lemieux, J., Topp, A., Chappell, H., Ennis, M., & Goodwin, P. J. (2006). Economic analysis of psychosocial group therapy in women with metastatic breast cancer. *Breast Cancer Research and Treatment, 100*(2), 183–190.

Lepore, S. J. (2001). A Social-cognitive processing model of emotional adjustment to cancer. In A. Baum & B. L. Andersen (Eds.), *Psychosocial interventions for cancer* (pp. 99–116). Washington, DC: American Psychological Association.

Lepore, S. J., Buzaglo, J. S., Lieberman, M. A., Golant, M., & Davey, A. (2011). Standard versus prosocial online support groups for distressed breast cancer survivors: A randomized controlled trial. *BMC Cancer, 11*, 379–379.

Lepore, S. J., & Coyne, J. C. (2006). Psychological interventions for distress in cancer patients: A review of reviews. *Annals of Behavioral Medicine, 32*(2), 85–92. doi: 10.1207/s15324796abm3202_2

Lepore, S. J., Helgeson, V. S., Eton, D. T., & Schulz, R. (2003). Improving quality of life in men with prostate cancer: A randomized controlled trial of group education interventions. *Health Psychology, 22*(5), 443–452. doi: 10.1037/0278-6133.22.5.443

Lerner, M. (1994). *Choices in healing: Integrating the best of conventional and complementary approaches to cancer*. Cambridge, MA: MIT Press.

LeShan, L. L. (1989). *Cancer as a turning point: A handbook for people with cancer, their families and health professionals*. New York, NY: Dutton.

Levy, K. N., Ellison, W. D., Scott, L. N., & Bernecker, S. L. (2011). Attachment style. *Journal of Clinical Psychology, 67*(2), 193–203.

Lewis, E. J., & Sharp, D. M. (2011). Relaxation and image based herapy. In M. Watson & D. Kissane (Eds.), *Handbook of psychotherapy in cancer care* (pp. 49–57). Chichester, UK: Wiley-Blackwell.

Lewis, F. M., Cochrane, B. B., Fletcher, K. A., Zahlis, E. H., Shands, M. E., Gralow, J. R., . . . Schmitz, K. (2008). Helping her heal: A pilot study of an educational counseling intervention for spouses of women with breast cancer. *Psycho-Oncology, 17*(2), 131–137.

Liberati, A., Altman, D. G., Tetzlaff, J., Mulrow, C., Gotzsche, P. C., Ioannidis, J. P., . . . Moher, D. (2009). The PRISMA statement for reporting systematic reviews and meta-analyses of studies that evaluate health care interventions: Explanation and elaboration. *Annals of Internal Medicine, 151*(4), W65–94. doi: 0000605-200908180-0 0136 [pii]

Lichtenthal, W. G., Prigerson, H. G., & Kissane, D. W. (2010). Bereavement: A special issue in oncology. In J. C. Holland (Ed.), *Psycho-Oncology* (Vol. 2, pp. 537–543). New York, NY: Oxford University Press.

Lipsey, M. W., & Wilson, D. B. (1993). The efficacy of psychological, educational, and behavioral treatment: Confirmation from meta-analysis. *American Psychologist, 48*(12), 1181–1209.

Lipsey, M. W., & Wilson, D. B. (2001). *Practical meta-analysis*. Thousand Oaks, CA: Sage.

Loscalzo, M., & Brintzenhofeszoc, K. (1998). Brief crisis counseling. In J. C. Holland (Ed.), *Psycho-Oncology* (pp. 662–675). New York, NY: Oxford University Press.

Low, C. A., Stanton, A. L., Bower, J. E., & Gyllenhammer, L. (2010). A randomized controlled trial of emotionally expressive writing for women with metastatic breast cancer. *Health Psychology, 29*(4), 460–466.

Luborsky, L., Singer, B., & Luborsky, L. (1975). Comparative studies of psychotherapies: Is it true that 'everyone has won and all must have prizes'? *Archives of General Psychiatry, 32*(8), 995–1008.

Lyles, J. N., Burish, T. G., Krozely, M. G., & Oldham, R. K. (1982). Efficacy of relaxation training and guided imagery in reducing the aversiveness of cancer chemotherapy. *Journal of Consulting and Clinical Psychology, 50*(4), 509–524.

Lyman, G. A., & Levine, M. (2012). Comparative effectiveness research in oncology: An Overview. *Journal of Clinical Oncology, 30*(34), 4181–4184.

Maier, T. (2012). Limitations to evidence-based practice. In P. Sturmey & M. Hersen (Eds.), *Handbook of evidence-based practice in clinical psychology* (Vol. 2, pp. 55–69). New York, NY: Wiley.

Manne, S., & Badr, H. (2008). Intimacy and relationship processes in couples' psychosocial adaptation to cancer. *Cancer, 112*(11,Suppl), 2541–2555. doi: 10.1002/cncr.23450

Manne, S. L., Ostroff, J. S., & Winkel, G. (2007). Social-cognitive processes as moderators of a couple-focused group intervention for women with early stage breast cancer. *Health Psychology, 26*(6), 735–744. doi: 10.1037/0278-6133.26.6.735

Manne, S. L., Winkel, G., Zaider, T., Rubin, S., Hernandez, E., & Bergman, C. (2010). Therapy processes and outcomes of psychological interventions for women diagnosed with gynecological cancers: A test of the generic process model of psychotherapy. *Journal of Consulting and Clinical Psychology, 78*(2), 236–248. doi: 10.1037/a0018223

Manne, S. L., & Andrykowski, M. A. (2006). Are psychological interventions effective and accepted by cancer patients? II. Using empirically supported therapy guidelines to decide. *Annals of Behavioral Medicine, 32*(2), 98–103. doi: 10.1207/s15324796abm3202_4

Manne, S. L., Kashy, D. A., Rubin, S., Hernandez, E., & Bergman, C. (2012). Therapist and patient perceptions of alliance and progress in psychological therapy for women diagnosed with gynecological cancers. *Journal of Consulting and Clinical Psychology, 80*(5), 800–810. doi: 10.1037/a0029158.supp

Manne, S. L., Kissane, D. W., Nelson, C. J., Mulhall, J. P., Winkel, G., & Zaider, T. (2011). Intimacy-enhancing psychological intervention for men diagnosed with prostate cancer and their partners: A pilot study. *Journal of Sexual Medicine, 8*(4), 1197–1209. doi: 10.1111/j.1743-6109.2010.02163.x

Manne, S. L., & Ostroff, J. S. (2008a). *Coping with breast cancer: A couples-focused group intervention, therapist guide*. New York, NY: Oxford University Press.

Manne, S. L., & Ostroff, J. S. (2008b). *Coping with breast cancer: Workbook for couples*. New York, NY: Oxford University Press.

Manne, S. L., Ostroff, J. S., Norton, T. R., Fox, K., Goldstein, L., & Grana, G. (2006). Cancer-related relationship communication in couples coping with early stage breast cancer. *Psycho-Oncology, 15*(3), 234–247. doi: 10.1002/pon.941

Manne, S. L., Ostroff, J. S., Winkel, G., Fox, K., Grana, G., Miller, E., . . . Frazier, T. (2005). Couple-focused group intervention for women with early stage breast cancer. *Journal of Consulting and Clinical Psychology, 73*(4), 634–646. doi: 10.1037/0022-006x.73.4.634

Manne, S. L., Rubin, S., Edelson, M., Rosenblum, N., Bergman, C., Hernandez, E., . . . Winkel, G. (2007). Coping and communication-enhancing intervention versus supportive counseling for women diagnosed with gynecological cancers. *Journal of Consulting and Clinical Psychology, 75*(4), 615–628. doi: 10.1037/0022-006X.75.4.615

Manne, S. L., Winkel, G., Rubin, S., Edelson, M., Rosenblum, N., Bergman, C., . . . Rocereto, T. (2008). Mediators of a coping and communication-enhancing intervention and a supportive counseling intervention among women diagnosed with gynecological cancers. *Journal of Consulting and Clinical Psychology, 76*(6), 1034–1045.

Markowitz, J. C., Kocsis, J. H., Bleiberg, K. L., Christos, P. J., & Sacks, M. H. (2005). A comparative trial of psychotherapy and pharmacotherapy for "pure" dysthymic patients. *Journal of Affective Disorders, 89*, 167–175.

Markowitz, J. C., Manber, R., & Rosen, P. (2008). Therapists' responses to training in brief supportive psychotherapy. *American Journal of Psychotherapy, 62*(1), 67–81.

McGlynn, E. A., Asch, S. M., Adams, J., Keesey, J., Hicks, J., DeCristofaro, A., & Kerr, E. A. (2003). The quality of health care delivered to adults in the United States. *New England Journal of Medicine, 348*(26), 2635–2645. doi: 10.1056/NEJMsa022615348/26/2635 [pii]

McHugh, R. K., & Barlow, D. H. (2012a). The reach of evidence-based psychological interventions. In R. K. McHugh & D. H. Barlow (Eds.), *Dissemination and implementation of evidence-based psychological interventions* (pp. 3–15). New York, NY: Oxford University Press.

McHugh, R. K., & Barlow, D. H. (Eds.). (2012b). *Dissemination and implementation of evidence-based psychological interventions*. New York, NY: Oxford University Press.

McHugh, R. K., & Barlow, D. H. (2012c). Training in evidence-based psychological interventions. In R. K. McHugh & D. H. Barlow (Eds.), *Dissemination and implementation of evidence-based psychological interventions* (pp. 43–60). New York, NY: Oxford University Press.

McHugh, R. K., & Barlow, D. H. (2012d). Dissemination and implementation of evidence-based psychological interventions: Current status and future directions. In R. K. McHugh & D. H. Barlow (Eds.), *Dissemination and implementation of evidence-based psychological interventions* (pp. 247–263). New York, NY: Oxford University Press.

McKibbon, A. (1999). *PDQ evidence-based principles and practice*. London: B.C. Decker.

McLean, L. M., & Jones, J. M. (2007). A review of distress and its management in couples facing end-of-life cancer. *Psycho-Oncology, 16*(7), 603–616.

McLean, L. M., Jones, J. M., Rydall, A. C., Walsh, A., Esplen, M. J., Zimmermann, C., & Rodin, G. M. (2008). A couples intervention for patients facing advanced cancer and their spouse caregivers: Outcomes of a pilot study. *Psycho-Oncology, 17*(11), 1152–1156. doi: 10.1002/pon.1319

McLean, L. M., & Nissim, R. (2007). Marital therapy for couples facing advanced cancer: Case review. *Palliat Support Care, 5*(3), 303–313.

McLean, L. M., Walton, T., Rodin, G., Esplen, M. J., & Jones, J. M. (2011). A couple-based intervention for patients and caregivers facing end-stage cancer: Outcomes of a randomized controlled trial. *Psycho-Oncology*. doi: 10.1002/pon.2046

McLeroy, K. R., Bibeau, D., Steckler, A., & Glanz, K. (1988). An ecological perspective on health promotion programs. *Health Education Quarterly, 15*(4), 351–377.

McMillan, S. C., Small, B. J., Weitzner, M., Schonwetter, R., Tittle, M., Moody, L., & Haley, W. E. (2006). Impact of coping skills intervention with family caregivers of hospice patients with cancer: A randomized clinical trial. *Cancer, 106*(1), 214–222. doi: 10.1002/cncr.21567

McQuaid, E. L., & Nassau, J. H. (1999). Empirically supported treatments of disease-related symptoms in pediatric psychology: Asthma, diabetes, and cancer. *Journal of Pediatric Psychology, 24*(4), 305–328.

McQuellon, R. P., Wells, M., Hoffman, S., Craven, B., Russell, G., Cruz, J., . . . Savage, P. (1998). Reducing distress in cancer patients with an orientation program. *Psycho-Oncology, 7*(3), 207–217.

Medscape. (2014). *eMedicine*. Retrieved February 8, 2014, from http://emedicine.medscape.com/

Meehl, P. E. (1954). *Clinical versus statistical prediction: A theoretical analysis and a review of the evidence*. Minneapolis: University of Minnesota Press.

Meijer, A., Roseman, M., Milette, K., Coyne, J. C., Stefanek, M. E., Ziegelstein, R. C., . . . Thombs, B. D. (2011). Depression screening and patient outcomes in cancer: A systematic review. *PLoS ONE, 6*(11). doi: 10.1371/journal.pone.0027181

Merckaert, I., Libert, Y., Messin, S., Milani, M., Slachmuylder, J. L., & Razavi, D. (2010). Cancer patients' desire for psychological support: Prevalence and implications for screening patients' psychological needs. *Psycho-Oncology, 19*(2), 141–149. doi: 10.1002/pon.1568

Meyer, T. J., & Mark, M. M. (1995). Effects of psychosocial interventions with adult cancer patients: A meta-analysis of randomized experiments. *Health Psychology, 14*(2), 101–108.

Meyers, F. J., Carducci, M., Loscalzo, M. J., Linder, J., Greasby, T., & Beckett, L. A. (2011). Effects of a problem-solving intervention (COPE) on quality of life for patients with advanced cancer on clinical trials and their caregivers: Simultaneous care educational intervention (SCEI): Linking palliation and clinical trials. *Journal of Palliative Medicine, 14*(4), 465–473. doi: 10.1089/jpm.2010.0416

Miller, B. F., Kessler, R., & Peek, C. J. (2011). *A national agenda for research in collaborative care: Papers from the Collaborative Care Research Network Research Development Conference.* (Publication No. 11-0067). Rockville, MD: Agency for Healthcare Research and Quality

Miller, S. D., & Duncan, B. L. (2004). *The outcome and session rating scales: Administration and scoring manual.* Chicago, IL: Institute for the Study of Therapeutic Change.

Miller, W. R., & Rollnick, S. (2002). *Motivational interviewing: Preparing people for change* (2nd ed.). New York, NY: Guilford Press.

Minami, T., Wampold, B. E., Serlin, R. C., Hamilton, E. G., Brown, G. S., & Kircher, J. C. (2008). Benchmarking the effectiveness of psychotherapy treatment for adult depression in a managed care environment: A preliminary study. *Journal of Consulting and Clinical Psychology, 76*(1), 116–124.

Mishel, M. H. (1990). Reconceptualization of the uncertainty in illness theory. *Image: Journal of Nursing Scholarship, 22*(4), 256–262.

Mishel, M. H., Germino, B. B., Gil, K. M., Belyea, M., Laney, I. C., Stewart, J., . . . Clayton, M. (2005). Benefits from an uncertainty management intervention for African-American and Caucasian older long-term breast cancer survivors. *Psycho-Oncology, 14*(11), 962–978. doi: 10.1002/pon.909

Mitchell, A. J. (2007). Pooled results from 38 analyses of the accuracy of distress thermometer and other ultra-short methods of detecting cancer-related mood disorders. *Journal of Clinical Oncology, 25*(29), 4670–4681. doi: JCO.2006.10.0438 [pii]10.1200/JCO.2006.10.0438

Mitchell, A. J. (2010a). Short screening tools for cancer-related distress: A review and diagnostic validity meta-analysis. *Journal of the National Comprehensiv Cancer Network, 8*(4), 487–494. doi: 8/4/487 [pii]

Mitchell, A. J. (2010b). Screening procedures for psychosocal distress. In J. C. Holland, W. Breitbart, P. B. Jacobsen, M. Lederberg, M. Loscalzo, & R. McCorkle (Eds.), *Psycho-Oncology* (2nd ed., pp. 389–396). New York, NY: Oxford University Press.

Moher, D., Liberati, A., Tetzlaff, J., & Altman, D. G. (2009). Preferred reporting items for systematic reviews and meta-analyses: The PRISMA statement. *Annals of Internal Medicine, 151*(4), 264–269, W264. doi: 0000605-200908180-00135 [pii]

Mokuau, N., Braun, K. L., Wong, L. K., Higuchi, P., & Gotay, C. C. (2008). Development of a family intervention for Native Hawaiian women with cancer: A pilot study. *Social Work, 53*(1), 9–19.

Moorey, S., Greer, S., Bliss, J., & Law, M. (1998). A comparison of adjuvant psychological therapy and supportive counselling in patients with cancer. *Psycho-Oncology, 7*(3), 218–228. doi: 10.1002/(SICI)1099-1611(199805/06)7:3<218::AID-PON308>3.0.CO;2-D

Morrow, G. R., & Morrell, C. (1982). Behavioral treatment for the anticipatory nausea and vomiting induced by cancer chemotherapy. *New England Journal of Medicine, 307*(24), 1476–1480. doi: 10.1056/NEJM198212093072402

Morrow, G. R., Roscoe, J. A., Kirshner, J. J., Hynes, H. E., & Rosenbluth, R. J. (1998). Anticipatory nausea and vomiting in the era of 5-HT3 antiemetics. *Supportive Care in Cancer, 6*(3), 244–247.

Morrow, G. R., & Rosenthal, S. N. (1996). Models, mechanisms and management of anticipatory nausea and emesis. *Oncology, 53*(Suppl 1), 4–7.

Mueser, K. T., Torrey, W. C., Lynde, D., Singer, P., & Drake, R. E. (2003). Implementing evidence-based practices for people with severe mental illness. *Behavior Modification, 27*, 387–411.

Mulcrow, D. D., & Oxman, A. D. (1997). *Cochrane collaboration handbook*. Oxford, UK: Oxford University Press.

Nathan, P. E., & Gorman, J. M. (1998). *A guide to treatments that work*. New York, NY: Oxford University Press.

Nathan, P. E., & Gorman, J. M. (2002). *A guide to treatments that work* (2nd ed.). New York, NY: Oxford University Press.

Nathan, P. E., & Gorman, J. M. (2007). *A guide to treatments that work* (3rd ed.). New York, NY: Oxford University Press.

National Association of Social Work (NASW). (2007). Evidence-based practice. Retrieved 12/23/2009, 2009, from http://www.socialworkers.org/research/naswresearch/0108evidencebased/default.asp

National Breast Cancer Centre and National Cancer Control Initiative. (2003). *Clinical practice guidelines for the psychosocial care of adults with cancer*. Retrieved May 6, 2015 from http://www.nhmrc.gov.au/guidelines-publications/cp90

National Comprehensive Cancer Network. (2014). *NCCN clinical practice guidelines in oncology for distress management*. Retrieved February 10, 2014, from http://www.nccn.org/professionals/physician_gls/f_guidelines.asp#supportive

National Consensus Project for Quality Palliative Care. (2009). Clinical practice guidelines for quality palliative care. In National Consensus Project for Quality Palliative Care (Ed.) (2nd ed.). Pittsburgh, PA.

National Institute for Clinical Excellence. (2004). *Improving supportive and palliative care for adults with cancer. The Manual*. London: National Institute for Clinical Excellence (NICE).

National Quality Forum. (2006). *A national framework and preferred practices for palliative and hospice care quality*. Washington, DC: Retrieved April 22, 2015, from http://www.qualityforum.org/Publications/2006/12/A_National_Framework_and_Preferred_Practices_for_Palliative_and_Hospice_Care_Quality.aspx

Newell, S. A., Sanson-Fisher, R. W., & Savolainen, N. J. (2002). Systematic review of psychological therapies for cancer patients: overview and recommendations for future research. *Journal of the National Cancer Institute, 94*(8), 558–584.

Nezu, A. M., Nezu, C. M., Friedman, S. H., Faddis, S., Houts, P. S. (1999). *Helping cancer patients cope: A problem-solving approach*. Washington, DC: American Psychological Association.

Nezu, A. M., Nezu, C. M., Felgoise, S. H., McClure, K. S., & Houts, P. S. (2003). Project Genesis: Assessing the efficacy of problem-solving therapy for distressed adult cancer patients. *Journal of Consulting and Clinical Psychology, 71*(6), 1036–1048. doi: 10.1037/0022-006x.71.6.1036

Nicholas, D. R. (1982). Prevalence of anticipatory nausea and emesis in cancer chemotherapy patients. *Journal of Behavioral Medicine, 5*(4), 461–463.

Nicholas, D. R., Aegisdottir, S., & Kruczek, T. (2006). Cultural and family issues. In M. J. Fisch & A. W. Burton (Eds.), *Cancer pain management* (pp. 163–175). New York, NY: McGraw Hill.

Nicholas, D. R., & Veach, T. A. (2000). The psychosocial assessment of the adult cancer patient. *Professional Psychology: Research and Practice, 31*(2), 206–215.

Norcross, J. C. (2002). *Psychotherapy relationships that work: Therapist contributions and responsiveness to patients.* New York, NY: Oxford University Press.

Norcross, J. C. (2011). *Psychotherapy relationships that work.* (2nd ed.). New York, NY: Oxford University Press.

Norcross, J. C., Hogan, T. P., & Koocher, G. P. (2008). *Clinician's guide to evidence-based practices: Mental health and the addictions.* New York, NY: Oxford University Press.

Norcross, J. C., Krebs, P. M., & Prochaska, J. O. (2011). Stages of change. *Journal of Clinical Psychology, 67*(2), 143–154.

Norcross, J. C., & Lambert, M. J. (2011). Evidence-based therapy relationships. In J. C. Norcross (Ed.), *Psychotherapy relationships that work* (2nd ed., pp. 3–21). New York, NY: Oxford University Press.

Northouse, L., Kershaw, T., Mood, D., & Schafenacker, A. (2005). Effects of a family intervention on the quality of life of women with recurrent breast cancer and their family caregivers. *Psycho-Oncology, 14*(6), 478–491. doi: 10.1002/pon.871

Northouse, L. L., & McCorkle, R. (2010). Spouse caregivers of cancer patients. In J. C. Holland (Ed.), *Psycho-Oncology* (pp. 516–521). New York, NY: Oxford University Press.

Northouse, L. L., Mood, D. W., Schafenacker, A., Montie, J. E., Sandler, H. M., Forman, J. D., . . . Kershaw, T. (2007). Randomized clinical trial of a family intervention for prostate cancer patients and their spouses. *Cancer, 110*(12), 2809–2818.

Novalis, P. N., Rojcewicz, S. J., & Peele, R. (1993). *Clinical manual of supportive psychotherapy.* Washington, DC: American Psychiatric Press.

O'Connor, A. M., Bennett, C. L., Stacey, D., Barry, M., Col, N. F., Eden, K. B., . . . Rovner, D. (2009). Decision aids for people facing health treatment or screening decisions. *Cochrane Database of Systematic Reviews, 3,* CD001431.

O'Hara, R. E., Hull, J. G., Lyons, K. D., Bakitas, M., Hegel, M. T., Li, Z., & Ahles, T. A. (2010). Impact on caregiver burden of a patient-focused palliative care intervention for patients with advanced cancer. *Palliative and Supportive Care, 8*(4), 395–404.

Ogles, B. M, Lambert, M. J., & Fields, S. A. (2002). *Essentials of outcome assessment.* Chichester, UK: Wiley.

Oncology Nursing Society. (2008a). *Putting evidence into practice (PEP): Anxiety.* Retrieved February 9, 2014, from http://www2.ons.org/Research/PEP/Anxiety

Oncology Nursing Society. (2008b). *Putting evidence into practice (PEP): Depression.* Retrieved February 9, 2014, from http://www2.ons.org/Research/PEP/Depression.

Oncology Nursing Society (ONS). (2009). Putting evidence into practice (PEP). Retrieved May 6, 2015 from https://www.ons.org/practice-resources/pep

OQ Measures. (2004). *OQ-Analyst user's guide.* Retrieved April 18, 2010, from http://www.oqmeasures.com/products/oq-analyst/

Orlinsky, D. E., & Howard, K. (1987). A generic model of psychotherapy. *Journal of Integrative and Eclectic Psychotherapy, 6,* 6–27.

Osborn, R. L., Demoncada, A. C., & Feuerstein, M. (2006). Psychosocial interventions for depression, anxiety, and quality of life in cancer survivors: Meta-analyses. *International Journal of Psychiatry in Medicine, 36*(1), 13–34.

Ost, L. G. (1987). Applied relaxation: Description of a coping technique and review of controlled studies. *Behaviour Research and Therapy, 25*(5), 397–409. doi: 10.1016/0005-7967(87)90017-9

Overington, L., & Ionita, G. (2012). Progress monitoring measures: A brief guide. *Canadian Psychology/Psychologie Canadienne, 53*(2), 82–92. doi: 10.1037/a0028017

Owen, J. E., Bantum, E. O., & Golant, M. (2009). Benefits and challenges experienced by professional facilitators of online support groups for cancer survivors. *Psycho-Oncology, 18*(2), 144–155.

Paul, G. L. (1967). Strategy of outcome research in psychotherapy. *Journal of Consulting Psychology*, 31(2), 109–118.

Park, C. L., & Folkman, S. (1997). Meaning in the context of stress and coping. *Review of General Psychology, 1*(2), 115–144. doi: 10.1037/1089-2680.1.2.115

Patel, D., Sharpe, L., Thewes, B., Bell, M. L., & Clarke, S. (2011). Using the Distress Thermometer and Hospital Anxiety and Depression Scale to screen for psychosocial morbidity in patients diagnosed with colorectal cancer. *Journal of Affective Disorders, 131*(1-3), 412–416. doi: 10.1016/j.jad.2010.11.014

Penedo, F. J., Molton, I., Dahn, J. R., Shen, B. J., Kinsinger, D., Traeger, L., . . . Antoni, M. (2006). A randomized clinical trial of group-based cognitive-behavioral stress management in localized prostate cancer: Development of stress management skills improves quality of life and benefit finding. *Annals of Behavioral Medicine, 31*(3), 261–270. doi: 10.1207/s15324796abm3103_8

Penedo, F. J., Traeger, L., Dahn, J. R., Molton, I., Gonzalez, J. S., Schneiderman, N., & Antoni, M. H. (2007). Cognitive behavioral stress management intervention improves quality of life in Spanish monolingual Hispanic men treated for localized prostate cancer: Results of a randomized controlled trial. *International Journal of Behavioral Medicine, 14*(3), 164–172.

Persons, J. B. (2005). Empiricism, mechanism, and the practice of cognitive-behavior therapy. *Behavior Therapy, 36*(2), 107–118.

Pinsker, H. (1997). *A primer of supportive psychotherapy*. Hillsdale, NJ: Analytic Press.

Pirl, W. F. (2010). Instruments in psycho-oncology. In J. C. Holland, W. Breitbart, P. B. Jacobsen, M. Lederberg, M. Loscalzo, & R. Mccorkle (Eds.), *Psycho-Oncology* (pp. 119–130). New York, NY: Oxford University Press.

Pitceathly, C., Maguire, P., Fletcher, I., Parle, M., Tomenson, B., & Creed, F. (2009). Can a brief psychological intervention prevent anxiety or depressive disorders in cancer patients? A randomised controlled trial. *Annals of Oncology, 20*(5), 928–934.

Plass, A., & Koch, U. (2001). Participation of oncological outpatients in psychosocial support. *Psycho-Oncology, 10*(6), 511–520. doi: 10.1002/pon.543 [pii]

Porter, J. F., Spates, C. R., & Smitham, S. (2004). Behavioral activation group therapy in public mental health settings: A pilot investigation. *Professional Psychology: Research and Practice, 35*(3), 297–301.

Porter, L. S., Keefe, F. J., Baucom, D. H., Hurwitz, H., Moser, B., Patterson, E., & Kim, H. J. (2009). Partner-assisted emotional disclosure for patients with gastrointestinal cancer: Results from a randomized controlled trial. *Cancer, 115*(18 Suppl), 4326–4338.

Porter, L. S., Keefe, F. J., Baucom, D. H., Hurwitz, H., Moser, B., Patterson, E., & Kim, H. J. (2012). Partner-assisted emotional disclosure for patients with GI cancer: 8-week follow-up and processes associated with change. *Supportive Care in Cancer, 20*(8), 1755–1762.

Prigerson, H. G., Maciejewski, P. K., Reynolds, C. F., 3rd, Bierhals, A. J., Newsom, J. T., Fasiczka, A., . . . Miller, M. (1995). Inventory of Complicated Grief: A scale to measure maladaptive symptoms of loss. *Psychiatry Research, 59*(1-2), 65–79.

Prochaska, J. O., & DiClemente, C. C. (2005). The transtheoretical approach. In J. C. Norcross & M. R. Goldfried (Eds.), *Handbook of psychotherapy integration* (2nd ed., pp. 147–171). New York, NY: Oxford University Press.

Rait, D., & Lederberg, M. S. (1990). The family of the cancer patient. In J. C. Holland & J. H. Rowland (Eds.), *Handbook of psychooncology* (pp. 585–598). New York, NY: Oxford University Press.

Rakovshik, S. G., & McManus, F. (2010). Establishing evidence-based training in cognitive behavioral therapy: A review of current empirical findings and theoretical guidance. *Clinical Psychology Review, 30*(5), 496–516. doi: 10.1016/j.cpr.2010.03.004

Rawl, S. M., Given, B. A., Given, C. W., Champion, V. L., Kozachik, S. L., Barton, D., . . . Williams, S. D. (2002). Intervention to improve psychological functioning for newly diagnosed patients with cancer. *Oncology Nursing Forum, 29*(6), 967–975.

Redd, W. H., Andresen, G. V., & Minagawa, R. Y. (1982). Hypnotic control of anticipatory emesis in patients receiving cancer chemotherapy. *Journal of Consulting and Clinical Psychology, 50*(1), 14–19.

Redd, W. H., & Andrykowski, M. A. (1982). Behavioral intervention in cancer treatment: Controlling aversion reactions to chemotherapy. *Journal of Consulting and Clinical Psychology, 50*(6), 1018–1029. doi: 10.1037/0022-006x.50.6.1018

Redd, W. H., Montgomery, G. H., & DuHamel, K. N. (2001). Behavioral intervention for cancer treatment side effects. *Journal of the National Cancer Institute, 93*(11), 810–823.

Rehse, B., & Pukrop, R. (2003). Effects of psychosocial interventions on quality of life in adult cancer patients: Meta analysis of 37 published controlled outcome studies. *Patient Education and Counseling, 50*(2), 179–186.

Rodolfa, E., Bent, R., E., E., Nelson, P., Rehm, L., & Ritchie, P. (2005). A cube model for competency development: Implications for psychology educators and regulators. *Professional Psychology: Research and Practice, 36*(4), 347–354.

Rogers, C. R. (1961). *On becoming a person: A therapist's view of psychotherapy*. Boston, MA: Houghton Mifflin.

Rolland, J. S. (2005). Cancer and the family: An integrative model. *Cancer, 104*(11 Suppl), 2584–2595.

Roscoe, J. A., Morrow, G. R., Hickok, J. T., Mustian, K. M., & Shelke, A. R. (2004). Biobehavioral factors in chemotherapy-induced nausea and vomiting. *Journal of the National Comprehensive Cancer Network, 2*(5), 501–508.

Rowland, J. H. (1989). Developmental stage and adaptation: Adult model. In J. C. Holland & J. H. Rowland (Eds.), *Handbook of psycho-oncology: Psychological care of the patient with cancer* (pp. 44–57). New York, NY: Oxford University Press.

Rubin, A., & Bellamy, J. (2012). *Practitioner's guide to using research for evidence-based practice.* (2nd ed.). Hoboken, NJ: Wiley.

Ruscio, A. M., & Holohan, D. R. (2006). Applying empirically supported treatments to complex cases: Ethical, empirical, and practical considerations. *Clinical Psychology: Science and Practice, 13*(2), 146–162. doi: 10.1111/j.1468-2850.2006.00017.x

Ruzek, J. I., Karlin, B. E., & Zeiss, A. (2012). Implementation of evidence-based psychological treatment in the Veterans Health Administration. In G. McHugh & D. H. Barlow (Eds.), *Dissemination and implementation of evidence-based psychological interventions* (pp. 78–96). New York, NY: Oxford University Press.

Sackett, D. L., Rosenberg, W. M., Gray, J. A., Haynes, R. B., & Richardson, W. S. (1996). Evidence based medicine: What it is and what it isn't. *British Medical Journal, 312*(7023), 71–72.

Sackett, D. L., Straus, S. E., Richardson, W. S., Rosenberg, W. M., & Haynes, R. B. (2000). *Evidence based medicine: How to practice and teach EBM*. London, UK: Churchill Livingstone.

Satterfield, J. M., Spring, B., Brownson, R. C., Mullen, E. J., Newhouse, R. P., Walker, B. B., & Whitlock, E. P. (2009). Toward a transdisciplinary model of evidence-based practice. *Milbank Quarterly, 87*(2), 368–390.

Savard, J., Simard, S., Giguere, I., Ivers, H., Morin, C. M., Maunsell, E., . . . Marceau, D. (2006). Randomized clinical trial on cognitive therapy for depression in women with metastatic breast cancer: Psychological and immunological effects. *Palliative and Supportive Care, 4*(3), 219–237.

Scheier, M. F., Helgeson, V. S., Schulz, R., Colvin, S., Berga, S., Bridges, M. W., . . . Pappert, W. S. (2005). Interventions to enhance physical and psychological functioning among younger women who are ending nonhormonal adjuvant treatment for early-stage breast cancer. *Journal of Clinical Oncology, 23*(19), 4298–4311.

Schildmann, E. K., & Higginson, I. J. (2011). Evaluating psycho-educational interventions for informal carers of patients receiving cancer care or palliative care: Strengths and limitations of different study designs. *Palliative Medicine, 25*(4), 345–356.

Schnur, J. B., & Montgomery, G. H. (2010). A systematic review of therapeutic alliance, group cohesion, empathy, and goal consensus/collaboration in psychotherapeutic interventions in cancer: Uncommon factors? *Clinical Psychology Review, 30*(2), 238–247.

Schoenwald, S. K. (2012). The transport and diffusion of multisystemic therapy. In G. McHugh & D. H. Barlow (Eds.), *Dissemination and implementation of evidence-based psychological interventions* (pp. 227–246). New York, NY: Oxford University Press.

Schoenwald, S. K., McHugh, K., & Barlow, David H. (2012). The science of dissemination and implementation. In R. K. McHugh & D. H. Barlow (Eds.), *Dissemination and implementation of evidence-based psychological interventions*. (pp. 16–42). New York, NY: Oxford University Press.

Schulz, K. F., Altman, D. G., & Moher, D. (2010). CONSORT 2010 statement: Updated guidelines for reporting parallel group randomized trials. *Annals of Internal Medicine, 152*(11), 726–732. doi: 0003-4819-152-11-201006010-00232 [pii]10.1059/0003-4819-152-11-201006010-00232

Scott, J. L., Halford, W. K., & Ward, B. G. (2004). United we stand? The effects of a couple-coping Intervention on adjustment to early stage breast or gynecological cancer. *Journal of Consulting and Clinical Psychology, 72*(6), 1122–1135. doi: 10.1037/0022-006x.72.6.1122

Scott, J. L., & Kayser, K. (2009). A review of couple-based interventions for enhancing women's sexual adjustment and body image after cancer. *Cancer Journal, 15*(1), 48–56. doi: 10.1097/PPO.0b013e31819585df

Scott, N. W., McPherson, G. C., Ramsay, C. R., & Campbell, M. K. (2002). The method of minimization for allocation to clinical trials: A review. *Controlled Clinical Trials, 23*(6), 662–674. doi: S0197245602002428 [pii]

Shadish, W. R., Matt, G. E., Navarro, A. M., Siegle, G., Crits-Christoph, P., Hazelrigg, M. D., . . . Weiss, B. (1997). Evidence that therapy works in clincally representative conditions. *Journal of Consulting and Clinical Psychology, 65*(3), 355–365.

Shadish, W. R., Navarro, A. M., Matt, G. E., & Phillips, G. (2000). The effects of psychological therapies under clinically representative conditions: A meta-analysis. *Psychological Bulletin, 126*(4), 512–529.

Shapiro, J. P. (2009). Integrating outcome research and clinical reasoning in psychotherapy planning. *Professional Psychology: Research and Practice, 40*(1), 46–53. doi: 10.1037/a0012596

Shear, K., Frank, E., Houck, P. R., & Reynolds, C. F. (2005). Treatment of complicated grief: A randomized controlled trial. *Journal of the American Medical Association, 293*(21), 2601–2608. doi: 10.1001/jama.293.21.2601

Sheard, T., & Maguire, P. (1999). The effect of psychological interventions on anxiety and depression in cancer patients: Results of two meta-analyses. *British Journal of Cancer, 80*(11), 1770–1780.

Sheldon, L. K., Swanson, S., Dolce, A., Marsh, K., & Summers, J. (2008). Putting evidence into practice: Evidence-based interventions for anxiety. *Clinical Journal of Oncology Nursing, 12*(5), 789–797.

Shimokawa, K., Lambert, M. J., & Smart, D. W. (2010). Enhancing treatment outcome of patients at risk of treatment failure: Meta-analytic and mega-analytic review of a psychotherapy quality assurance system. *Journal of Consulting and Clinical Psychology, 78*(3), 298–311.

Siegel, R., Ma, J., Zou, Z., & Jemal, A. (2014). Cancer statistics, 2014. *CA: A Cancer Journal for Clinicians, 64*(1), 9–29. doi: 10.3322/caac.21208

Simpson, J. A., Carlson, L. E., & Trew, M. E. (2001). Effect of group therapy for breast cancer on healthcare utilization. *Cancer Practice, 9*(1), 19–26. doi: 10.1046/j.1523-5394.2001.91005.x

Sjoqvist, S. (2007). On the history of supportive therapy. *Nordic Psychology, 59*(2), 181–188.

Smith, M. L., & Glass, G. V. (1977). Meta-analysis of psychotherapy outcome studies. *American Psychologist, 32*, 752–760.

Spanier, G. B., & Filsinger, E. E. (1983). The dyadic adjustment scale. In E. E. Filsinger (Ed.), *Marriage and family assessment: A sourcebook for family therapy.* (2nd ed., pp. 155–168). Beverly Hills, CA: Sage.

Spencer, S. M., Carver, C. S., & Price, A. A. (1998). Psychological and social factors in adaptation. In J. C. Holland (Ed.), *Psycho-Oncology* (pp. 211–222). New York, NY: Oxford University Press.

Spengler, P. M., Strohmer, D. C., Dixon, D. N., & Shivy, V. A. (1995). A scientist-practitioner model of psychological assessment: Implications for training, practice and research. *Counseling Psychologist, 23*(3), 506–534.

Spiegel, D. (2012). Mind matters in cancer survival. *Psycho-Oncology, 21*(6), 588–593. doi: 10.1002/pon.3067

Spiegel, D., Bloom, J. R., Kraemer, H. C., & Gottheil, E. (1989). Effect of psychosocial treatment on survival of patients with metastatic breast cancer. *Lancet, 2*(8668), 888–891.

Spiegel, D., Butler, L. D., Giese-Davis, J., Koopman, C., Miller, E., DiMiceli, S., . . . Kraemer, H. C. (2007). Effects of supportive-expressive group therapy on survival of patients with metastatic breast cancer: A randomized prospective trial. *Cancer, 110*(5), 1130–1138. doi: 10.1002/cncr.22890

Spiegel, D., & Classen, C. (2000). *Group therapy for cancer patients: A research-based handbook of psychosocial care.* New York, NY: Basic Books.

Spiegel, D., & Spira, J. (1991). *Supportive-expressive group therapy: A treatment manual of psychosocial intervention for women with recurrent breast cancer.* Stanford, CA: Stanfod University School of Medicine.

Spira, J. L., & Casden, D. R. (2010). Group psychotherapy for persons with cancer. In J. C. Holland, W. Breitbart, P. B. Jacobsen, M. S. Lederberg, M. Loscalzo, & R.

McCorkle (Eds.), *Psycho-Oncology* (2nd ed., pp. 408–414). New York, NY: Oxford University Press.

Spitzer, R. L., Kroenke, K., & Williams, J. B. (1999). Validation and utility of a self-report version of PRIME-MD: The PHQ primary care study. Primary care evaluation of mental disorders. Patient health questionnaire. *Journal of the American Medical Association, 282*(18), 1737–1744. doi: joc90770 [pii]

Spitzer, R. L., Williams, J. B., Gibbon, M., & First, M. B. (1992). The Structured Clinical Interview for DSM-III-R (SCID). I: History, rationale, and description. *Archives of General Psychiatry, 49*(8), 624–629.

Spring, B. (2007). Evidence-based practice in clinical psychology: What it is: Why it matters: What you need to know. *Journal of Clinical Psychology, 63*(7), 611–631.

Spring, B., Pagoto, S., Kaufmann, P. G., Whitlock, E. P., Glasgow, R. E., Smith, T. W., . . . Davidson, K. W. (2005). Invitation to a dialogue between researchers and clinicians about evidence-based behavioral medicine. *Annals of Behavioral Medicine, 30*(2), 125–137. doi: 10.1207/s15324796abm3002_5

Stanton, A. L., Danoff-Burg, S., Sworowski, L. A., Collins, C. A., Branstetter, A. D., Rodriguez-Hanley, A., . . . Austenfeld, J. L. (2002). Randomized, controlled trial of written emotional expression and benefit finding in breast cancer patients. *Journal of Clinical Oncology, 20*(20), 4160–4168.

Stehl, M. L., Kazak, A. E., Alderfer, M. A., Rodriguez, A., Hwang, W. T., Pai, A. L. H., . . . Reilly, A. (2009). Conducting a randomized clinical trial of a psychological intervention for parents/caregivers of children with cancer shortly after diagnosis. *Journal of Pediatric Psychology, 34*(8), 803–816.

Steketee, G. S. (1996). *Treatment of obsessive compulsive disorder.* New York, NY: Guilford Press.

Stephen, J. E., Christie, G., Flood, K., Golant, M., Rahn, M., Rennie, H., . . . Turner, J. (2011). Facilitating online support groups for cancer patients: The learning experience of psycho-oncology clinicians. *Psycho-Oncology, 20*(8), 832–840. doi: 10.1002/pon.1791

Straus, S. E., Richardson, W. S., Glasziou, P., & Haynes, R. B. (2005). *Evidence-based medicine: How to practice and teach EBM* (3rd ed.). Edinburgh, UK: Elsevier.

Straus, S. E., Tetroe, J., & Graham, I. (2009). Defining knowledge translation. *CMAJ, 181*(3-4), 165–168. doi: cmaj.081229 [pii]10.1503/cmaj.081229

Stricker, G., & Trierweiler, S. J. (1995). The local clinical scientist: A bridge between science and practice. *American Psychologist, 50*(12), 995–1002.

Stroebe, M., & Schut, H. (1999). The dual process model of coping with bereavement: Rationale and description. *Death Studies, 23*(3), 197–224. doi: 10.1080/074811899201046

Strong, V., Waters, R., Hibberd, C., Murray, G., Wall, L., Walker, J., . . . Sharpe, M. (2008). Management of depression for people with cancer (SMaRT oncology 1): A randomised trial. *Lancet, 372*(9632), 40–48. doi: S0140-6736(08)60991-5 [pii] 10.1016/S0140-6736(08)60991-5

Strong, V., Waters, R., Hibberd, C., Rush, R., Cargill, A., Storey, D., . . . Sharpe, M. (2007). Emotional distress in cancer patients: The Edinburgh Cancer Centre symptom study. *British Journal of Cancer, 96*(6), 868–874. doi: 10.1038/sj.bjc.6603626

Stroup, D. F., Berlin, J. A., Morton, S. C., Olkin, I., Williamson, G. D., Rennie, D., . . . Thacker, S. B. (2000). Meta-analysis of observational studies in epidemiology: A proposal for reporting. Meta-analysis of Observational Studies in Epidemiology (MOOSE) group. *Journal of the American Medical Association, 283*(15), 2008–2012. doi: jst00003 [pii]

Substance Abuse Mental Health Systems Administration (SAMHSA). (n.d.). *National registry of evidence-based programs and practices (NREPP).* Retrieved December 20, 2014, from http://www.nrepp.samhsa.gov/

Sue, D. W. (2001). Multidimensional facets of cultural competence. *The Counseling Psychologist, 29*(6), 790–821.

SUMSearch. (2014). [online database]. Retrieved February 8, 2014, from http://www.sumsearch.org

Taylor, S. E., Falke, R. L., Shoptaw, S. J., & Lichtman, R. R. (1986). Social support, support groups, and the cancer patient. *Journal of Consulting and Clinical Psychology, 54*(5), 608–615. doi: 10.1037/0022-006x.54.5.608

Thornicroft, G., Lempp, H., & Tansella, M. (2011). The place of implementation science in the translational medicine continuum. *Psychological Medicine, 41*(10), 2015–2021. doi: 10.1017/s0033291711000109

Trierweiler, S. J., & Stricker, G. (1998). *The scientific practice of professional psychology.* New York, NY: Plenum Press.

TRIP database. (2014). [database online]. Retrieved February 8, 2014, from http://www.tripdatabase.com/

Tuinman, M. A., Gazendam-Donofrio, S. M., & Hoekstra-Weebers, J. E. (2008). Screening and referral for psychosocial distress in oncologic practice: Use of the distress thermometer. *Cancer, 113*, 870–878.

Turnbull, G., Baldassarre, F., Brown, P., Hatton-Bauer, J., Li, M., & Lebel, S. (2012). *Psychosocial health care for cancer patients and their families.* (Program in evidence-based care evidence-based series number 19-3). Toronto, ON: Cancer Care Ontario.

UpToDate. (2014). [database online]. Retrieved February 3, 2014, from Wolters Kluwer Health http://www.uptodate.com/home

Valentine, A. D. (2010). Central nervous system tumors. In J. C. Holland, W. Breitbart, P. B. Jacobsen, M. Lederberg, M. Loscalzo, & R. McCorkle (Eds.), *Psycho-Oncology* (pp. 131–134). New York, NY: Oxford University Press.

van Scheppingen, C., Schroevers, M. J., Smink, A., van der Linden, Y. M., Mul, V. E., Langendijk, J. A., . . . Sanderman, R. (2011). Does screening for distress efficiently uncover meetable unmet needs in cancer patients? *Psycho-Oncology, 20*, 655–663. doi: 10.1002/pon.1939

VandeCreek, L., Knapp, S., & Brace, K. (1990). Mandatory continuing education-for licensed psychologists: Its rationale and current implementation. *Professional Psychology: Research and Practice, 21*(2), 135–140. doi: 10.1037/0735-7028.21.2.135

Veach, T. A., Nicholas, D. R., & Barton, M. A. (2002). *Cancer and the family life cycle.* New York, NY: Brunner-Routledge.

von Bertalanffy, L. (1968). *General systems theory.* New York, NY: George Braziller.

von Elm, E., Altman, D. G., Egger, M., Pocock, S. J., Gotzsche, P. C., Vandenbroucke, J. P., & STROBE Initiative. (2007). The Strengthening the Reporting of Observational Studies in Epidemiology (STROBE) statement: Guidelines for reporting observational studies. *Annals of Internal Medicine, 147*(8), 573–577.

Walsh, F. (2003). Family resilience: A framework for clinical practice. *Family Process, 42*(1), 1–18. doi: 10.1111/j.1545-5300.2003.00001.x

Walsh, K., Jones, L., Tookman, A., Mason, C., McLoughlin, J., Blizard, R., & King, M. (2007). Reducing emotional distress in people caring for patients receiving specialist palliative care. Randomised trial. *British Journal of Psychiatry, 190*, 142–147.

Wampold, B. E. (2008). *The great psychotherapy debate: Models, methods, and findings.* New York, NY: Routledge.

Wampold, B. E., Mondin, G. W., Moody, M., Stich, F., Benson, K., & Ahn, H. (1997). A meta-analysis of outcome studies comparing bona fide psychotherapies: Empiricially, "all must have prizes." *Psychological Bulletin, 122*(3), 203–215.

Watson, M., & Kissane, D. (2011). *Handbook of psychotherapy in cancer care.* Chicester, UK: Wiley-Blackwell.

Weir, H. K., Thun, M. J., Hankey, B. F., Ries, L. A., Howe, H. L., Wingo, P. A., . . . Edwards, B. K. (2003). Annual report to the nation on the status of cancer, 1975-2000, featuring the uses of surveillance data for cancer prevention and control. *Journal of the National Cancer Institute, 95*(17), 1276–1299.

Weisman, A. D., & Worden, J. W. (1976). The existential plight in cancer: Significance of the first 100 days. *International Journal of Psychiatry in Medicine, 7*(1), 1–15.

Weissman, M. M., Markowitz, J. C., & Klerman, G. L. (2000). *Comprehensive guide to interpersonal psychotherapy.* New York, NY: Basic Books.

Wellisch, D. K. (1995). A family systems approach to coping with cancer. In R. H. Mikesell, D-D. Lusterman & S. H. McDaniel (Eds.), *Integrating family therapy: Handbook of family psychology and systems theory* (pp. 389–403). Washington, DC: American Psychological Association.

Wellisch, D. K. (2000). Family issues and palliative care. In H. M. Chochinov & W. Breitbart (Eds.), *Handbook of psychiatry in palliative medicine* (pp. 275–289). New York, NY: Oxford University Press.

Wolpe, J. (1958). *Psychotherapy by reciprocal inhibition.* Palo Alto, CA: Stanford University Press.

Yalom, I. D. (1980). *Existential psychotherapy.* New York, NY: Basic Books.

Zabora, J. R., Brintzenhofeszoc, K, Curbow, K., Hooker, C., & Piantadosi, S. (2001). The prevalence of distress by cancer site. *Psycho-Oncology, 10*, 19–28.

Zaider, I. Z., & Kissane, D. (2010). Psychosocial interventions for couples and families coping with cancer. In J. C. Holland, W. S. Breitbart, P. B. Jacobsen, M. S. Lederberg, M. Loscalzo, & R. McCorkle (Eds.), *Psycho-Oncology* (2nd ed., pp. 483–487). New York, NY: Oxford University Press.

Zainal, N. Z., Booth, S., & Huppert, F. A. (2013). The efficacy of mindfulness-based stress reduction on mental health of breast cancer patients: A meta-analysis. *Psycho-Oncology, 22*(7), 1457–1465.

Zigmond, A., & Snaith, R. (1983). The hospital anxiety and depression scale. *Psychiatrica Scandinavia, 67*, 361.

ABOUT THE AUTHOR

Donald R. Nicholas, PhD, is a professor of psychology in the Department of Counseling Psychology at Ball State University. For over 25 years he has been involved in providing psychological services to cancer patients and their families in affiliation with I.U. Health Ball Memorial Cancer Center in Muncie, Indiana. He has also served on the Palliative and Supportive Care Editorial Board of the National Cancer Institute; has researched and published multiple articles on psychosocial oncology, including a special issue on psycho-oncology in *The Counseling Psychologist*; and coauthored the book *Cancer and the Family Lifecycle* (Brunner-Routledge, 2002). He is a recent recipient of the Dorothy Booz Black Award for Counseling Health Psychology, awarded by the Society of Counseling Psychology of the American Psychological Association.

INDEX

Page numbers followed by *b, t,* or *f* indicate boxes, tables, or figures, respectively. Numbers followed by n indicate footnotes.

www.ingramcontent.com/pod-product-compliance
Lightning Source LLC
Chambersburg PA
CBHW051150180926
51611CB00001B/8
* 9 7 8 0 1 9 9 7 4 4 4 4 2 *